Psychopharmacology

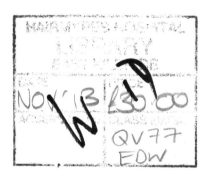

Psychopharmacology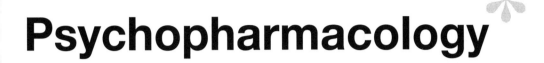

Practice and Contexts

Karen-leigh Edward

Chris Alderman

OXFORD
UNIVERSITY PRESS
AUSTRALIA & NEW ZEALAND

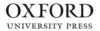

OXFORD
UNIVERSITY PRESS

Oxford University Press is a department of the University of Oxford.

It furthers the University's objective of excellence in research, scholarship, and education by publishing worldwide. Oxford is a registered trademark of Oxford University Press in the UK and in certain other countries.

Published in Australia by
Oxford University Press
253 Normanby Road, South Melbourne, Victoria 3205, Australia

National Library of Australia Cataloguing-in-Publication data

Author: Edward, Karen-leigh.
Title: Psychopharmacology : practice and contexts / Karen-leigh
Edward; Chris Alderman.

ISBN: 9780195519631 (pbk.)
Notes: Includes index.

Subjects: Psychopharmacology.
Other Authors/Contributors: Alderman, Chris.

Dewey Number: 615.78

Reproduction and communication for educational purposes
The Australian *Copyright Act 1968* (the Act) allows a maximum of one chapter or 10% of the pages of this work, whichever is the greater, to be reproduced and/or communicated by any educational institution for its educational purposes provided that the educational institution (or the body that administers it) has given a remuneration notice to Copyright Agency Limited (CAL) under the Act.

For details of the CAL licence for educational institutions contact:

Copyright Agency Limited
Level 15, 233 Castlereagh Street
Sydney NSW 2000
Telephone: (02) 9394 7600
Facsimile: (02) 9394 7601
Email: info@copyright.com.au

Edited by Joy Window
Typeset by diacriTech, India
Proofread by Carol Goudie
Indexed by Julie King
Printed by Sheck Wah Tong Printing Press Ltd

Links to third party websites are provided by Oxford in good faith and for information only. Oxford disclaims any responsibility for the materials contained in any third party website referenced in this work.

This book is dedicated to the millions of people around the world whose lives are touched every day by mental illness.

Mental illness and subsequent medication regimens can be experienced differently by individuals as described in this poem providing a consumer's perspective ...

Medicated

Roll up, roll up
Join me on the medication trolley
I've been on it for years
I've been Largactiled with bitter syrup
I've been Pimozided & Mellarilled & numbed
I was so Stelazined I was like a cat on a hot tin roof
I've been Modectated into a shuffle
& Clozapined into a stupor
I was Seranaced to sleep
& Abilifyed to sleeplessness
When I was Risperidoned I lactated like a cow
They Cogentined me to stop the look ups but I kept looking up
I was Lithiumed & Epilimed to even my pendulum
I've been Imipramined, Prothiadened, Lexaproed
Effexored & Zolofted to happiness
I was Valiumed & Ativaned into tranquility
Now I'm Zyprexaed & ravenous & fuzzled
I'm Lamotrigined & balanced
& Seroquelled
Yes indeedy, I'm medicated & dedicated to
The medication trolley
Here's looking at you pill bottles.

Sandy Jeffs 2012

Contents

List of Abbreviations and Acronyms   xii
Preface   xiv
Acknowledgments   xvi

Part 1: Practice

1 Psychotropic Drug Use: History and Context   3

Introduction   4
Psychological treatment   5
Biological treatment   6
A brief history of modern psychotropic drug treatment   6
Major changes in psychotropic prescribing: the last 20 years   9
Australian National Medicinal Drug Policy and
     Quality Use of Medicines   11
New Zealand Drug Policy   15
Medication-related problems   16
Multidisciplinary care and psychotropic pharmacotherapy   18
Recovery framework for mental health service provision   20

2 Law, Ethics and Accountability   25

Introduction   26
The legal and strategic context for mental disorders   27
Involuntary treatment   28
Seclusion and restraint   33
Ethical principles   34
Ethical decision-making and ethical theories   36

3 Pharmacokinetics   46

Introduction   47
Pharmacokinetics – the science of drug movements   47
Pharmacokinetics and nursing practice   54

4   Pharmacodynamics   **59**

Introduction   60
Pharmacodynamics – the science of drug actions   60
Pharmacodynamics and nursing practice   70

5   Medication Administration and Calculations   **78**

Introduction   79
Basic mathematical skills   79
Drug calculations   81
Medication administration   83
Patient/client and carer education   104

Part 2: Context

6   Mood Disorders   **111**

Introduction   112
The spectrum of mood disturbance   113
Non-pharmacological treatment of mood disorders   118
Pharmacotherapy for mood disorders   123
General principles of treatment for bipolar disorder   138

7   Anxiety Disorders   **150**

Introduction   151
Anxiety is part of life, not always an illness   151
Non-pharmacological treatment of anxiety disorders   154
General principles of pharmacotherapy for anxiety disorders   156
Commonly encountered anxiety disorders and their treatment   160

8   Schizophrenia and Other Psychoses   180

Introduction   181
Psychosis – a set of symptoms, not a disease   181
Schizophrenia   183
Antipsychotic medications   187
Adverse effects of antipsychotic drugs   194
Drug interactions with antipsychotics   200
Adherence and antipsychotic drug treatment   201

9   Substance Use Disorders   212

Introduction   213
What are substance disorders and how do they
     relate to those with mental illness?   213
Care considerations for people with substance use disorders   227

10   Mental Illness in Children and Adolescents   238

Introduction   239
Special issues in child and adolescent psychiatry   239
Attention deficit/hyperactivity disorder   242
Autism spectrum disorders   250
Tic disorders   250
General psychiatry for children   251

11   Older People   257

Introduction   258
The physical effects of ageing   258
Multiple diseases – multiple medicines   260
Cognitive disorders (including dementia)   260
Other comorbidities   262

Increasing susceptibility to side effects of medicines   264

Beers list (medication list)   265

Drugs and falls in the older person   271

12 Mental Illness in Special Populations   280

Introduction   281

Eating disorders   281

Personality disorders   283

Sleep disorders   285

Drug-induced psychiatric syndromes   290

Pain and psychiatry   297

Complementary medicines   298

Drugs in pregnancy and lactation   298

Part 3: Advanced Practice and Context

13 Adherence and Concordance   305

Introduction   306

The global burden of disability of chronic conditions   306

Adherence versus compliance   312

Concordance   313

The student nurse's experience of medication management   316

Some considerations regarding medicines and adherence or
   non-adherence   321

**14 Nurse Practitioner and Other Advanced
Practice Roles   326**

Introduction   327

Advanced practice   327

Nurse practitioners 327
Nurse practitioner competency standards 328
Prescribing medications as an advanced nursing
    practice for NPs 329
Medicare Benefits Scheme and Pharmaceutical
    Benefits Scheme for the nurse practitioner 330
A person–centred approach to NP prescribing in the
    context of mental illness 334

Test Yourself Answers 339

Glossary of Terms 341

Index 348

List of Abbreviations and Acronyms

ADHD	attention deficit with hyperactivity disorder
ADR	adverse drug reaction
bd	*bis in die* (twice daily)
BPRS	Brief Psychiatric Rating Scale
CBT	cognitive behavioural therapy
CNS	central nervous system
CMI	Consumer Medicines Information
COPD	chronic obstructive pulmonary disease
COX	cyclooxygenase
CPAP	continuous positive airway pressure
CSA	central sleep apnoea
CVD	cardiovascular disease
DDD	daily defined dose
DMMR	Domiciliary Medication Management Review
DUSC	Drug Utilisation Sub-Committee
ECG	electrocardiogram
ECT	electroconvulsive therapy
ED	emergency department
FDA	Food and Drug Administration (US)
GABA	gamma aminobutyric acid
GAD	generalised anxiety disorder
GAF	Global Assessment of Functioning
GI	gastrointestinal
GP	general practitioner
HIV	human immunodeficiency virus
HMR	Home Medicines Review
HPOS	Health Professional Online Service
IH	inhalation
IM	intramuscular
IMI	intramuscular injection
MAOI	monoamine oxidase inhibitor

MBS	Medicare Benefits Scheme
MDI	metered dose inhaler
MDMA	3,4-methylenedioxy-N-methylamphetamine, 'Ecstasy'
NEB	nebulised
NP	nurse practitioner
NSAID	non-steroidal anti-inflammatory drug
NIMC	National Inpatient Medication Chart
NMDA	N-methyl-D-aspartic acid
OCD	obsessive-compulsive disorder
OSA	obstructive sleep apnoea
PANSS	Positive and Negative Syndrome Scale
PBAC	Pharmaceutical Benefits Advisory Committee
PBS	Pharmaceutical Benefits Scheme
PHARMAC	Pharmaceutical Management Agency (New Zealand)
PPE	personal protective equipment
prn	*pro re nata* (as needed)
PO	*per oral* (by mouth)
POM	patient's own medicines
PTSD	post-traumatic stress disorder
QUM	Quality Use of Medicines
RPBS	Repatriation Pharmaceutical Benefits Scheme
RMMR	Residential Medication Management Review
SAPS	Scale for the Assessment of Positive Symptoms
SANS	Scale for the Assessment of Negative Symptoms
SNRI	serotonin/noradrenaline reuptake inhibitor
SSRI	selective serotonin reuptake inhibitor
SL	sublingual
TCA	tricyclic antidepressant
TGA	Australian Therapeutic Goods Administration
THC	delta-9 tetra hydro-cannabinol
TP	topical

Preface

Thank you for choosing this book ...

Almost all people who experience mental illness will at some stage of their lives use medication. The effects of mental disorder can be profound, affecting almost all aspects of a person's life: relationships, employment, and even the private moments that individuals spend with themselves in their own thoughts. In this context, medication can be a source of hope for people, providing the opportunity to reduce or even eliminate the symptoms of mental disorder that interrupt personal thoughts, goals and dreams. Even so, it is important to recognise that psychotropic medications also have considerable potential to cause drug-related harm, and as such it is very important that practitioners have an appropriate understanding of treatment monitoring and risk minimisation strategies. The vital role of nurses and other health professionals in helping people manage mental health conditions holistically was an important consideration in the approach to the development of this textbook.

This work resulted from an idea of a publishing manager and an experienced nurse clinician, both of whom had seen that an opportunity existed to serve the needs of those who seek a deeper understanding of the biological treatment of people with mental illness. From this was born a partnership between two clinicians and academics who strongly believe that the context of care is a fundamental consideration when framing a more complete understanding of the principles governing the selection, implementation and monitoring of medication therapy for people living with mental illnesses. The book combines two specialised and complementary perspectives on psychotropic pharmacotherapy – that of an experienced mental health nursing clinician with a background in academic sciences, and that of a specialist clinical pharmacist with decades of diverse experience in the field of psychiatric pharmacy and a background in medication safety research. This textbook brings together the many years of the authors' experience and interprets available evidence to introduce the complex considerations needed in the care of people who are to be prescribed and administered psychotropic medications. The book is oriented around the various groups of mental disorders, allowing the reader to assimilate information related to medication in the context of the mental health disorders that people experience. Each chapter begins with the information needed to build knowledge that can be applied later in thoughtful analysis of the numerous case vignettes throughout the book. The book is designed to allow readers to develop insight into the great variability in the ways in which individuals experience mental health disorders, and the equally variable fashion in which each person has the potential to experience both benefit and harm as a result of drug treatment. In this way, the reader can establish a linked understanding of the medications.

The blended perspectives provided in this text are intended to allow a holistic basis for nurses and other health providers looking to achieve insight and understanding into the way in which medications can assist in the treatment of mental disorders, and the strategies that can be used to reduce the likelihood of iatrogenic harm related to the use of psychotropic drugs.

We wish you well in your journey in learning and practice in health care.

Karen-leigh Edward
Chris Alderman
Jan 2013

Acknowledgments

The authors would like to acknowledge the staff at Oxford University Press for their commitment and support in the development of the book. In particular, thank you to Debra James and her team for professional leadership, support and commitment in the publication of this book.

The author and the publisher wish to thank the following copyright holders for reproduction of their material.

American Geriatric Society for Table 11.2 'An abridged version of the AGS Beers Criteria for Potentially Inappropriate Medication Use in Older Adults', adbridged from Beers M. H., Ouslander J. G., Rollingher I., Reuben D. B., Brooks J. & Beck J. C. (1991). 'Explicit criteria for determining inappropriate medication use in nursing home residents' *Archives of Internal Medicine* 151(9): 1825; American Psychiatric Association for Table 9.1 'Diagnoses associated with class of substances'; Australian Commission on Safety and Quality in Healthcare for Figure 5.1 'The National Inpatient Medication Chart (NIMC)' and Table 5.3 'Recommended terms'; Figure 1.2 'The medicines management pathway cycle' is reproduced with permission from Journal of Pharmacy Practice and Research, 2004: 34, p. 294; The Annals of Pharmacotherapy for Table 1.3 'Professional roles in medicines management and psychotropic Pharmacotherapy', (d) the Harvey Whitney Books Company.

Every effort has been made to trace the original source of copyright material contained in this book. The publisher will be pleased to hear from copyright holders to rectify any errors or omissions.

Part 1

Practice

Chapter 1

Psychotropic Drug Use: History and Context

Chapter overview

This chapter covers the following topics:

* evolution of the understanding of the basis of mental illness
* aspects of the history of psychotropic drug use
* context of medicinal drug use – the Australian National Medicinal Drug Policy and principles of Quality Use of Medicines
* drug-related problems.

Chapter learning objectives

After reading this chapter, you should be able to:

* describe aspects of the history of psychotropic drug development and use
* outline the salient features of the Australian National Medicinal Drug policy and principles of Quality Use of Medicines, and relate these to the concept of drug-related problems.

Key terms

Drug-related problems
Medicinal drug policy
Psychotropic drugs
Quality Use of Medicines

Introduction

Mental illness is not a new phenomenon, having affected humankind for thousands of years. There is evidence to suggest that in the prehistoric era people suffered from mental illnesses that may have been similar to those affecting people today. When our ancestors observed unusual or irrational behaviours that we would now understand to arise from a mental illness, a common response would be to attribute the behaviour to the influence of an external force or power, with conceptual models such as demonic possession or religious influences invoked in many cases. Only relatively recently has the biological basis for mental illness been recognised and embraced as a basis for management interventions, and the role of biological interventions in psychiatry, in particular drug therapy, continues to evolve as new scientific and clinical information becomes available. Although the response to mental illness today is very different from responses recorded in the early history of humankind, substantial stigma is still associated with mental disease.

It was Hippocrates, regarded by most as the forefather of modern medicine, who first proposed that mental illness was due to an imbalance of the four 'humours', suggesting that there was some form of biological basis and internal locus for the origins of mental illness, rather than a reflection of external influences. Although the metaphor that was used by Hippocrates did not prove to be an accurate one, this model foreshadowed a movement from mysticism to a paradigm whereby psychopathology could be regarded as the effects of a disease of the brain, rather than demonic possession or the effects of an intervention from a deity. A quotation from the work of Hippocrates, *On the Sacred Disease*, provides insight into the extent of his understanding of normal human emotion and the processes of mental illness, rendered all the more remarkable by the fact that this passage was compiled so long ago.

Figure 1.1: Hippocrates – the first proponent of the organic basis for mental illness (Hippocrates, 400 BCE)

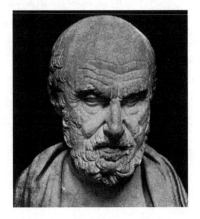

Men ought to know that from nothing else but the brain come joys, delights, laughter and sports, and sorrows, griefs, despondency, and lamentations. And by this, in an especial manner, we acquire wisdom and knowledge, and see and hear, and know what are foul and what are fair, what are bad and what are good, what are sweet, and what unsavory; some we discriminate by habit, and some we perceive by their utility. By this we distinguish objects of relish and disrelish, according to the seasons; and the same things do not always please us. And by the same organ we become mad and delirious, and fears and terrors assail us, some by night, and some by day, and dreams and untimely wanderings, and cares that are not suitable, and ignorance of present circumstances, desuetude, and unskilfulness. All these things we endure from the brain, when it is not healthy, but is more hot, more cold, more moist, or more dry than natural, or when it suffers any other preternatural and unusual affection. And we become mad from its humidity. For when it is more moist than natural, it is necessarily put into motion, and the affection being moved, neither the sight nor hearing can be at rest, and the tongue speaks in accordance with the sight and hearing … In these ways I am of the opinion that the brain exercises the greatest power in the man.

Broadly, the treatments that are used for the management of mental disorders are usually categorised as either 'psychological' or 'biological'.

Psychological treatment

Psychological therapies include such approaches as cognitive therapy, behavioural therapy, family focused therapy or psychoanalysis. Often based around counselling, these techniques are known to be effective for the management of many mental disorders, and in some cases are the preferred forms of treatment of many conditions. Over time, and in the backdrop of research findings, psychological treatments can be conceptualised in the context of mental disorders – for example, in the case of bipolar affective disorder there is moderate to strong support for such interventions as psychoeducation and cognitive therapy (for the mania episode of the disorder). For the depressive episode of bipolar affective disorder psychoeducation, family focused therapy and interpersonal therapy is preferred. In the psychological treatment of schizophrenia there is moderate to strong support of social skills training, cognitive behavioural therapy, assertive community treatment, family focused therapy, supported employment, social learning, cognitive remediation and adaptation therapy, and illness management and recovery-based interventions. Although psychological therapies do not have the same potential to cause adverse effects as biological therapies (e.g. the side effects of drugs), they are not universally effective, may not be suitable for more severe forms of mental illness, and can be expensive and difficult to access for **patients/clients**. Various aspects of psychological therapies are addressed elsewhere in this text, in chapters dealing with a range of disorders.

Biological treatment

Biological therapy for mental disorders can take a number of forms, but generally involves the use of some form of physical intervention (such as **pharmacotherapy**). Psychosurgery was once more widely practised than is the case now, and involves surgery to specific parts of the brain with a view to addressing the symptoms of various psychiatric disorders. **Electroconvulsive therapy (ECT)** remains an effective treatment for some mental disorders, in particular **mood disorders** such as major depression. The place in the management of mental illness is less clear for other non-drug biological interventions such as transcranial electromagnetic therapy and bright light therapy.

The bulk of biological therapy for mental disorders is undertaken using medications, which are very often prescribed by clinicians who are not psychiatrists (approximately 80% of all antipsychotics are prescribed in primary care settings by GPs). The medicines most commonly used in the management of mental disorders are often referred to as **psychotropic drugs**, because of their specific abilities to produce effects upon emotion and behaviour. This area of **pharmacology** is also known as psychopharmacology.

A brief history of modern psychotropic drug treatment

The most significant changes in psychotropic drug pharmacoepidemiology in the Australasia/Pacific region and elsewhere have taken place in two waves. The first of these occurred with the introduction of the first truly effective psychotropic drugs: chlorpromazine as a treatment for **psychosis**, and the tricyclic **antidepressants** (TCAs) and non-selective monoamine oxidase inhibitors (MAOIs) in the early 1950s. The introduction of these drugs heralded truly revolutionary developments in the management of mental illness, in that effective pharmacological treatment options were available to patients/clients who had disorders that were, until that time, refractory to most interventions.

Thereafter followed the exploration of the pharmacological potential of RO 50690, which eventually came to be known as chlordiazepoxide, later to be marketed under the brand name Librium®, a reference used to imply that is was capable of engendering a sense of equilibrium. Then, in 1963 the same company that produced Librium® oversaw the introduction of diazepam into clinical therapeutics. Marketed as Valium® (after the Latin *vale*, denoting 'strong' or 'well'), diazepam would eventually become the most prescribed drug of all time. It is worth noting that although the history of the benzodiazepines (such as diazepam) has been marked by controversy, these drugs are actually much safer than many other agents that are widely used in the community, and it is often overlooked that the benzodiazepines replaced the barbiturates as pharmacological options for the management of **anxiety** and **insomnia**. Although the place of the benzodiazepines relative to safer non-drug alternatives can be debated, the increased safety relative to barbiturates has probably prevented many deaths that would have otherwise been attributable to barbiturate-associated suicides.

A second wave of major change in agents has altered the landscape of psychotropic pharmacoepidemiology profoundly. After a resolution in the US Senate in late 1989 the 1990s came to be known as the 'decade of the brain'. The decade of the brain was an initiative undertaken by the Library of Congress (USA) and the National Institute of Mental Health (USA) to enhance public awareness of the benefits of brain research and was from the period 1990–99. Since 1990, there have been extraordinarily significant changes, arguably major improvements, in the pharmacological treatment options for psychotic disorders, affective disorders (including both major depression and bipolar affective disorder), **anxiety disorders** and substance use disorders. Important developments have included the introduction of the atypical antipsychotics, along with the selective serotonin reuptake inhibitors (SSRIs) and other new generation antidepressants.

With the advent of these new treatment options pharmacoepidemiology of psychotropic drug usage in Australia has altered radically, accompanied by important pharmacoeconomic and public health changes. Entirely new concerns regarding different patterns of **adverse drug reactions** and **drug interactions** have arisen, and the role that various clinicians can play in the detection, investigation, management and prevention of medication-related harm in the context of pharmacological treatment of mental illness has been enhanced considerably. Relatively new agents that have achieved significant and rapid uptake in recent times are now widely prescribed, although prescribers of these agents have less familiarity with the safety profiles of these drugs. The proportion of subjects in each cohort using hypnosedatives and tranquilisers is approximately similar, implying that awareness of the disadvantages of these drugs (e.g. potential for tolerance, **dependence** and withdrawal reactions; contribution to falls among the elderly; increased likelihood of motor vehicle accidents) has probably not increased in the decade since 1995. Therefore it is apparent that the principles for the safe and effective use of psychotropic drugs continue to become more complex. With this in mind, the validity of a role for a psychotropic pharmacotherapy expert in the context of multidisciplinary care is emphasised, and this function can logically be performed by specialist psychiatry pharmacists with appropriate training and experience.

Australian Statistics on Medicines (ASM) is published periodically by the Drug Utilisation Sub-Committee of the Pharmaceutical Benefits Advisory Committee. The data presented are estimates of aggregate community use of prescription medicines in Australia, and are drawn from the Health Insurance Commission records of prescriptions submitted for payment of a subsidy under the Pharmaceutical Benefits and Repatriation Pharmaceutical Benefits Schemes (PBS/RPBS), as well as an ongoing survey of a representative sample of community pharmacies (used to estimate non-subsidised use of prescription medicines). It is important to note that complete data on prescription medicines **dispensed** to inpatients in public hospitals are not yet available, but plans are in progress to allow this. The units of measurement for the presentation of the data are the prescription rate and the defined daily dose per 1000 population per day (DDD/1000 population/day). The defined daily dose is established by the World Health Organization Collaborating Centre for Drug Statistics Methodology on the basis of the assumed average dose per day of the medication, used for its main indication by adults. Although this system is imperfect, particularly in the context of off-label medication usage, it is an internationally recognised comparative system that is widely used for pharmacoepidemiology research purposes. Readers who are interested to more fully understand the evolution of Australian prescribing trends for psychotropic drugs can find great detail of the changes of prescribing patterns that have been observed in recent times by referring to the publicly available information that is disseminated at the ASM website.

Major changes in psychotropic prescribing: the last 20 years

The variety of psychotropic drugs at the disposal of modern clinicians has expanded enormously in recent years from the relatively small range that was available as recently as the early 1990s. Until the 1990s prescribers worked for many years with the tricyclic antidepressants (TCAs), irreversible, non-selective monoamine oxidase inhibitors MAOIs, the conventional antipsychotics (chlorpromazine, haloperidol and related drugs), lithium, benzodiazepines and barbiturates. From this relatively small array of choices prescribers provided drug therapy for a broad array of mental disorders, recognising the limitations arising from the 'broad spectrum' nature of the drugs' clinical pharmacology and the complexity of the agents' pharmacokinetic profiles.

Since the early 1990s the range of drug treatments for mental disorders has expanded enormously, with the introduction of new classes of antidepressants, the development of the atypical **antipsychotic drugs**, and the novel use of drugs not traditionally regarded as psychotropic agents all profoundly influencing the ways in which mental illness is treated. With the introduction of these changes there has been an accompanying change in the dynamics of the ways in which psychotropic drug prescribing is undertaken: clinicians are no longer dealing with a relatively small and circumscribed group of agents with which they are familiar. Instead, doctors treating mental disorders must grapple with a large range of complex drugs that have an evolving profile of adverse effects and drug interactions. The subtle effects of these drugs remain poorly understood, and in the postmarketing surveillance phase (where the drugs are prescribed in vast quantities to enormous numbers of patients worldwide) clinicians continue to encounter difficulties and limitations that may not have been initially anticipated. The increase in the complexity of choice in prescribing in this field is exemplified in Table 1.1, which illustrates the changes in available drug therapy for the management of major depression.

Table 1.1: Drug therapy for major depression (Australia) – 1990 versus 2012

Treatment options 1990	Treatment options 2012
Tricyclic antidepressants	*Tricyclic antidepressants*
Amitriptyline	Amitriptyline
Clomipramine	Clomipramine
Desipramine	Dothiepin
Dothiepin	Doxepin
Doxepin	Imipramine
Imipramine	Nortriptyline
Nortriptyline	Trimipramine
Protriptyline	
Trimipramine	
Monoamine oxidase inhibitors	*Monoamine oxidase inhibitors*
Phenelzine	Phenelzine
Tranylcypromine	Tranylcypromine
	Moclobemide
	Serotonin reuptake inhibitors
	Citalopram, escitalopram
	Fluoxetine
	Fluvoxamine
	Paroxetine
	Sertraline
	Serotonin/noradrenaline reuptake inhibitors
	Venlafaxine/desvenlafaxine
	Duloxetine
	Noradrenaline reuptake inhibitors
	Reboxetine
	Other antidepressants
	Bupropion
	Mirtazapine
	Agomelatine

In addition to the increased range of psychotropic medications that are now available for use in the management of mental illness, there is a considerably larger range of other medication therapy available and in use for the management of non-psychiatric illness. Given the high frequency of medical comorbidities that exists among patients/clients with mental illness, it is logical that there will be substantial potential for interactions between psychotropic medications and other agents used for the management of general medical conditions. Given the highly specialised nature of psychiatry as a discipline in medicine, it is not necessarily reasonable to expect that psychiatrists will have a full working knowledge of drug therapy used in other areas of medicine, and thus the input of other specialist clinicians (e.g. pharmacists) in this regard could be expected to improve the overall safety of patient management by decreasing the potential for drug interactions or drug-induced exacerbations of coexisting medical illnesses. The increased range of new psychotropic pharmacotherapy options has been accompanied by a wave of promotional activities that is unprecedented in the field of psychiatry. Multinational pharmaceutical companies invest billions of dollars in efforts to influence the prescribing behaviour of psychiatrists and other medical practitioners who are involved in the management of psychotropic medication therapy for patients/clients with mental illness. The quality of the information promulgated, the objectivity of the promotional literature distributed, and the ability of busy clinicians to selectively interpret the materials may all be less than what is required to ensure that prescribing decisions are made in a fashion that is likely to ensure that **Quality Use of Medicines** principles are applied in the decision-making processes.

Australian National Medicinal Drug Policy and Quality Use of Medicines

In 1992 Australian Health Ministers adopted the *National Mental Health Policy and Plan*, and this document in concert with the National Statement of Rights and Responsibilities endorsed earlier forms the National Mental Health Strategy, a commitment by state, territory and Commonwealth governments to improve the lives of people with a mental illness. The stated objective was to provide a blueprint for the future delivery of mental health services in Australia. The fundamental aims of the strategy are: to promote the mental health of the Australian community, prevent the development of mental health problems and mental disorders where possible, reduce the impact of mental disorders on individuals, families and the community; and to advocate the rights of people with mental disorders. Inherent to the promotion of mental health in Australia is the notion that appropriate treatments should be available, accessible and affordable for those affected by these disorders. This key principle is consistent with the area of focus for Australia's National Medicinal Drug Policy (Department of Health and Ageing, 2010).

The four central objectives of the National Medicinal Drug Policy are: the facilitation of timely access to required medicines at a cost that individuals and the community can afford; ensuring that medicines meet appropriate quality, safety and efficacy standards; the maintenance of a responsible and viable medicines industry in Australia; and the achievement of Quality Use of Medicines (QUM). As result, a natural progression has been the development of the Australian National Strategy for QUM, a strategy designed to embrace the use of all medicines, including prescription, non-prescription and complementary therapies. Integral to the national QUM strategy is a range of objectives that include involvement in QUM activities by health care providers and health educators (Department of Health and Ageing, 2002).

Underpinning the national QUM strategy are five key principles that have been developed in consultation with all key stakeholders; and as a consequence these principles are relevant to the work of all stakeholders involved in the provision of psychotropic drug treatment for patients/clients, regardless of the setting in which it is provided.

In summary, these principles include:

* the recognition of the primacy of consumers and their views

* the notion of partnership between key participants (e.g. between providers and patients/clients, between providers)

* the need for consultation and collaboration in the design, implementation and evaluation of QUM initiatives

* support for existing QUM activities and initiatives

* the need to adopt and embrace system-based approaches that foster an environment and behaviours that support QUM.

Overall, the national QUM strategy is based on the premise that to achieve Quality Use of Medicines, it is necessary to address a range of objectives, both in a policy sense (at a local and national level), as well as in the interaction between health care providers and the individual patient. In terms of the latter, it is evident that there are many aspects of the work of multidisciplinary teams involved in mental health care that can address key the issues outlined in the definition of QUM that is provided in the national strategy document. These include:

* judicious selection of management options (considering the place of medicines in treating illness and maintaining health, and recognising the possibility that no treatment, or a non-drug treatment, may be appropriate to manage a particular situation)

* appropriate selection of a suitable medication, if a medicine is considered necessary – this will involve consideration of the characteristics of the individual patient, the clinical condition, risks and benefits associated with treatment options, the dosage and duration of treatment, coexisting conditions, other therapies, monitoring considerations, and costs for the individual, the community and the health system as a whole

* safe and effective use of medications to achieve optimal health outcomes through monitoring, minimising misuse, overuse and underuse of medications; and ensuring that the patient or their carer has the knowledge and skills to use medicines and solve problems related to the use of medications.

The existence of the National Medicinal Drug Policy has guided initiatives at research, policy and practice levels in Australia. For example, research addressing medication-related problems in the community and in aged-care facilities, and funded through the QUM policy area in the federal Department of Health and Ageing, led to federal funding for medical and pharmacy practitioners to conduct collaborative medication management services for people at risk of medication misadventure. Funding from the same source enabled research that addressed the high prevalence of medication-related problems along the continuum of care from hospital to community settings. The Council of Australian Health Ministers, through their Pharmaceutical Reforms agenda, has made the adoption of models arising from the research a condition of health care reform funds being made available to the states.

These models involve collaborative processes aimed at improving the relaying of medicines and patient care information between hospital and community-based health workers.

Federal government policy initiatives have also funded key building blocks of QUM, such as sources of independent medicines information for health care providers. National therapeutic guidelines covering a range of major therapeutic areas are available and regularly updated. The *Australian Medicines Handbook* (Rossi, 2012) is funded as an independent, regularly updated medicines formulary and *Australian Prescriber* is funded as an independent quarterly medicines bulletin. Independent medicines information for consumers is available through Consumer Medicines Information leaflets, which are produced for all prescription medicines available in Australia and provided to consumers free of charge at the point of consultation with their doctor and pharmacist. The federal government also funds and provides support for major national service delivery initiatives such as the National Prescribing Service. These initiatives use evidence-based strategies such as academic detailing, and audit and feedback, to deliver independent information on medicines and health care to health professionals and consumers. In addition, best practice has been supported through other means, such as the development of practice guidelines and standards. Federally endorsed guidelines, for example, have been prepared in the areas of medication management along the continuum of care and in aged care.

The fundamental elements of the **Australian National Medicinal Drug Policy** are:

* timely access to required medicines at a cost affordable to individuals and the community

* medicines of appropriate quality, safety and efficacy

* a responsible and viable medicines industry in Australia

* achievement of Quality Use of Medicines (QUM):

  - judicious selection of treatment options

  - appropriate selection of a suitable medication regimen, if considered necessary

- safe and effective use of medications through monitoring, minimising misuse

- ensuring that patients/carers have knowledge and skills to use medicines safely.

Although much of the responsibility for establishment and maintenance of a National Medicinal Drug Policy and attaining Quality Use of Medicines can rest with funding agencies, governments and the health administration sector (at national, regional and local levels), there are many others with significant roles to play. For example, consumer agencies, professional organisations and health advocacy bodies can all contribute. The combined efforts of all of those involved have great potential to improve the lives of people affected by mental illness and requiring psychotropic drug therapy.

New Zealand Drug Policy

In common with Australia, the government of New Zealand has invested in developing extensive infrastructure that is targeted at optimising the safe and effective use of medicines in the community. PHARMAC, the Pharmaceutical Management Agency of New Zealand, determines the range of medicines and related products that are subsidised for use in the community and in public hospitals. The roles undertaken by PHARMAC include management of the schedule of government-subsidised community pharmaceuticals, and promoting optimal use of medicines. The work of PHARMAC includes the development and implementation of public information campaigns, monitoring expenditure and usage patterns of drugs, and facilitating access to drugs with limited availability of clinical trials.

Ask yourself!

1   What professional groups have key responsibilities in clinical teams that can allow QUM principles to be used to optimise treatment outcomes for those with mental illness?

2   What tools might be used to help optimise psychotropic pharmacotherapy by facilitating QUM?

3   What are the positive and negative roles played by the pharmaceutical industry in the QUM effort?

Medication-related problems

In Australia and around the world, considerable and justifiable attention has been directed to medical and psychiatric problems associated with the use of tobacco, alcohol and illicit drugs. Adverse outcomes arising from the use of **medicinal drugs** have not necessarily been highlighted to the same extent. An understanding of medication-related harm that focuses exclusively on adverse drug reactions and drug–drug interactions cannot provide a comprehensive description of the nature and scope of the various problems encountered with the use of pharmacotherapy. It has become clear that health care professionals, including those involved with the care of people with significant mental illness, have needed a framework that can help to develop a much more complete picture of the scope of the problems associated with medicinal drugs. This is even more critical when dealing with vulnerable populations such as older people and children. The most widely adopted system for categorisation of **medication-related problems** is that developed by Strand et al., who proposed eight categories of medication-related problems to define circumstances where people may be exposed to actual or potential medication-related harm. This system defines a medication-related problem as 'any undesirable event experienced by the patient that involves or is suspected to involve drug therapy and that actually or potentially interferes with a desired patient outcome' (Strand et al., 1990, p. 1094). The eight categories of drug-related problems used in this system are outlined in Table 1.2, accompanied by illustrative example.

Table 1.2: Categorisation of medication-related problems

Indication without medication therapy
There is an indication for medication use but patient/client is not receiving a drug for the indication.
Example: Heavy alcohol drinker is not prescribed thiamine to prevent Wernicke's encephalopathy.
Medication use without indication
Patient is taking a medication for which there is no medically valid indication.
Example: Patient/client with acute agitation in hospital (that has resolved) continues antipsychotics after discharge.

Improper medication selection

The patient/client has a medication indication but is taking the wrong drug.

Example: Patient/client with history of prostatic hypertrophy and urinary retention is prescribed highly anticholinergic tricyclic antidepressant.

Subtherapeutic dosage

The patient/client has a medical problem that is being treated with too little of the correct medication.

Example: A diabetic inpatient treated with an antipsychotic develops serious hyperglycaemia but the insulin dosage is not adjusted to accommodate this.

Over-dosage

The patient/client has a medical problem that is being treated with too much of the correct medication.

Example: Patient/client is prescribed a very large dose of an antidepressant drug; the magnitude of the dosage does not create additional antipsychotic benefit but generates severe adverse effects.

Adverse drug reaction (ADR)

The patient/client has a medical problem that is the result of an ADR or adverse effect.

Example: The patient/client develops sexual dysfunction as a result of treatment with an antidepressant.

Drug interaction

Medication–medication, medication–laboratory, or medication–food interaction.

Example: Elevated serum theophylline concentration with toxicity secondary to fluvoxamine treatment.

Failure to receive a medication

Medical problem resulting from not receiving medication intended as part of designed treatment.

Example: The patient/client is prescribed expensive, non-subsidised drug therapy but does not have the prescription filled and does not adhere to the established treatment plan.

Adapted from: Strand et al. (1990)

The use of this framework by teams involved in the management of pharmacotherapy for people with mental illness allows a structured and systematic approach to preventing **iatrogenic illness** and facilitating optimal treatment outcomes.

Multidisciplinary care and psychotropic pharmacotherapy

Given the complexity of the processes surrounding psychotropic drug therapy, it is not surprising that all of the essential elements that need to be addressed to achieve optimal outcomes and the prevention of drug-related harm (iatrogenic illness) cannot necessarily be addressed completely by any one professional group working in isolation. The complexity of the medication management process is represented in Figure 1.2.

Figure 1.2: The medicines management pathway cycle

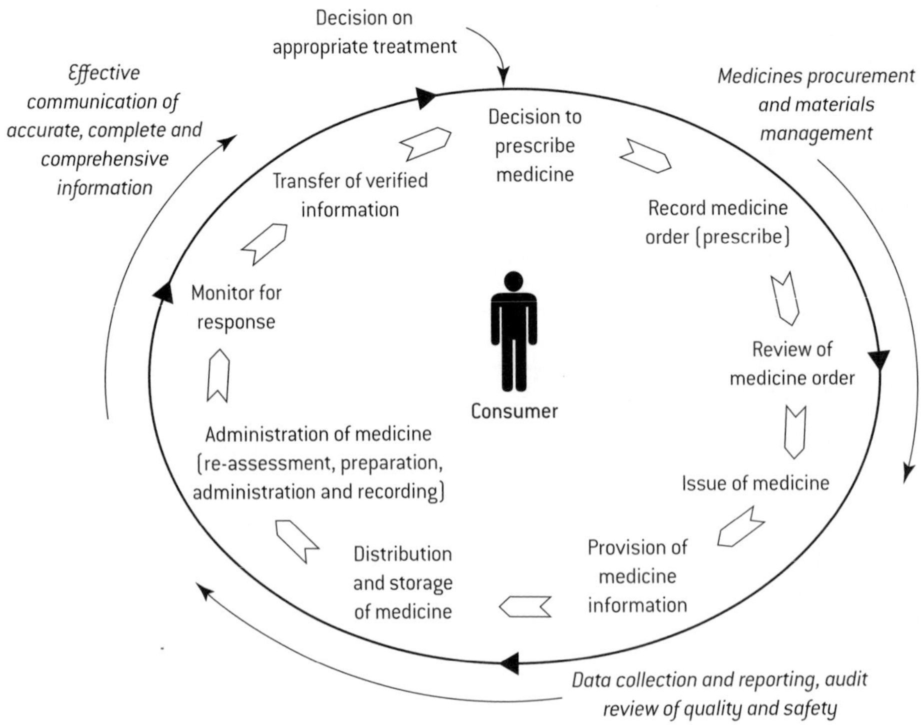

The key professional groups that are potentially involved in the use of psychotropic drugs in the treatment of people with mental illness are medical, nursing and pharmacy staff, supported by other professional groups including social workers, psychologists and occupational therapists. Each of these professions has key parts to play, but it is also clear that there is considerable overlap between professional roles, necessitating effective interprofessional communication in the interest of patient care. Examples of these roles are outlined in Table 1.3, although the extent of the roles and responsibilities outlined is not intended to be comprehensive.

Table 1.3: Professional roles in medicines management and psychotropic pharmacotherapy

Medical staff:
Recognise/identify need for pharmacotherapy: prescribe safely and in accordance with legislation.
Monitor for adverse effects and efficacy.
Communicate and discuss with consumers and carers regarding benefits and risks of therapy.
Combine drug therapy with non-pharmacological approaches.
Understand and manage comorbid general medical/surgical and substance use issues.
Participate in audit/research and investigations to advance knowledge.
Nurses:
Recognise/identify need for pharmacotherapy. Where within scope of practice and qualifications, prescribe safely and in accordance with legislation.
Administer treatment to patients/clients, safely and in accordance with legislation.
Monitor for adverse effects and efficacy.
Communicate and discuss with consumers and carers regarding benefits and risks of therapy.
Combine drug therapy with non-pharmacological approaches.
Contribute to management of comorbid general medical/surgical and substance use issues.
Participate in audit/research and investigations to advance knowledge.

(Continued)

Table 1.3: Professional roles in medicines management and psychotropic pharmacotherapy *(Continued)*

Pharmacists:
Recognise/identify need for pharmacotherapy. Advocate and facilitate safe prescribing in accordance with legislation.
Oversee procurement, storage and distribution of treatments to points of care.
Act as authoritative resource for other team members needing information about drugs.
Monitor for adverse effects and efficacy.
Communicate and discuss with consumers and carers regarding benefits and risks of therapy.
Contribute to management of comorbid general medical/surgical and substance use issues.
Participate in audit/research and investigations to advance knowledge.

Other staff:
Provide information to other team members that will assist in processes that allow recognition of the need for pharmacotherapy, and the design of an appropriate treatment approach.
Monitor for adverse effects and efficacy.
Combine drug therapy with non-pharmacological approaches.
Contribute to management of comorbid general medical/surgical and substance use issues.
Participate in audit/research and investigations to advance knowledge.
Overall, it is evident that cooperation between professional groups and open communication between the treating team and the patient/client and/or carers is paramount to achieving high quality outcomes for people with mental illness where pharmacotherapy is to be considered.

Recovery framework for mental health service provision

The **recovery framework** is central to all mental health services and the interventions that mental health workers utilise when working with people who experience mental illness. Mental health promotion is an important part of recovery since mental health promotion incorporates aspects such as prevention and early intervention and in this context is relevant to all consumers of mental health services. Recovery-orientated practice can be viewed as incorporating early intervention, self-care management strategies, **relapse** prevention and rehabilitation (also known as disability support). These types of interventions ensure routine practice is flexible, hopeful, respectful and meaningful and should underpin such activities as developing care plans with consumers and other stakeholders, therapeutic interventions and organisational policies and procedures. The guiding principles of the recovery framework include:

* working within a recovery framework

* facilitation of recovery and wellness

* working within a philosophy of hope and partnership with consumers and their carers

* understanding consumers in the context of their whole self and not just their illness/disorder

* protecting people's rights and working with people in the context of respect and equity

* ensuring consumers set their own goals and are enabled through the clinical contact to measure their own success

* focusing on strengths rather than symptoms

* facilitation of timely treatment and timely discharge from services

* working in a culturally and gender sensitive manner.

MARY'S STORY

Mary is an 81-year-old woman with a history of ischaemic heart disease and severe osteoarthritis. She was admitted to hospital after a high lethality suicide attempt involving a medication overdose. She takes various medications for her heart (including perhexiline and metoprolol) and has frequent episodes of angina which are partially relieved with sublingual nitrate spray. She undergoes a course of ECT and at a multidisciplinary meeting plans for her subsequent drug therapy are discussed.

During the case conference:

- Her doctor enquires about neurovegetative features and the quality of her interpersonal interactions on the inpatient unit. There is a subsequent decision to prescribe an antidepressant.

- The nurses involved with caring for Mary identify significant sleep disturbance and loss of weight. At handover it is reported that she has significant bradycardia and hypotension that appears to have developed after the introduction of an SSRI.

- A pharmacist contacts nursing and medical staff to report concerns about a drug interaction resulting in beta blocker toxicity – the antidepressant is subsequently changed.

- The unit occupational therapist visits Mary after discharge and find that she is unable to manage her medications at home – the arthritis in her hands is so severe that she cannot even open the packaging. The report from a neuropsychologist indicates that she has significant cognitive impairment, in keeping with the clinical observations of nursing and medical staff. The pharmacist makes arrangements for her medicines to be packed in a dosage administration aid.

Ask yourself!

In relation to Mary's case:

1   Could effective pharmacotherapy be designed and delivered by one discipline alone?

2   What systems can be used to summarise clinical information and facilitate interprofessional care?

3   What aspects of Mary's circumstances mean that multidisciplinary care is likely to assist?

From the consumer's perspective – *How does this feel for me?*

Hospital admissions can be a confusing time – although many people speak to a consumer, it is not always clear to the consumer who undertakes what role.

Although many processes of professional care may be running in the background, to a consumer these may not always be visible and it may seem that there is little progress.

'Why are all of these people asking me all of these questions?'

Summary

Psychotropic drug therapy is clearly among the most important of the treatment modalities available for the management of serious mental illness. A review of the history of psychotropic drug development indicates that the evolution of new treatment strategies in psychiatry has been rapid in recent times, possibly outpacing the rate at which understanding and knowledge about treatment options is developing. All of this underscores the importance of a truly multidisciplinary approach to drug treatment for mental illness, where a range of practitioners contribute the skills and experience of their disciplines as a part of a comprehensive approach to management. To achieve this, a broad view of the issues relating to the safety and efficacy of drug treatment is required, incorporating attention to all aspects of care where drug-related problems can be observed.

Discussion questions

1   What is meant by the term 'drug-related problem?'

2   Discuss examples whereby various health professionals may contribute specific expertise in designing and implementing pharmacotherapy for those with mental illness.

Test yourself (answers at the back of the book)

1   The first effective antipsychotic drug to be introduced into widespread clinical practice was:

   A   clozapine

   B   chlorpromazine

   C   clomipramine

   D   cetirazine

2   Which of the following statements is true with respect to psychological treatments for mental disorders?

   A   They are frequently associated with significant biological side effects.

   B   They are usually inexpensive and easy to access.

   C   There is evidence to support use in a range of clinical settings.

   D   They are always less effective than biological treatments.

3   Which of the following is an example of a non-drug form of biological treatment for mental disorders?

   A   Cognitive behavioural therapy

   B   Psychoeducation

   C   Lithium augmentation

   D   Transcranial electromagnetic therapy

4 An initiative by the Library of Congress (USA) and the National Institute of Mental Health (USA) to enhance public awareness of the benefits of brain research, the 'decade of the brain' spanned the period:

A 1950–59

B 1960–69

C 1900–99

D 2000–09

5 Established in collaboration with the World Health Organization, a unit of measurement of drug usage used in pharmacoepidemiology is:

A defined daily dose/1000 population/day

B drug mass/prescription

C mg/kg/day

D mg/month/1 000 000 people

Useful websites

Australian Statistics on Medicine (2009) available at <www.health.gov.au/internet/main/publishing.nsf/content/nmp-quality.htm>

Quality and Medicines Mapping (2007) available at

References

Department of Health and Ageing. (2002). *The National Strategy for Quality Use of Medicines*. Canberra, Australia.

Department of Health and Ageing. (2010). National Medicines Policy available at <www.health.gov.au/internet/main/publishing.nsf/Content/National+Medicines+Policy-1>, accessed 30 July 2012.

Hippocrates. (400 BCE). *On the Sacred Disease*, translated by Francis Adams (2009) available at <www.classics.mit.edu/hippocrates/sacred.html>, accessed 30 July 2012.

Rossi S. (2012). *Australian Medicines Handbook*. Adelaide, South Australia: AMH Pty Ltd.

Strand L. M. et al. (1990). 'Drug-related problems: their structure and function' *Dicp* 24(11): 1093–1097.

Chapter 2

Law, Ethics and Accountability

Chapter overview

This chapter covers the following topics:

* mental health law
* involuntary treatment
* ethical theories
* ethical principles
* seclusion and restraint (physical and chemical).

Chapter learning objectives

After reading this chapter, you should be able to:

* understand the legal context for treatment in mental health services
* identify key components of the mental health law in your own context
* understand and discuss what ethics is and what ethics is not.

Key terms

Autonomy
Beneficence
Ethical decision-making
Ethical principles
Involuntary treatment
Justice
Mental Health Act
Non-maleficence

Introduction

In this chapter you will explore mental health laws in Australia and New Zealand, the legal context for mental illness, **involuntary treatment** and **ethical principles**, and how these may influence consent, confidentiality and **ethical decision-making**.

In each state and territory of Australia and in New Zealand, legislative requirements are in place for health care workers to practise the care of people who experience mental disorders. These legislative requirements apply across the care continuum from assessment, review and transport to hospitalisation or community care. While there are discrete differences in mental health legislation in various jurisdictions, there are many similarities that underpin the principles for the protection of people with mental illness and the improvements to mental health care (see Table 2.1).

Table 2.1: Mental health laws in Australia and New Zealand

Country	State/territory	Mental Health Act
Australia	Victoria	*Mental Health Act 1986*
	Tasmania	*Mental Health Act 1996*
		On 21 June 2012, The Minister for Health, Michelle O'Byrne, tabled a Bill in Parliament to introduce a new Mental Health Act for Tasmania. The Mental Health Bill 2012 aims to bolster the rights of mental health consumers by ensuring that treatment for people with a mental illness reflects a human rights approach.
	South Australia	*Mental Health Act 1993*
	Western Australia	*Mental Health Act 1996*
	Northern Territory	*Mental Health and Related Services Act 2004*
	Queensland	*Mental Health Act 2000*
	New South Wales	*Mental Health Act 2007*
	Australian Capital Territory	*Mental Health (Treatment and Care) Act 1994*

New Zealand	*Mental Health (Compulsory Assessment and Treatment) Act 1992*
	The Mental Health Act sets out eleven basic patient rights:
	the right to information
	respect for cultural identity
	the right to an interpreter
	the right to treatment
	the right to be informed about treatment
	the right to refuse video recording
	the right to independent psychiatric advice
	the right to legal advice
	the right to company
	the right to have visitors and make telephone calls
	the right to send and receive mail.

Note: Legislative Acts relating to mental illness and addictions in New Zealand can be located on the New Zealand Ministry of Health website. The following Acts are included:
- *Alcoholism and Drug Addiction Act 1966*
- *Criminal Procedure (Mentally Impaired Persons) Act 2003*
- *Intellectual Disability (Compulsory Care and Rehabilitation) Act 2003*
- *Mental Health (Compulsory Assessment and Treatment) Act 1992*
- *Mental Health (Compulsory Assessment and Treatment) Amendment Act 1999*
- *Misuse of Drugs Act 1975.*

The legal and strategic context for mental disorders

In Australia, the *Fourth National Mental Health Plan: An Agenda for Collaborative Government Action in Mental Health 2009–2014* was launched. This document sets out a plan for joint government action in mental health for five years from 2009, offering a framework to build up a system of care that is able to intervene early, and one that provides direction to governments in considering future funding priorities for mental health and mental health services.

In 2005, the New Zealand government launched *Te Tāhuhu – Improving Mental Health 2005–2015: The Second New Zealand Mental Health and Addiction Plan*. The Te Tāhuhu Plan was developed to provide direction for the ongoing development and contemporary nature of the mental health and addiction sector in New Zealand. In order to ensure the New Zealand government priorities expressed in the Te Tāhuhu were actioned, *Te Kōkiri: New Zealand Mental Health and Addiction Action Plan 2006–2015* was launched.

Within each of the above strategic plans for mental health services, the basic human rights of people are a major priority. Human rights are also the foundation for mental health legislation, especially in the context of involuntary care and treatment, consent, negligence, guardianship and confidentiality.

Involuntary treatment

Most people will be treated in primary care by GPs or by a private psychiatrist, psychologist or allied health professional for mental illness. However, for the minority their mental condition is impaired to an extent that their capacity to understand the disorder is compromised and the disorder may affect the person's judgment and safety. The individual who is experiencing mental illness may also present a risk to themselves and/or others, for example deliberate self-harm, self-injurious behaviour, suicide; homicidal ideation; and danger arising from impaired judgment secondary to the effects of the illness and/or treatment.

Involuntary treatment is an option of care for a person who meets certain criteria in the relevant mental health Act. The legislation is highly variable and frequently updated between the states and territories of Australia and you should refer to the legislation that pertains to your area for greater detail.

By way of illustration, in Victoria (Australia) the criteria that need to be fulfilled so that a person might be committed for involuntary treatment are:

1. if they appear to be mentally ill; and

2. the person's mental illness requires immediate treatment and that treatment can be obtained by the person being subject to an involuntary treatment order; and

3. because of the person's mental illness, involuntary treatment of the person is necessary for their health or safety (whether to prevent a deterioration in the person's physical or mental condition or otherwise) or for the protection of members of the public; and

4. the person has refused or is unable to consent to the necessary treatment for the mental illness; and

5. the person cannot receive adequate treatment for the mental illness in a manner less restrictive of their freedom of decision and action.

Involuntary admission for mental illness is initiated when someone makes a 'request' that a person is to be examined by a medical practitioner to see if they meet the grounds for an involuntary order. If the medical practitioner decides that the person meets the grounds for an involuntary order, they may make a 'recommendation' that the person be further examined either at a mental health service or in the community. Within 72 hours a medical practitioner or a mental health practitioner will further examine the person after which they decide whether to issue an interim involuntary treatment order (either as an inpatient or in the community). The authorised psychiatrist or their delegate then must examine the person within 24 hours of the interim involuntary treatment order being made and confirm or reject the involuntary treatment order. Within an eight-week period of the involuntary treatment order being made, the Mental Health Review Board reviews the order to determine if the person meets the criteria for involuntary treatment at that time. The order will automatically expire after 12 months unless extended by the authorised psychiatrist. The Mental Health Review Board must review any extension.

In New South Wales (Australia) the *Mental Health Act 2007* states that involuntary treatment should occur only when a person's condition seriously impairs their judgment and is causing serious problems, such as disturbed mood, abnormal experiences or disturbed behaviour, and there is no other available way of preventing serious harm occurring to the person themselves or to another person.

In Tasmania (Australia) the *Mental Health Act 1996* provides for a person's involuntary admission to an approved hospital by way of an Initial Order, a Continuing Care Order or an Authorisation for Temporary Admission.

Initial Orders are made by a medical practitioner on the application of an Authorised Officer (nurse, social worker etc.) or person responsible (a guardian, spouse or de facto, carer, or close friend or relative). Initial Orders must be confirmed by an approved medical practitioner (generally, a psychiatrist), and are effective for up to 72 hours. An Initial Order provides authority for a person to be detained in an approved hospital for the purposes of assessment. A person who is already subject to an Initial Order, a Community Treatment Order or an Authorisation for Temporary Admission can be placed on a Continuing Care Order. Continuing Care Orders are made by two medical practitioners, at least one of whom must be an approved medical practitioner, who have each separately examined the person.

In the Northern Territory (Australia) involuntary treatment is initiated when the doctor has examined the patient/client either in person or by videoconference and, in addition, is satisfied that the person has either refused or is unable to consent to necessary treatment and that there is no less restrictive treatment option. Within 24 hours (mental illness) or 72 hours (mental disturbance), the patient will be examined by another doctor. If the second doctor agrees with the first, the patient may be detained for up to 14 days (mental illness) or a further seven days (mental disturbance). During this time the case will be reviewed by the Mental Health Review Tribunal. When a person is admitted to a mental health facility as an involuntary patient on the grounds of mental illness or mental disturbance, Mental Health Services must notify the tribunal of the admission. The tribunal will conduct a hearing within seven days from the date of admission and make a decision about whether the person should remain an involuntary patient.

In Queensland (Australia) in all cases involuntary treatment must be authorised or confirmed by a psychiatrist. The Act also recognises the importance of videoconference facilities in providing greater access to specialist mental health services for people in rural or remote locations.

The *South Australian Mental Health Act 1993* is designed to protect the autonomy and freedom of the mentally ill and emphasises treatment is to be received in the least restrictive environment. There is also an emphasis on recognising the role of the family and carers in the treatment, and initial detention orders may be implemented by non-medical personnel.

In Western Australia a person who is referred under section 29 for examination by a psychiatrist in an authorised hospital is to be received into the hospital and may be detained there for up to 24 hours from the time of reception.

In the ACT the *Mental Health (Treatment and Care) Act 1994* is underpinned by the objective to provide treatment, care, rehabilitation and protection for mentally dysfunctional or mentally ill persons in a manner that is least restrictive of their human rights.

Confidentiality in relation to those in psychiatric care also varies with legislation. For instance, the Victorian *Mental Health Act 1986* prohibits any staff member of a psychiatric service from providing information about people who are, or have been, in receipt of psychiatric services (some exceptions apply within this section of the Act). While the New Zealand *Mental Health (Compulsory Assessment and Treatment) Act 1992* requires mandatory consultation with the family/whānau of a person held, under section 7A of the Act, unless it is indicated it is not in the person's best interest.

Involuntary treatment and care for people who experience mental illness creates many situations where health care workers may feel conflicted in a moral, legal and ethical contexts. One example is when a person is placed on an involuntary or compulsory treatment order under the **Mental Health Act** but is required to pay for medicines that the person does not want to take. Another example is when an individual is admitted to the mental health ward involuntarily and is adamant about not taking their prescribed medication, consideration must be made of the legislation, ethical principles and the individual's basic human rights according to *The United Nations Principles for the Protection of Persons with Mental Illness*.

In 1991, the United Nations developed the *Principles for the Protection of Persons with Mental Illness and for the Improvement of Mental Health Care*. The first of the principles outlined relates to fundamental freedoms and basic rights (United Nations, 1991, p. 92):

1. All persons have the right to the best available mental health care, which shall be part of the health and social care system.

2. All persons with a mental illness, or who are being treated as such persons, shall be treated with humanity and respect for the inherent dignity of the human person.

3. All persons with a mental illness, or who are being treated as such persons, have the right to protection from economic, sexual and other forms of exploitation, physical or other abuse and degrading treatment.

4. There shall be no discrimination on the grounds of mental illness. 'Discrimination' means any distinction, exclusion or preference that has the effect of nullifying or impairing equal enjoyment of rights. Special measures solely to protect the rights, or secure the advancement, of persons with mental illness shall not be deemed to be discriminatory. Discrimination does not include any distinction, exclusion or preference undertaken in accordance with the provisions of these Principles and necessary to protect the human rights of a person with a mental illness or of other individuals.

5. Every person with a mental illness shall have the right to exercise all civil, political, economic, social and cultural rights as recognized in the Universal Declaration of Human Rights, the International Covenant on Economic, Social and Cultural Rights, the International Covenant on Civil and Political Rights, and in other relevant instruments, such as the Declaration on the Rights of Disabled Persons and the Body of Principles for the Protection of All Persons under Any Form of Detention or Imprisonment.

6. Any decision that, by reason of his or her mental illness, a person lacks legal capacity, and any decision that, in consequence of such incapacity, a personal representative shall be appointed, shall be made only after a fair hearing by an independent and impartial tribunal established by domestic law. The person whose capacity is at issue shall be entitled to be represented by a counsel. If the person whose capacity is at issue does not himself or herself secure such representation, it shall be made available without payment by that person to the extent that he or she does not have sufficient means to pay for it. The counsel shall not in the same proceedings represent a mental health facility or its personnel

and shall not also represent a member of the family of the person whose capacity is at issue unless the tribunal is satisfied that there is no conflict of interest. Decisions regarding capacity and the need for a personal representative shall be reviewed at reasonable intervals prescribed by domestic law. The person whose capacity is at issue, his or her personal representative, if any, and any other interested person shall have the right to appeal to a higher court against any such decision.

7. Where a court or other competent tribunal finds that a person with mental illness is unable to manage his or her own affairs, measures shall be taken, so far as is necessary and appropriate to that person's condition, to ensure the protection of his or her interest.

Ask yourself!

1 What legislative requirements would you consider when a person has been involuntarily detained in the mental health unit and refuses to receive their medication?

2 Why are these considerations important?

3 What are the person's basic human rights and are you at risk of violating these if you adhere to the legislative requirements? If not, explain your rationale.

Seclusion and restraint

Seclusion is a form of isolation but is generally known (in mental health services) to be the confinement of the mental health patient/client at any time of the day or night, alone, in a room or area from which free exit is stopped. Restraint is also a limitation to an individual's freedom and can mean physical restraint (the restriction of the person's freedom of movement by physical means) and chemical restraint (when medication that has a sedating effect is prescribed and administered to control the individual's behaviour as contrasted to providing treatment) (Gaynor, 2009).

Despite a lack of evidence that seclusion and restraint offer positive clinical and health outcomes for patients/clients of mental health services, health care workers continue to engage in these practices on a daily basis. The ongoing practices of seclusion and restraint often subject the recipient to trauma, contribute to the broader community's fear of treatments in mental health facilities and contribute to the stigma attached to mental illness and mental health care. However, with a strong focus on safety of self, others and property in all mental health legislations, and the shift of acute mental health service care to emergency departments and public hospitals (and associated acute mental health care wards or units), seclusion and restraint have become regarded as accepted contemporary clinical practices in these overcrowded, highly accessible and under-resourced areas.

Ethical principles

Beauchamp and Childress (1991, 2001) define four main ethical principles: respect for **autonomy**, **beneficence**, **non-maleficence** and **justice**. Although there are more ethical virtues to consider (such as compassion, discernment, trustworthiness, virtue and integrity), only the four main principles mentioned above will be discussed here in regard to professional life. Ethical theories underpinned by ethical principles are important to consider when making decisions in health, and these can provide a framework when trying to make a correct ethical decision.

What ethics is not…

Ethics and legislation are not the same!

Actions can be…

ethical and legal

unethical and illegal

ethical and illegal

unethical and legal

Source: Bennett & Bennett (2011), p. 98

Autonomy

The ethical principle of autonomy relates to allowing people to 'self-rule' and make decisions for themselves that allow self-determination in life. There are two ethical theories with which to view the principle of autonomy – a paternalistic view or a libertarian view. Paternalism relates to making decisions for people who are considered to have a limit in their capacity to act voluntarily. The libertarian view prioritises the person's wishes over their apparent best interests, and the person has control over their own life choices. This view, while respectful of the person's choices, does not prevent the person making decisions that may be harmful rather than beneficial. The principle of autonomy relates to consent and the choice of treatment (or not). In mental health, and given that mental illness is episodic in nature, individuals may be still able to make decisions for themselves even during periods of acute illness.

Beneficence

The principle of beneficence relates to 'doing good'. The principle of beneficence relates to the ethical theory of utilitarianism. Utilitarianism maintains that we should strive to achieve the greatest amount of good because most people would benefit. There are two types of utility – act utilitarianism and rule utilitarianism. These are respectively the performance of an act or acts to benefit the most people, regardless of the individual's feelings or community constraints, and to benefit the most people but through the fairest means.

Non-maleficence

Derived from Hippocrates and from the Latin term *primum non nocere*, 'first do no harm', the concept of non-maleficence means to 'do no harm'. In bioethics there is an inherent obligation to not inflict harm when dealing with issues of the vulnerable, sick and injured. In the care of a person who is experiencing mental illness and is subject to compulsory care, we can justify doing good and not doing harm if the paradigm we use is a hard paternalist view, that is, overriding the person's voluntary and autonomous choices when their ability to make those choices is impaired and the person is at significant risk of preventable harm and the action outweighs the risks.

Justice

The ethical principle of justice relates to the concepts of equity and fairness. In essence, when treating patients/clients that are alike, there must be extenuating circumstances and a significant divergence from the norm to explain inconsistent decisions made with regard to treatment. This ethical principle relates to such matters such as non-discriminatory actions when care is provided or offered and includes the concepts of fairness, equity and non-discrimination.

Ethical decision-making and ethical theories

There are many ethical theories that form a specific theoretical framework to provide the health care worker with general strategies for defining the ethical actions to be taken in any given situation – for example, deontology, teleology (which includes utilitarianism, existentialism and pragmatism), natural law, and transcultural principles. The principles in these ethical theories can assist a health care worker to unpack the ethical principles that pertain to any given situation faced.

Under the deontological ethical theory, an action is right or wrong according to whether it follows pre-established criteria and is viewed as a 'must do', a rule, an absolute. This is an ethic based upon duty. The principles in the deontological ethical theory for ethical decision-making include the following:

* People should always be treated as ends and never as means.

* Human life has value.

* Always to tell the truth.

* Do no harm.

* All people are of equal value.

The teleological ethical theories or 'consequential ethics' are outcome-based and the focus is not the motive that causes one to act ethically, but the consequences of that action.

Natural law ethics, also known as the virtue system of ethics, considers actions as morally or ethically right if they are in harmony with the end purpose of human nature and human goals.

Transcultural ethical theory is an ethical system that centres on the diversity of cultures and beliefs.

Another important consideration is that health care professionals generally occupy a privileged position in society, and are obliged to perform their duties in a fashion that (based on ethical principles) will not facilitate or passively allow outcomes that may compromise the rights or safety of others. These considerations may relate to financial and interpersonal issues beyond the construct of individual patient care. For example:

✳ A health care worker must act ethically and honestly when interacting with the pharmaceutical industry, and must not accept direct or indirect financial inducements that can influence decision-making.

✳ A health care worker must never engage in an intimate or sexual relationship with a patient.

✳ If a health care worker becomes aware that a colleague is practising while impaired, they must take steps to ensure that this does not create a danger for people under the care of that practitioner.

✳ It is necessary to preserve confidentiality in all respects of a patient's care.

✳ Research must always be conducted in a fashion that protects the interests of subjects above all else, as well as guaranteeing academic integrity, good clinical practice, and freedom from the influence of undue inducements.

COLIN'S STORY

Colin owns two restaurants in the city business district. He is a 40-year-old married man with two children, aged 14 and 16 (both girls). He has been using marijuana recreationally to try to relax after his stressful days managing the businesses. Colin begins to feel suspicious and thinks there are people 'out to get him'. His paranoid thoughts are firm, fixed beliefs that are not supported by any evidence that these thoughts are true. He complains that he has jumbled thinking from time to time and believes the television is speaking directly to him when he is home. Colin starts to become fearful for himself and locks himself in his bedroom. His wife contacts the general practitioner who attends the home. After some discussion, with a member of the crisis team for the mental health service, he attends Colin's home to assess Colin's mental state and refers him for further mental health assessment in the hospital's mental health ward. Colin is assessed by the psychiatrist who determines that his mental illness requires immediate treatment, and that treatment can be obtained by an involuntary treatment order; and because of Colin's mental illness, involuntary treatment of Colin is necessary for his health and safety. Colin has refused the necessary treatment for the mental illness and he was assessed as not being in a position where he could receive adequate treatment for the mental illness in a manner less restrictive. Colin continues to refuse treatment when in hospital and his fear is mounting. He attempts to leave the ward and is stopped by the staff who attempt to engage Colin in treatment. Colin begins yelling and thrashing out at the staff. He is very frightened and just wants to leave so that he can protect his family and home from the threat he believes is happening. Colin is restrained physically by the staff, given a sedative to calm him and placed in a more secure part of the ward – the high-dependency area.

Care Plan

The following is an example care plan for the patient/client presented in this chapter. The areas of daily living that are considered include bio-psycho-social factors and the plan is mapped out using the nursing process (Assessment; Planning; Implementation; Evaluation). Remember: the success is in the detail, so be specific about *who, when and what* in the collaborative plan; never include someone in the plan if they were not consulted in the planning process; and always work within a recovery-orientated framework (refer to Chapter 1).

Date: 30 July 2012

Name: Colin   Case manager: To be appointed after discharge

Areas of daily living	Assessment of current situation	Goal	Plan (undertaken with patient/client)	Implementation	Who is responsible? (Include only those who have been consulted in the planning process)	Evaluation/review date
Mental health	Drug-induced psychosis with paranoid ideas	Minimise the adverse effects of the psychotic symptoms.	Colin has been admitted involuntarily to the mental health unit.	Provide Colin and his family with information related to rights and responsibilities. Monitor Colin's acute symptoms and revise care plans as symptoms abate.	Primary nurse on the ward	Each shift change
Social	Colin manages two restaurants in the city district. Colin is married with two teenage daughters.	Work with Colin to facilitate support as appropriate for Colin's wife and children while Colin is in hospital.	Arrange a family meeting to be held on the ward with the psychiatrist, primary nurse and allied health/ social worker.	Meeting to be scheduled.	Primary nurse on the ward	31/7/12

(Continued)

Date: 30 July 2012 *(Continued)*

Name: Colin

Case manager: To be appointed after discharge

Areas of daily living	Assessment of current situation	Goal	Plan (undertaken with patient/client)	Implementation	Who is responsible? (Include only those who have been consulted in the planning process)	Evaluation/review date
Biological	Commenced on antipsychotic medication.	Monitor desired and unwanted effects of medication.	Baseline observations to monitor the potential negative physical effects of antipsychotic medications.	Undertake baseline observations related to: • blood pressure • temperature • pulse • respiration • weight • waist measurement • cholesterol levels • thyroid function test, full blood examination, liver function test, white blood cell count, etc. • oral health.	Primary nurse on the ward	30/7/12

	Monitor efficacy of medications.	Minimise ADRs.	Use the Positive and Negative Syndrome Scale (PANSS). See also: • Brief Psychiatric Rating Scale (BPRS) • Scale for the Assessment of Positive Symptoms (SAPS) • Scale for the Assessment of Negative Symptoms (SANS).	Positive and negative symptoms Weight gain Hyperprolactinaemia Sedation Hyperlipidaemia Postural hypotension Other cardiovascular effects Hyperglycaemia	Primary nurse on the ward. 30/7/12
Environmental	Lives independent with family. Self-employed.	None identified.			
Substance using behaviours	Uses cannabis daily.	To reduce the risks associated with cannabis use	Explore Colin's motivations and beliefs related to cannabis use.	Work together to reduce cannabis use or cannabis cessation.	Colin and primary nurse. Referral for case management post discharge for follow-up. 1/8/12

(Continued)

Date: 30 July 2012 *(Continued)*

Name: Colin

Case manager: To be appointed after discharge

Areas of daily living	Assessment of current situation	Goal	Plan (undertaken with patient/client)	Implementation	Who is responsible? (Include only those who have been consulted in the planning process)	Evaluation/ review date
Risk behaviours	Colin is fearful, wants to leave to ward and is aggressively thrashing out at staff.	Minimise risk of injury (to staff and Colin) from aggressive thrashing out.	Provide a safe environment and appropriate level of supervision. Maximise the potential for building a therapeutic relationship to facilitate trust and engagement for Colin.	Monitor in the High Dependency Unit until Colin's symptoms abate and aggressive thrashing out at staff ceases. Allocate a primary nurse to increase continuity of care and maximise opportunities for building a therapeutic relationship.	Primary nurse and consultant psychiatrist.	Constant observation from admission. Reviewed every hour for re-entry into the general ward environment.

Ask yourself!

As Colin's health care worker:

1   What ethical considerations will you make when caring for Colin?

2   What legislative requirements do you need to adhere to in Colin's care?

3   How can you ensure the ethical principles of beneficence and non-maleficence are carried out in this scenario?

4   What ethical theories can you apply when making ethical decisions and does this affect your care decision?

From the consumer's perspective – *How does this feel for me?*

'I'm going to sue you all for holding me against my will!'

'You have to help me, call the police! Why won't you call the police?'

'You have no right to hold me here! I want to go home!'

Consider your responses to Colin's concerns keeping in mind the ethical and legal responsibilities you have to adhere to in the conduct of care. Can you justify ethically and legally holding Colin against his will and administering medication that he does not want or think he needs?

Summary

In this chapter you explored the legal and ethical dimensions of mental health care provision in the context of the strategic directions for mental health services. The challenges presented in this chapter (although not exhaustive) provide a framework for conceptualising the law, ethics and personal accountability in caring for those who experience mental disorder, and in particular for those who have an involuntary status. Treatment in care for the mentally ill incorporates many challenges with the administration of medications in a variety of different situations, and these can challenge your own ethical and moral values. However, care for this vulnerable group in our community needs to be conceptualised and informed by a theoretical and evidence-based framework and not merely based on personal beliefs (which can vary from clinician to clinician).

Discussion questions

1   *How* can you ensure that you are conducting your interventions for another in mental health services in a legal and ethical manner?

2   *Who* can request and assess/admit someone for involuntary treatment in your state, territory or country?

3   *What* lessons can be learned from Colin's story? How can you ensure your accountability while acting in a legal and ethical manner in the care of Colin?

Test yourself (answers at the back of the book)

1   Which of the following is true with respect to mental health law statutes in Australia and New Zealand?

A   Laws are virtually identical in each jurisdiction.

B   Laws apply only in the context of community-based care.

C   Laws apply only in the context of institutional care.

D   Laws protect those where mental illness may impair judgment or safety.

2   When used in psychiatric practice, the term 'seclusion' refers to:

A   providing a quiet environment that the patient can use to reflect upon events

B   isolation in response to antisocial behaviour necessitating a sanction

C   prevention of transmissible diseases

D   confinement to an area from which free exit is not possible

3   Which of the following is regarded as a fundamental ethical principle relevant to psychiatry?

A   Confidentiality must be maintained.

B   Clients with severe illness have treatment decisions made on their behalf.

C   Never deal with the pharmaceutical industry under any circumstances.

D   Patient seclusion can only be undertaken under the parameters of a court order.

4   With respect to the relationship between ethics and the law, actions can conceivably be:

A   both ethical and legal

B   both ethical and illegal

C   both unethical and legal

D   all of the above

5   With respect to ethical aspects of relationships between patient/client and health care worker:

   A   it is reasonable to have an intimate relationship if both are consenting adults

   B   it is not reasonable to establish an intimate or sexual relationship

   C   it is reasonable to establish an intimate relationship with a family member

   D   it is routine to form close platonic relationships with patients/clients

Useful websites

AustLII (2012) Australian Legal Information Institute available at <www.austlii.edu.au>

Australian Department of Health and Ageing available at <www.health.gov.au//internet/main/publishing.nsf/Content/Home>

Principles for the Protection of Persons with Mental Illness and for the Improvement of Mental Health Care available at <www.un.org/documents/ga/res/46/a46r119.htm>

New Zealand Ministry of Health available at <www.health.govt.nz>

References

Beauchamp T. L. & Childress J. F. (1991). 'Principles of biomedical ethics' *International Clinical Psychopharmacology* 6(2): 129.

Beauchamp T. L. & Childress J. F. (2001). *Principles of Biomedical Ethics.* USA: Oxford University Press.

Bennett B. & Bennett A. (2011). 'Laws, ethics and mental health nursing'. In Edward K., Munro I., Robins A. & Welch A. (eds). *Mental Health Nursing. Dimensions of praxis*, pp. 80–120. Melbourne, Australia: Oxford University Press.

Gaynor N. J. (2009). 'Clinical management of acute behavioural disturbance associated with volatile solvent intoxication' *Australasian Emergency Nursing Journal* 12(2): 55–58.

United Nations. (1991). *Principles for the Protection of Persons with Mental Illness and for the Improvement of Mental Health Care.* A/RES/46/119. Geneva, Switzerland: Office of the United Nations High Commissioner for Human Rights.

Chapter 3

Pharmacokinetics

Chapter overview

This chapter covers the following topics:

✳ basic principles of pharmacokinetics

✳ detailed information about each of the major pharmacokinetic processes.

Chapter learning objectives

After reading this chapter, you should be able to:

✳ describe the factors influencing the basic aspects of drug product formulation

✳ outline the processes by which drugs enter and are eliminated from the body

✳ apply pharmacokinetic knowledge in the care process.

Key terms

Absorption
Administer
Drug distribution
Drug elimination
Half-life
Metabolism
Pharmacodynamics
Pharmacokinetics
Receptors
Renal clearance

Introduction

This chapter addresses the basic science of the ways in which drugs enter, move around and are eliminated from the human body. Nurses and other health care professionals need to understand these processes to be able to safely **administer** drugs to patients/clients, and to be able to interpret the effects that medications produce in clinical practice. Many psychotropic drugs have quite distinctive pharmacokinetic profiles that will profoundly influence the individual's response to treatment.

Pharmacokinetics – the science of drug movements

Pharmacokinetics is a pharmacological science addressing the disposition of drugs and their metabolites in the human body. All drugs have a distinct pharmacokinetic profile that is influenced by various factors; these factors characterise the entry of the drug into the body, the reversible movements of the drug between internal sites, and the final elimination of the drug from the body. The basic characteristics of drug action are profoundly influenced by the pharmacokinetics of the agent, and an understanding of pharmacokinetics is critical to the formulation of drug treatment regimens. To be truly useful, the application of pharmacokinetics must be combined with an understanding of the mechanism and characteristics through which drugs produce physiological and biochemical effects (**pharmacodynamics**). The consideration of both pharmacokinetics and pharmacodynamics facilitates individualisation of drug therapy, optimising the efficacy of treatment and reducing the likelihood of toxicities.

Various parameters determine the characteristics of the movement of drugs within the body. The means by which the drug enters the body (**absorption**), its movements after absorption (distribution), and the way it ultimately leaves the body (elimination, which can be further subdivided to consider drug **metabolism** and excretion) are all important processes that must be understood if you wish to have a working knowledge of clinical pharmacokinetics.

The usual situation is that after the drug is administered absorption, distribution and elimination actually occur simultaneously for at least part of the duration of the drug's effects.

Practical applications of pharmacokinetics will guide the rational selection of the best drug delivery route, will influence the size of the dose administered and the frequency of administration, and may also form the basis for aspects of the formulation of the drug product. Many factors influence **drug elimination**, and these will have critical influences upon the treatment regimen. Aspects of the distribution of the drug within the body also directly influence its elimination.

Drug absorption

A drug can produce a therapeutic effect only after it has entered the body and reached the site of action. For most drugs, this is after the medication moves into the systemic circulation, and is subsequently transported to its site of action. In some specific situations drugs act at the site they are delivered to – for example, when applied to the skin. However, for most drugs and all psychotropic agents, the medication needs to be absorbed (undergo absorption), which involves movement across a barrier structure and into the body's internal environment. In all cases where a drug is administered with the intention of achieving a systemic effect, the product must be formulated in a way that allows it to cross the barrier to absorption. In some circumstances, the route of administration involves direct introduction into systemic circulation. This may be because the drug is altered in nature during its passage (this is the case for proteins or polypeptides such as insulin). Delivery directly into the systemic circulation usually intensifies the effects of the medication and/or decreases the time for the onset of action (e.g. intravenous administration of antipsychotic drugs).

Drugs can be administered by a variety of routes. For most situations, the best route is oral administration, because of its convenience, reliability and tolerability; this is the route most commonly used for the administration of psychotropic drugs. Orally and rectally administered drugs need to be absorbed into the systemic circulation to produce a therapeutic effect. Drug absorption after oral administration largely involves the small intestine, and involves several steps. Most psychotropic drugs are administered as tablets or capsules; these must break down in the environment of the gastrointestinal tract and, notably, this breakdown can be modified by the way a drug product is formulated (e.g. sustained release or enteric coated formulations). Some tablets have a layer which is resistant to acidic environments – for example, enteric-coated preparations do not release the drug until reaching the intestine, where the pH is higher than in the stomach. This approach protects acid-labile drugs from gastric acid, or alternatively may be used to protect the gastric mucosa from the irritant effects of some drugs.

After a tablet or capsule disintegrates, the drug must dissolve in the gastrointestinal fluids to allow absorption across the mucosa. In some cases chemical reactions in the gut may inactivate the drug pharmacologically – for example, proteins administered orally are digested and the original properties of the compound are lost (e.g. insulin, which cannot be administered orally). In addition, drugs undergo gut-wall metabolism (see below), and some or all of the original drug is lost before reaching the systemic circulation. Not all orally administered drugs undergo gut-wall metabolism, but in some cases the loss of active compound at this step is so great that the efficacy of the drug is severely diminished.

After moving across the gut mucosa, drugs then diffuse into small blood vessels close to the gut lining. These blood vessels form a part of the hepatic portal circulation system, and from here drugs are transported directly to the liver before entering the general systemic circulation. For some drugs most of the orally administered dose is chemically modified into metabolites before accessing the systemic circulation. In this situation the drug is said to undergo a significant first pass effect, and only a relatively small proportion of the drug reaches the site of action. A first pass effect is also known as presystemic metabolism. An alternative route of administration may be required under these circumstances – for example, asenapine, an antipsychotic drug, has a significant first pass effect and is usually administered sublingually, bypassing the hepatic portal circulation. Another approach is to increase the dose of the drug when administered orally to compensate for the small proportion reaching the systemic circulation. An example is morphine: the oral dose is much higher than the dose of morphine used intravenously.

Under some circumstances oral drug administration is not practical or possible and the drug may be administered by injection (parenterally). In this case, the drug is dissolved and introduced via a needle or cannula. Drugs may be injected directly into a vein, or can be delivered to other sites from which there is absorption into the general circulation. After intravenous administration the drug has direct access to the systemic circulation: the intensity of effect is usually greater when this route of administration is used, and the onset of action may also be quicker. An alternative parenteral route (such as subcutaneous or intramuscular injections) can be used to allow the administration of the drug to a site from which general systemic absorption can occur. Subcutaneous injections are placed into the tissue close to the dermal layer of the skin – from here the medication is transported into the vasculature found in the subcutaneous tissue. The intramuscular route of administration is very commonly used. The medication is injected into a muscle mass such as the gluteal or deltoid, and is absorbed into the systemic circulation through the blood vessels supplying the muscle. In some cases (e.g. depot formulations of antipsychotic drugs), intramuscular injections are deliberately formulated for slow release from the injection site, in order to achieve sustained action.

Drug distribution

Following absorption, further movements of the drug occur within the body. The term **drug distribution** describes the reversible movements of a drug within the body, usually from one compartment to another. Some drugs are poorly soluble in water, and are distributed to sites outside of the general circulation. Drugs produce their therapeutic effects by binding to an appropriate receptor. In the case of psychotropic agents the targeted **receptors** are found in the central nervous system. Drug distribution to an extravascular site (located or occurring outside a blood or lymph vessel) is reversible – having been transferred from the intravascular site to the brain, the drug will eventually distribute back into the blood or plasma, from which it will ultimately be removed from the body. Drugs usually distribute to several areas within the body at once, and simultaneous transfer between a number of compartments may occur. It is not normally possible to measure the concentration of a drug at its site of action. Instead, its concentration in the blood or plasma is measured, and this information is considered in relation to the known pharmacokinetic characteristics of the drug.

When a drug is extensively distributed to sites outside of the plasma, the plasma concentration does not truly reflect the total amount of drug in the body. The term 'volume of distribution' is used to describe that volume which would be consistent with the known amount of drug in the body, and the observed concentration in the plasma. For drugs where distribution to sites outside of the plasma does not occur, the volume of distribution will be close to plasma volume (about 3 litres), but for drugs extensively distributed to sites outside of the plasma, the volume of distribution (which is an imaginary figure) may be considerably greater than 3 litres. In the case of many psychotropic agents the volume of distribution can be very large indeed (the volume of distribution for haloperidol is normally in excess of 500 litres). Many drugs bind to proteins found circulating in the plasma; such proteins are very large molecules that cannot cross intact biological membranes. Even when the drug is highly bound to plasma proteins, a small proportion remains unbound. Only an unbound drug can distribute to extravascular sites. Drug distribution has a critical influence upon the characteristics of the drug's actions. Drugs act at specific receptor sites, and where drug distribution to these sites is slow or limited, this will be reflected in the drug's action. Drugs can be metabolised or excreted only in the unbound state, and thus the properties of the drug's distribution will in part determine the duration of the effect.

Figure 3.1: Drug absorption and distribution

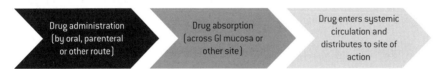

Drug administration (by oral, parenteral or other route)

Drug absorption (across GI mucosa or other site)

Drug enters systemic circulation and distributes to site of action

Drug metabolism and elimination

Elimination collectively refers to the various ways in which a drug irreversibly leaves the body, and can be subdivided into the processes of drug excretion (whereby the drug is transported out of the body's internal environment) and drug metabolism (where the drug is converted into a different chemical). The new compound produced during drug metabolism is called a metabolite.

The term used to define drug elimination is 'clearance'. The clearance is measured in units of volume per unit time – if a drug has a plasma clearance of 5 litres per hour, this means that 5 litres of plasma are cleared of that drug each hour. If the concentration of the drug in the plasma is 20 mg per litre, then the rate of elimination for that drug will be 100 mg per hour. Factors that influence clearance have a profound impact on drug action.

The two major mechanisms by which a drug is eliminated from the body are renal excretion and metabolic elimination (commonly referred to as drug metabolism). Most drugs are organic chemicals and are not soluble in water. To allow drug excretion, drug metabolism requires a reaction that changes the structure of the parent drug, producing a new chemical compound which is more soluble in water. Drug metabolism takes place at various organs but the most important of all is in the liver. Metabolism usually results in the creation of a metabolite with less pharmacological activity than the parent compound. Drug metabolism often involves several steps – for example, a drug may undergo oxidation followed by conversion to a glucuronide metabolite. Several types of metabolism may take place simultaneously, with different paths of metabolism competing.

Hepatic drug elimination

Drug metabolism is achieved by enzyme systems located primarily in the liver. Under certain circumstances the activity of these enzymes may be increased, meaning that metabolism will occur at a faster rate (hepatic enzyme induction). If enzyme activity is induced while the rate and extent of drug absorption remains constant, the plasma level of the drug will normally decrease. Hepatic enzyme induction usually occurs as a result of the influence of a chemical

Figure 3.2: Drug metabolism pathways

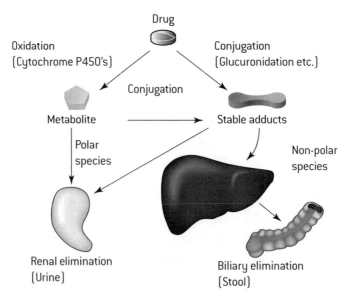

Drug

Oxidation
(Cytochrome P450's)

Conjugation
(Glucuronidation etc.)

Conjugation

Metabolite

Stable adducts

Polar
species

Non-polar
species

Renal elimination
(Urine)

Biliary elimination
(Stool)

compound from outside of the body (called an inducing agent). For example, cigarette smoking significantly increases the rate of clozapine metabolism, causing decreased plasma levels.

Some drugs have the effect of decreasing the rate of hepatic drug metabolism. This process is called hepatic enzyme inhibition, and may also give rise to important drug interactions. Provided that drug absorption and distribution are unchanged, and that hepatic metabolism is the main route of elimination, then enzyme inhibition will cause an increase in plasma drug levels, possibly resulting in clinical toxicity.

Renal drug excretion

The kidneys are another important site for the elimination of drugs from the body. Drug elimination may be achieved through filtration at the glomerulus in the kidney, and the drug excreted into the urine.

In addition to filtration, drugs can be actively secreted into the urine, and thus **renal clearance** can actually exceed the glomerular filtration rate. There may also be reabsorption, where the drug is reabsorbed from the filtrate back into the systemic circulation. The overall nature, extent and rate of renal clearance will be a composite of filtration, secretion and reabsorption.

Figure 3.3: Parts of the nephron

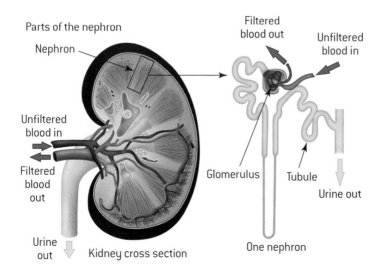

To be renally cleared a drug must be transported in solution to the kidney. Drugs which are poorly soluble in water are usually not excreted unchanged by the kidney to any significant extent – these drugs usually undergo conversion to metabolites which are more water soluble. For some drugs such as lithium, most of a dose is excreted unchanged in the urine. In the example of lithium, a significant decline in renal function will cause increased drug levels, sometimes causing toxicity.

Elimination half-life

Clearance determines the rate of decline of plasma drug levels. The elimination **half-life** of a drug is defined as the time required for the plasma concentration to decrease by 50% from an original value. If the plasma level decreases from 20 mg/L to 10 mg/L after a period of 12 hours, then the apparent half-life of the drug is said to be 12 hours. For most drugs, steady state plasma concentrations are not attained until the drug has been administered for a period of time approximately equivalent to six times the half-life of the drug. Similarly, the time taken to remove almost all of a drug from the body after a single dose (or after stopping a maintenance dose) is roughly six times the half-life of the drug.

Ask yourself!

1   What factors influence the onset of drug action after oral administration, and how might these be changed by individual clinical circumstances?
2   What does the term 'volume of distribution' describe?

Pharmacokinetics and nursing practice

Assessment

The nursing process consists of assessment, planning, intervention and evaluation. In terms of addressing possible pharmacokinetic issues for patients/clients your nursing assessment should include screening for factors which may alter oral drug absorption. These might include gastrointestinal pathology (such as gastroenteritis), a variety of acute and chronic illnesses (such as diabetes, cardiac failure and renal impairment), and interacting drug therapy.

Perhaps your assessment suggests that oral administration is not practical or effective, and so alternative routes of administration need to be considered. Assessment should also include consideration of factors that may influence drug elimination. Relevant considerations include the presence of cardiac failure, hepatic or renal impairment, or the administration of interacting drugs.

Evaluation

As serious adverse effects may arise as a result of alterations in the pharmacokinetics of some drugs, continuous nursing evaluation is necessary to allow early intervention where clinical toxicity or lack of therapeutic effect has serious clinical ramifications. These evaluations need to be planned for at the assessment stage or other appropriate time in the clinical continuum, and where possible involve the active participation of the patient/client in the therapeutic relationship or therapeutic alliance.

Drug administration

The correct method of administration should be used to enhance the therapeutic effectiveness of drugs, and in some cases to minimise the incidence of untoward effects. Areas for attention should include the correct order of administration of oral drugs in relation to food or other drugs, maintenance of the integrity of sustained release or enteric coated oral dose forms, and the correct use of alternative administration routes where the oral route is ineffective, inconvenient or impractical in any particular clinical situation.

Education

Educating patients/clients and their 'significant others' is an important daily role for the health professional. Importantly with drug therapies, nurses need to ensure that people are aware of the signs and symptoms of drug accumulation which can lead to drug toxicity. Patients/clients and their 'significant others' also should be made aware of the correct actions to take in the event of suspected toxicity. Education materials using contemporary evidence in the form of plain language statements about drug accumulation for various drugs are important in drug education.

MATTHEW'S STORY

Matthew is a 23-year-old man who lives with his family. He has a known history of schizophrenia and has had several admissions to hospital since his diagnosis. He has recently had a significant exacerbation of his illness in the context of repeatedly forgetting his medications and using cannabis heavily. He was admitted in an agitated state and required intramuscular antipsychotic medication to settle him. His mental state has now improved considerably and the clinical team is contemplating the next steps for his medication treatment.

Ask yourself!

As a nurse involved with caring for Matthew:

1 Why was intramuscular medication initially preferred to oral treatment options?
2 What can be done to design a treatment regimen that will help to keep his symptoms more stable?
3 How could an alternative route of medication administration help Matthew?

From the consumer's perspective – *How does this feel for me?*

It may not always be immediately obvious to a client/consumer why a particular route of drug administration has been chosen, and why two people treated with the same drug for the same illness may need different dosage regimens. Dosage requirements may change with the introduction of new drugs or after smoking cessation. Patients/clients might want to seek reassurance.

'Why do I need to have injections of this medication – can't I just taken tablets?'

'Why are they giving me a different dose of this medication now? The old dose seemed to work OK.'

'Why should the dose of my medication change because I gave up smoking?'

Summary

The clinical effects of all drugs used in the treatment of mental illness are profoundly influenced by pharmacokinetic parameters that govern the absorption, distribution, metabolism and elimination of the medications. Each drug has a unique pharmacokinetic profile, and the interaction with individual circumstances must be taken into account when selecting treatment and evaluating the therapeutic and adverse effects in the clinical setting. Nurses involved in the administration of drugs or monitoring of the effects of medications need a working knowledge of pharmacokinetics.

Discussion questions

1   Discuss the factors that significantly influence the absorption of drugs after oral administration.

2   Outline the reasons that drugs generally undergo metabolism prior to elimination.

3   Describe some fundamental applications of pharmacokinetics that can be used in the nursing assessment and evaluation processes.

Test yourself (answers at the back of the book)

1   Which of the following are mechanisms for drug elimination?

A   Renal excretion

B   Hepatic metabolism

C   Protein binding

D   A and B only

2   The route of administration that is usually preferred form most psychotropic drugs under usual circumstances is:

A   intravenous

B   oral

C   subcutaneous

D   rectal

3   The process whereby a drug is metabolised in the liver after transport via the portal vein and prior to systemic access is referred to:

A   hepatic filtration

B   first pass metabolism

C   high extraction filtration

D   drug distribution

4   With respect to the effects of drug metabolites:

A   all are inactive

B   all are active

C   they are generally referred to as pro-drugs

D   most are produced after transformation of a drug in the liver

5   The elimination half-life of a drug:

A   is determined by the rate of elimination

B   is influenced only by hepatic biotransformation

C   is the time taken for all of the drug to be eliminated after a dose

D   is never related to drug distribution characteristics

Useful website

Merck Manual: Overview of Pharmacokinetics available at

<www.merckmanuals.com/professional/clinical_pharmacology/
pharmacokinetics/overview_of_pharmacokinetics.html>

References

Birkett D. J. (2002). *Pharmacokinetics Made Easy*. Sydney: McGraw-Hill Australia Pty Ltd.

Brunton L. L., Chabner B. A. & Knollmann, B. C. (2010). Chapter 2 Pharmacokinetics: the dynamics of drug absorption, distribution, metabolism, and elimination, in *Goodman & Gilman's The Pharmacological Basis of Therapeutics*, 12th edn., China: McGraw-Hill Professional, McGraw-Hill Medical.

Chapter 4

Pharmacodynamics

Chapter overview

This chapter covers the following topics:

* basic principles of dynamics
* detailed information addressing major pharmacokinetic processes.

Chapter learning objectives

After reading this chapter, you should be able to:

* describe factors influencing the ways in which drugs produce pharmacological effects
* discuss underlying mechanisms for drug interactions and adverse drug reactions
* outline factors which may influence the individual response to drug therapy.

Key terms

Adverse drug reaction
Anticholinergic
Drug dependence
Drug interaction
Extrapyramidal side effects
Mechanism of action
Mood stabilisers
Pain
Receptors

Introduction

This chapter focuses on the mechanisms by which drugs produce pharmacological effects in the human body. Nurses and other health care professionals need insight into these principles to understand and interpret the therapeutic and adverse effects that medications produce in clinical practice. The pharmacodynamics of psychotropic drugs are especially complex and will govern the individual response to treatment. In this chapter you will first unpack the science behind drug actions including receptors and factors influencing drug response. You will also learn more detail about the unwanted effects of drugs (adverse drug reactions), and how these can arise in clinical practice. As many patients/clients are prescribed two or more drugs as part of a treatment regimen, interactions may arise where one drug decreases the metabolism of another drug, having implications for care. Finally, in this chapter you will be able to explore care considerations for patients/clients in the context of pharmacodynamics.

Pharmacodynamics – the science of drug actions

Pharmacodynamics, derived from the ancient Greek words for 'drug' and 'power', is the name of the scientific discipline used to understand the effects of drugs in the body. Aspects of pharmacodynamics include the mechanisms by which a drug produces any pharmacological action, either therapeutic or harmful, as well as the effects that may be produced by the concurrent administration of more than one drug. The science of pharmacodynamics is complementary to that of pharmacokinetics. Pharmacodynamic principles are used to understand the influence of person-specific factors such as age and body mass upon the acute and chronic effects of drug therapy. An understanding of the pharmacodynamic characteristics of drugs used in the treatment of an individual patient/client allows tailoring of drug therapy for maximum therapeutic benefit with minimum likelihood of unwanted reactions. Health care professionals need to be familiar with these characteristics as part of person-centred care within a multidisciplinary context as each episode of care will be different to the next for any one patient/client.

Drugs produce their effects through a variety of complex mechanisms. Understanding of the **mechanism of action** allows the application of this knowledge in designing a drug treatment regimen with best possible efficacy, and minimised toxicity. In some cases, the ultimate mechanism of drug action remains unclear, and the knowledge of the effects of the drug within the body is based largely on individual observations and population data. In some cases a beneficial effect and an adverse reaction may arise through different paths; for example, an antidepressant may produce its therapeutic effect by modulating the concentration of neurotransmitters in the brain, but independently may cause a rash that is thought to be a result of an allergic reaction.

Receptors

For many drugs, effects within the body happen through the interaction of the drug and cellular structures called receptors.

For example, a brain cell (also known as a neuron) is made up of a cell body, dendrites, an axon and axon terminals. Dendrites pick up information from other neurons and move it along to the cell body. From this point the axon moves the information onto the axon terminals where it is transmitted to

Figure 4.1: The space between two neurons (synaptic cleft) where neurotransmitters transport information

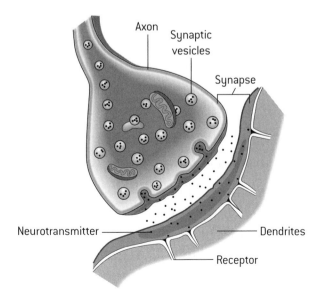

another neuron. The information is transmitted via neurotransmitters that are released and these travel across a synaptic cleft (the space between two neurons) and ultimately connect with receptor sites on the dendrites of another neuron. The process is repeated from neuron to neuron.

Table 4.1: Neurotransmitters, receptors and functions

Neurotransmitter	Receptors	Function
Acetylcholine	Muscarinic (M_1–M_5) and nicotinic	Memory function, sensory processing, motor coordination, autonomic nervous system
Norepinephrine	Alpha$_1$ and alpha$_2$; beta$_1$, beta$_2$ and beta$_3$	Central nervous system (CNS) sensory processing, cerebellar function, sleep, mood, learning, memory, anxiety
Dopamine	D_1–D_5	Motor regulation, reinforcement, olfaction, mood, concentration, hormone control
Serotonin (5-HT)	5-HT$_1$–5-HT$_8$	Emotional processing, mood, appetite, sleep, pain processing, hallucinations, and reflex regulation
Glutamate	NMDA (N-methyl-D-aspartic acid)	Memory and excitory function in CNS
Gamma aminobutyric acid (GABA)	GABA	Major inhibitory neurotransmitter in the CNS
Histamine	H1 and H2	Sleep, sedation and temperature regulation

Compounds such as hormones or neurotransmitters are the chemicals that would normally bind to receptors and produce a physiological effect. In the case of the endogenous compounds (internally derived compounds such as those found in cells), this interaction modifies a physiological or biochemical process, altering the rate, extent or nature of the function concerned. For example, when the neurotransmitter acetylcholine binds to its receptors on muscle tissue, the result is the contraction of the muscle fibres. However, even when producing therapeutic effects, the stimulation of other receptors can also produce a decrease in the rate or extent of a physiological process. The foundation for drug design is sometimes based upon observation of the physiological or biochemical effects arising from the actions of the endogenous compounds. In some cases the drug bears little resemblance in structure to the endogenous compound known to interact with the receptor. Those drugs which produce similar or synergistic effects to the endogenous compound are referred to as 'agonists', and those which produce an opposite effect 'antagonists'. In many cases, particularly in relation to psychotropic drugs, it has been established that subclasses of a number of receptors exist, and that under certain circumstances a given drug may act as both a receptor agonist and antagonist.

Not all drugs exert actions through direct binding to a receptor site. Enzymes are proteins found throughout the body, and facilitate chemical reactions. Enzymes usually facilitate the conversion of one chemical compound to another. In some cases the chemical is converted from an active compound into one with little or no pharmacological activity. Enzymatic degradation generally inactivates neurotransmitters, diminishing their effects. Remember that neurotransmitters are the chemicals that would normally bind to receptors and produce a physiological effect. However, drugs such as the cholinesterase inhibitors prolong and augment the activity of the neurotransmitter because they help preserve the ability of a neuron to transmit information.

The inhibition of enzymes may occur on a reversible basis and the administration of a sufficient dose of receptor antagonist (these block the binding of an agonist at a receptor molecule, inhibiting the signal produced by a receptor) will reverse the net pharmacological effect. For example, the administration of atropine (an antagonist of acetylcholine) can reverse the cholinergic effects arising from the administration of the anticholinesterase drugs such as donepezil. Enzyme inhibition can also be irreversible: some monoamine oxidase inhibitors (MAOIs) produce irreversible inhibition of the enzymes responsible for the degradation of neurotransmitters in the central nervous system, thus producing antidepressant effects. The body must make new monoamine oxidase enzymes before the effects of the inhibitor are diminished – this process (called 'washout' time) usually takes 14–21 days, and is commonly recommended before the commencement of potentially interacting drug therapy.

Factors influencing drug response

Many factors influence the response of an individual to a specific drug treatment regimen. Although some of the interindividual variation in response is explained by pharmacokinetic differences, this is not the full picture. Two people with identical drug plasma levels may have different therapeutic responses and adverse effects. In some cases the observed response will depend on the *disease state* being treated. Advanced or chronic conditions may not respond in the same fashion, nor to the same drugs for the same disease where active intervention has been instituted at an early stage.

Disease states may predispose the patient/client to drug effects not seen in other patients/clients. For instance, people with Lewy body dementia are especially susceptible to the parkinsonian effects of antipsychotic drugs. Another consideration includes drugs such as tricyclic antidepressants, which can cause tachycardia or bradycardia, and should be avoided if possible in the patient/client who has recently suffered a myocardial infarction, when disturbances in heart rate may precipitate potentially serious ventricular arrhythmias. Additionally, the influence of *age* on individual drug response is often profound. This may in part be explained by pharmacokinetic changes. Even so, older people are generally much more sensitive to the effects of central nervous system drugs, and this is also the case for children.

In some cases, drug dosage is estimated on the basis of body weight, but adjustments may be needed in the context of obesity, fluid overload, cachexia (a complex metabolic syndrome also known as a wasting syndrome, often associated with conditions such as AIDS and palliative conditions) and other circumstances. Dosage adjustments are particularly important for drugs where the therapeutic dose is close to that dose which produces significant toxicity – these are commonly called drugs of *low therapeutic index*.

The influence of *psychological factors* on drug response is poorly understood. For example, the treatment of depression for a patient/client with chronic **pain** may facilitate better pain relief. Similarly, anxiety states may also influence the outcome of drug therapy. These responses may be understood as placebo effects of drugs. The placebo response rate in clinical research involving psychotropic drugs is high, creating complications in the interpretation of the findings of these studies.

Adverse drug reactions (ADRs)

Drugs used for therapeutic purposes almost always carry some degree of risk for unexpected and potentially adverse effects. These effects are most commonly called *side effects or adverse drug reactions (ADRs)*. During clinical trials (prior to the marketing of any drug), a screening process is used to help to establish a profile of the adverse effects of the drug, although not all reactions come to attention during this stage and are subsequently understood during the postmarketing surveillance process. The postmarketing surveillance process uses such means as event monitoring, health records and other health databases to further confirm or deny the relative safety of the drug after it has been used in the general population. This type of survelliance is important since the subjects included in the clinical trials undertaken prior to the release of a drug into the general population are not necessarily completely representative of the broader population in which the drug may later be used – older people, children, pregnant women and people with multiple medical comorbidities may not be included in clinical trials. This means that the profile of ADRs observed for these people may not be the same as that seen in the research setting. Finally, some ADRs are very rare, and may not necessarily be revealed in clinical trials, as the number of subjects in clinical trials is smaller than would be needed to reliably observe a particularly uncommon event. For these reasons, it is very important that health professionals look carefully for ADRs and report these to regulatory authorities, allowing a more comprehensive picture of the real profile of adverse effects to be established.

ADRs can arise through mechanisms related to the manner in which the drug produces its therapeutic effects. In this context, the drug administered for a therapeutic effect may produce a response of unexpected or excessive intensity.

Ask yourself!

Antidepressant drugs can cause episodes of abnormally elevated mood (mania).

1   Is this ADR common and predictable?

2   How can this ADR be prevented? Or managed?

In other cases the ADR is not an excessive therapeutic response, but the effect may be predicted in terms of the known spectrum of the drug's pharmacological action. For example, antipsychotic drugs are known to block dopaminergic transmission in the brain. However, the extent of the dopaminergic blockade is relatively non-specific, and adverse effects such as **extrapyramidal side effects** may result. In terms of your care considerations prior knowledge of the mechanisms of drug action can be used to predict and manage adverse effects. This type of reaction is more likely when two drugs with similar ADR profiles are concurrently administered and may need to be managed through dose reductions for one or both drugs.

Sometimes ADRs arise through pharmacological properties of the drug which are unrelated to the intended therapeutic actions of the drug. In the case of the tricyclic antidepressants, although the beneficial effects on mood are thought to be mediated through increased synaptic concentrations of noradrenaline and serotonin, postsynaptic blockade of muscarinic receptors causes **anticholinergic** effects that are manifest as adverse reactions such as tachycardia, urinary hesitancy and constipation.

In many cases the adverse effects of drug therapy cannot be predicted from a prior knowledge of the drug's pharmacology. Idiosyncratic adverse effects are also quite common in clinical practice, sometimes relatively minor (e.g. minor skin rash) but at other times serious in nature (e.g. drug-induced hepatitis associated with some anticonvulsants used as **mood stabilisers**). In many cases an idiosyncratic ADR is reproducible upon rechallenge, a very undesirable outcome if in relation to a serious ADR. This emphasises the need for clear documentation of previous ADRs in medical records.

Person-specific factors may predispose an individual to an ADR, and the disease state being treated may directly contribute to the risk of side effects. For instance, elderly patients/clients appear more sensitive to the CNS effects of many commonly used drugs. Additionally, personal genetic variations in drug metabolism may increase the likelihood of ADRs for some drugs – for example, the incidence of extrapyramidal side effects with some antipsychotics is higher in a person who is a slow metaboliser, an inherited genetic characteristic. The risk of ADRs increases with the number of drugs in the treatment regimen, and older people who are often treated with multiple drugs (commonly seen in clinical practice) are at special risk for ADRs.

Figure 4.2: Stevens–Johnson syndrome, a serious dermatological ADR associated with
some psychotropic drugs

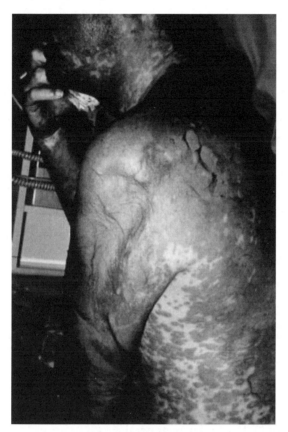

Under some circumstances, an adverse effect which is of relatively minor
significance assumes greater importance. For example, postural hypotension will
be of greater significance for the elderly people with osteoporosis, as a fall may
result in a fracture and further morbidity. The considerable range and diversity
of the nature of adverse reactions to drugs precludes an exhaustive discussion
here, and for further information it is useful to refer to specialist texts or a drug
information centre.

The Naranjo questionnaire is a useful tool that may be used by health care
workers in establishing the likelihood that a clinical syndrome may represent an
ADR (see below) (Naranjo et al., 1981).

Naranjo questionnaire

1. Are there previous conclusive reports on this reaction?

   Yes (+1) No (0) Do not know or not done (0)

2. Did the adverse event appear after the suspected drug was given?

   Yes (+2) No (−1) Do not know or not done (0)

3. Did the adverse reaction improve when the drug was discontinued or a specific antagonist was given?

   Yes (+1) No (0) Do not know or not done (0)

4. Did the adverse reaction appear when the drug was readministered?

   Yes (+2) No (−1) Do not know or not done (0)

5. Are there alternative causes that could have caused the reaction?

   Yes (−1) No (+2) Do not know or not done (0)

6. Did the reaction reappear when a placebo was given?

   Yes (−1) No (+1) Do not know or not done (0)

7. Was the drug detected in any body fluid in toxic concentrations?

   Yes (+1) No (0) Do not know or not done (0)

8. Was the reaction more severe when the dose was increased, or less severe when the dose was decreased?

   Yes (+1) No (0) Do not know or not done (0)

9. Did the patient have a similar reaction to the same or similar drugs in any previous exposure?

   Yes (+1) No (0) Do not know or not done (0)

10. Was the adverse event confirmed by any objective evidence?

   Yes (+1) No (0) Do not know or not done (0)

Scoring

> 9 = definite ADR

5–8 = probable ADR

1–4 = possible ADR

0 = doubtful ADR

Ask yourself!

1   What factors influence the likelihood of adverse reactions to psychotropic drugs?

2   Why are older people at greater risk of developing ADRs when receiving drug treatment for a mental illness?

Drug interactions

The use of two or more drugs in a treatment regimen may give rise to alterations to the therapeutic properties or adverse effect profile for one or more of the drugs involved. When the effects of one drug are altered by the concurrent administration of another, this is referred to as a 'drug interaction'. Drug interactions may be of minor or major significance, and like ADRs arise through a variety of mechanisms. Because of the variation in individual response to drug therapy, certain combinations of drugs may be used without ill effects in some patients/clients, whereas in others the same combination may cause a serious adverse reaction.

Pharmacodynamic drug interactions usually result from the compound pharmacological effects common to both drugs involved. These effects may be additive, or may work in opposition, thus producing either intensification or diminution of therapeutic or adverse effects. For example, when tricyclic antidepressants are combined with some antipsychotic drugs, the hypotensive effects will be additive. Conversely, the anticholinergic effect of psychotropic drugs can antagonise the therapeutic effect of cholinesterase inhibitors that are used for those with dementia illnesses.

Drug interactions may also arise from an alteration in the *pharmacokinetic* properties of one drug by another, and some of the most important drug interactions result from the influence of one drug on the elimination of another. In many cases the concurrent administration of a drug may affect the hepatic metabolism of a second drug. The administration of some anticonvulsant drugs such as carbamazepine or primidone commonly leads to an increase in the rate of hepatic drug metabolism. This effect is referred to as 'hepatic enzyme induction', and through increasing the rate of metabolic elimination can lead to decreased plasma levels of the second drug, with possible loss of therapeutic effects. A potential hazard to be aware of is that the dose of the second drug is sometimes increased to compensate for the loss of therapeutic effect. If the interacting drug therapy is later ceased, the dose must be reduced to previous levels in order to avoid inadvertent overtreatment. Drug interactions also may cause a decrease in the rate of hepatic metabolism of another drug (known as 'hepatic enzyme inhibition'), and the plasma levels of the second drug may rise, producing unintended toxicity. Concurrent treatment with fluvoxamine can produce hepatic enzyme inhibition, and may increase the plasma level of other drugs such as carbamazepine or methadone, predisposing to serious toxicity. Drug interactions may also result from alterations in the renal excretion of a compound. An important example of this type of interaction is the decrease in renal clearance of lithium caused by the addition of a non-steroidal anti-inflammatory drug (NSAID), increasing serum lithium levels.

Drug interactions can be clinically relevant for a wide range of medications, and the nature and extent of the interaction in the individual patient/client may vary considerably. The drugs most likely to be implicated in important interactions tend to be those of low therapeutic index, such as anticonvulsants, opioids and lithium. Again, for a more comprehensive discussion of specific drug interactions it is necessary to contact a drug information centre or refer to appropriate specialist texts.

Pharmacodynamics and nursing practice

For nurses in practice, when working with patients/clients who are prescribed and taking medications it is important to keep the nursing process in mind in order to consider desired effects and drug response, ADRs, drug interactions and the potential for idiosyncratic responses to medications.

Assessment

As a part of assessment, planning, intervention and evaluation, nurses need to be aware of and incorporate consideration of factors that may affect the pharmacodynamics of drug response. The assessment should include screening for potential ADRs and drug interactions that might arise from the initial treatment or planned adjustments to the drug regimen. Important questions relate to previous ADRs and current sensitivities. Particular attention to this consideration is needed for older people and those treated with extensive pharmacotherapy. Assessment should also include any complementary medicines that the person may be taking. Often patients/clients take complementary medicines (such as vitamins and over-the-counter medicines) and when asked whether they are on other medications they may not consider these to be notable enough to tell you.

Evaluation

Continuous nursing evaluation is necessary to detect the adverse effects of psychotropic pharmacotherapy. In some cases, after evaluation it may be necessary to advocate the discontinuation of a specific drug or drugs. If an adverse effect is relatively minor, early detection and counselling or reassurance may assist with subsequent **adherence** to the planned treatment approach. Nurses need to be aware of the value of the information provided by the patient/client and also by their carers, as the lived experience of the person provides a unique perspective on the effects of pharmacotherapy.

Education

It is a fundamental practice in health care that patients/clients and, where appropriate, carers and staff of assisted living facilities are provided with education about the potential adverse effects and drug interactions that might be expected to be associated with drugs used for the management of mental illness. The early detection of problems may prevent progression to serious toxicity or even death, and this educative role should be regarded as a routine task for all health professionals. The provision of plain language Consumer Medicines Information (CMI) may assist you with this educative role, and is best undertaken in a cooperative approach that should ideally involve members of the multidisciplinary team – nurses, medical staff and pharmacists.

BILL'S STORY

Bill is a 77-year-old man who lives with his wife in their own home. He has a history of bipolar affective disorder with periodic episodes of both mania and serious depression. His treatment includes both lithium 250 mg twice daily and fluoxetine 40 mg daily. He also has widespread osteoarthritis and recently commenced treatment with paracetamol 1000 mg four times daily and diclofenac 50 mg twice daily. He has now been brought to the emergency department by his son – he presents with nausea, tremor and drowsiness. Routine blood tests reveal that the serum lithium concentration is 2.1 mmol/L and that he also has significant hypothyroidism.

Care Plan

The following is an example care plan for the patient/client presented in this chapter. The areas of daily living that are considered include bio-psycho-social factors and the plan is mapped out using the nursing process (Assessment; Plan; Implementation; Evaluation). Remember: the success is in the detail, so be specific about *who, when and what* in the collaborative plan; never include someone in the plan if they were not consulted in the planning process; and always work within a recovery-orientated framework (refer to Chapter 1).

Date: 31 July 2012

Clients name: Bill

Case manager: TBC; presenting at the Emergency Department (ED)

Areas of daily living	Assessment of current situation	Goal	Plan (undertaken with patient/client)	Implementation	Who is responsible? (Include only those who have been consulted in the planning process)	Evaluation/ review date
Mental health	Diagnosis of bipolar affective disorder.	Review current treatment regimen.	Pathology examinations Physical examination Review mental state.	Mental state examination Blood test for thyroid function test, serum Li, full blood examination, etc.	Triage nurse, mental health nurse and registrar in ED.	On admission to ED
Social	Married	Keep spouse informed of progress.	Organise a family meeting.	Family meeting	Triage nurse, mental health nurse and registrar in ED.	Once Bill is stabilised
Biological	Presenting with nausea, tremor and drowsiness.	Stabilise symptoms.	Stabilise symptoms and preserve life.	Cease lithium.	Triage nurse, mental health nurse and registrar in ED.	Constant observation

(Continued)

Date: 31 July 2012						
Clients name: Bill		Case manager: TBC; presenting at the Emergency Department (ED)				
Areas of daily living	Assessment of current situation	Goal	Plan (undertaken with patient/client)	Implementation	Who is responsible? (Include only those who have been consulted in the planning process)	Evaluation/ review date
	Lithium toxicity detected through routine bloods (usual therapeutic range in adults is 0.4–1.0mmol/L and 0.3–0.8 mmol/L in older people). Lacks knowledge of possible drug interactions involving lithium.	Provide education to address knowledge gap regarding drug interactions.		Admit to hospital for physical monitoring. Rehydrate with an increased sodium intake. Monitor cardiac function to assess rhythm disturbances. Monitor renal function. Monitor nausea. Provide education to Bill and his family regarding knowledge gap.		
Environmental	Lives with wife in his own home.	None identified	N/A	N/A	N/A	N/A
Substance using behaviours	None identified	N/A	N/A	N/A	N/A	N/A
Risk behaviours	Physical risk due to lithium toxicity	Stabilise symptoms.	Stabilise symptoms and preserve life.	As above (see biological)	Triage nurse, mental health nurse and registrar in ED.	Constant observation

Ask yourself!

As a nurse involved with caring for Bill:

1   What might account for the clinical symptoms that Bill has developed?

2   Which drugs are known to interact with lithium, and how might these interactions be managed?

3   Could the hypothyroidism represent an adverse drug reaction, and if so which drug is implicated?

From the consumer's perspective – *How does this feel for me?*

Consumers are often wary about the possible side effects of medications and, given the chronic nature of many mental illnesses and the need for ongoing treatments, many will have experienced side effects before. Sometimes it is difficult to understand the need for concurrent treatment with a number of psychotropic drugs. Previous experience of ADRs is often a negative influence upon adherence to medication treatment.

Health care workers with experience in mental illness often hear the same complaints many times over from patients/clients:

'I take so many pills, I'll start to rattle.'

'I think that the medicine is worse than the depression.'

'Won't all these pills fight with one another?'

'I'm not taking all this when I go home; I'll just take some until I feel better.'

'Medication is not for me; I believe that vitamins work better than these tablets.'

Summary

All drugs used in the treatment of mental illness have the potential to cause adverse drug reactions and to be involved in drug interactions. Older people, those with multiple comorbidities and those treated with complex pharmacotherapy regimens are at greatest risk, and it is important to bear in mind that psychotropic drugs can affect medical conditions through adverse effects, or can interact with drugs used in the management of medical illnesses. Nurses and other health professionals have an ideal opportunity to monitor patients/clients to detect and document these issues, and to be involved in strategies to resolve them and prevent recurrences.

Discussion questions

1 Describe two different types of adverse drug reaction.

2 What effects might be expected when a drug interaction alters the hepatic metabolism or renal elimination of a drug?

3 What is meant by the term 'drug of low therapeutic index?'

Test yourself (answers at the back of the book)

1 Two people with identical drug plasma levels:

A will always exhibit the same response to the drug

B may have different therapeutic responses

C will have the same adverse effects

D A and C only

2 The profile of adverse effects associated with a drug:

A is always predictable on the basis of the pharmacology of the drug

B is never predictable on the basis of the pharmacology of the drug

C may reflect the pharmacology of the drug

D never reflect the pharmacology of the drug

3 Which of the following groups are most often under-represented in clinical trial cohorts?

A Premenopausal women

B Postmenopausal women

C Pregnant women

D Women unable to have children

4 With respect to the pharmacokinetic drug interactions:

A all involve hepatic enzyme induction

B all involve hepatic enzyme inhibition

C these may involve altered elimination of one drug caused by another

D none of the above

5 Excessive sedation after the combined use of benzodiazepines and antipsychotics probably reflects:

A a pharmacodynamic drug interaction

B a pharmacokinetic drug interaction

C reduced hepatic metabolism

D reduced renal excretion

Useful websites

The *Merck Manual: Overview of Pharmacodynamics* available at <www. merckmanuals.com/professional/clinical_pharmacology/ pharmacodynamics/overview_of_pharmacodynamics.html>

World Health Organization: *Adverse Drug Reactions Monitoring* available at

<www.who.int/medicines/areas/quality_safety/safety_efficacy/ advdrugreactions/en>

Healthline: *Drug Interactions* available at

<www.healthline.com/druginteractions>

References

Edwards I. R. & Aronson J. K. (2000). 'Adverse drug reactions: definitions, diagnosis, and management' *Lancet* 356(9237): 1255–1259.

Dukes M. & Aronson, J. (2006). *Meyler's Side Effects of Drugs: The International Encyclopedia of Adverse Drug Reactions and Interactions*. Amsterdam: Elsevier.

Naranjo C. A., Busto U., Sellers E. M. et al. (1981). 'A method for estimating the probability of adverse drug reactions' *Clin Pharmacol Ther* 30 (2): 239–245. DOI:10.1038/clpt.1981.154. PMID 7249508.

Tatro D. S. et al. (2003), *Drug Interaction Facts*. St Louis: J. B. Lippincott Company.

Chapter 5

Medication Administration and Calculations

Chapter overview

This chapter covers the following topics:

* basic mathematics
* drug calculations
* administration of medication and the nurse's role
* medication education for patients/clients and carers.

Chapter learning objectives

After reading this chapter, you should be able to:

* undertake basic mathematics for medication administration
* describe the nurse's role in administration of medication
* facilitate patient/client and carer education related to your knowledge of medication therapy.

Key terms

Adverse events
Medication administration
Medication calculations
Nurse practitioner
Nurse's role in administration of medication

Introduction

In this chapter you will explore basic mathematical skills, **medication administration**, and your role in administering drugs for treatment, monitoring the efficacy of medicines, and patient/client and carer education related to medication therapy.

Basic mathematical skills

Medication errors are common in health and can have dire consequences for the patient/client and for the nurse. Often these may occur because the nurse is distracted, or because of inadequate checking or errors in **medication calculations**.

As a health care worker who prepares and administers medications you will need to possess basic mathematical skills. Basic mathematics involves *addition*, *subtraction*, *multiplication* and *division*. These mathematical processes can be performed with whole numbers or decimals and fractions. It is important to have a good understanding of the basic principles of mathematics that underpin drug calculations. The safest approach is to use an electronic calculator, and to always check your calculations at least twice to ensure that an error has not arisen because of a data entry inaccuracy.

Some rules for mathematical calculations are fundamental to your medication calculation knowledge. For example, addition is commutative, meaning it can be performed in any order; for example 22 + 3 is the same as 3 + 22. However, subtraction is not commutative since 22 − 3 is *not* the same as 3 − 22. Additionally, in medication management and administration you will need to know about *factors* to be able to convert some measurements in drug calculations. For example, in practice a nurse will often need to convert grams to milligrams or milligrams to micrograms.

The two following definitions are useful to know:

Definition of milligram

The SI prefix (metric prefix) 'milli' represents a factor of 10^{-3}.

So 1 milligram = 10^{-3} grams (g)

Therefore 1 gram = 1000 milligrams (mg)

Definition of microgram

The SI prefix 'micro' represents a factor of 10^{-6}.

So 1 microgram = 10^{-6} grams

Therefore 1 gram = 1 000 000 micrograms (mcg)

Some drug calculations require you to convert different volumes or weights into the same unit or value.

To convert smaller units to larger ones, the smaller is divided by 1000:

* grams to kilograms (kg) = g/1000

* milligrams to grams = mg/1000

* micrograms to milligrams = micrograms/1000

* nanograms (ng) to micrograms = ng/1000

* millilitres to litres = mL/1000.

To convert larger units to smaller ones, the larger is multiplied by 1000:

* kilograms (kg) to grams (g) = kg × 1000

* grams to milligrams (mg) = g × 1000

* milligrams to micrograms (mcg) = mg × 1000

* micrograms to nanograms (ng) = mcg × 1000

* litres (L) to millilitres (mL) = L × 1000.

Nurses and other health care workers who are able to administer medications work with decimals when considering the amount of medication for an individual. It is important to note that two decimals can be multiplied together in the same way as two whole numbers are. In this case you carry out the multiplication ignoring the decimal points.

Example: 3.5 × 0.05 becomes 35 × 5, which equals 175.

Then count up the number of digits after the decimal point in both numbers and add them together.

1 + 2 = 3 decimal places

Finally, insert the decimal point in the result three places back from the right-hand digit, adding zeroes in front of it if necessary.

The answer in this case is 0.175.

When dividing numbers with decimals by whole numbers, the only essential rule is to place the decimal point in the answer exactly where it occurs in the decimal number.

For example: $0.333 \div 8 = 0.0416$

Percentages are simply fractions with a denominator of 100. In order to convert a percentage into a decimal, divide by 100.

The dosage of some medications is based upon the actual or ideal body weight of the person who will be administered the medication. Reflecting on the amount prescribed is an important practice as you will need to ensure any potential error is not an error in the prescription written by the doctor or **nurse practitioner**. Weight considerations are particularly important with medication administration to children, adolescents and older people.

Drug calculations
Correct formulae

Drug calculations are an important aspect of nursing practice (and for other health care professionals who are able to administer medications as part of their scope of practice). There is great variation in undergraduate curricula relating to the extent drug calculations education is covered. On the whole, and for many students, the education related to drug calculations is not comprehensive. Drug calculations need to be undertaken so that the accurate dose of drugs to administer to patients/clients is found. Important aspects relating to teaching drug calculations are the mathematical concepts, teaching the drug calculation formulae and then practising the skills in the clinical setting (Wright, 2005). In Australia in 1970, the metric system, also called the International System of Units (SI), was introduced. Basic units in this system include weight (grams), liquids (litres) and length (metres), with the symbols 'g', 'L' and 'm' respectively. Common variations to these measurements are one-millionth (micro), one-thousandth (milli) and one-thousand times (such as kilograms in weight measurement) and kilometres (length measurement). The mathematical skills required for drug calculations include conceptual skills (to enable you to set up the calculation problem and apply an appropriate solution) and computational skills (to enable you to calculate the solution using decimals, percentages, ratios, fractions and conversions between the various units of measurement). You will need to organise your drug calculations information using the desired dose, concentration and the volume on hand. You need to follow drug formulae when you begin your calculations, as follows:

$$\frac{\text{required dose}}{\text{stock dose}} \times \frac{\text{volume}}{\text{stock dose}} = \text{volume to be given}$$

Example 1

The patient is prescribed fluoxetine for their mood disorder at a dose of 20 mg bd. You have available in stock fluoxetine solution where the concentration is 20 mg/5 mL. What is the volume to be given to the patient?

    Answer: 5 mL bd

Example 2

The patient is prescribed venlafaxine XR for depression and prescribed 75 mg per day in divided doses (at breakfast and dinner). You have in stock 37.5 mg capsules. What is the volume to be given to the patient?

    Answer: 1 capsule bd

Example 3

How many tablets containing 62.5 mcg will be required to give a dose of 0.125 mg?

    Answer: 2 tablets

Example 4

A patient is ordered 150 mg of aspirin. 300 mg aspirin tablets are available in stock. How many tablets would you give?

    Answer: 0.5 tablet

Example 5

The patient is prescribed fluphenazine decanoate 25 mg per fortnight IMI (intramuscular injection). You have in stock 12.5 mg/0.5 mL. What volume should be given?

    Answer: 1 mL per IMI

Medication administration

Checking before administering drugs

The Six Rights

Before administering medication the single most important thing to do is to safeguard the patient and yourself by washing your hands and donning appropriate personal protective equipment if required. Additionally, when preparing the medication for administration:

1. Check the prescription label against the medication order and make sure they match.

2. Check the patient's name and any other identifying information (hospital number, photograph, etc.) against the prescription order and the prescription label and make sure they match.

When giving any medication, even those that a patient/client has been taking for a long time, you must adhere to the Six Rights. The Six Rights is a systematic procedure to minimise the potential risk of medication administration error. The Six Rights are often undertaken with a health care colleague (another nurse) as follows:

1. Right individual

   Prepare medication for one patient/client at a time and give the medication to the patient as soon as you prepare it.

2. Right medication

   Read medication label carefully in conjunction with the medication order, ensuring the medication order matches the label.

3. Right dose

   Read the strength of the medication on the medication label and ensure the patient is given the amount that is prescribed. This is where you may need to use calculations to provide the accurate dose. For example:

Example A – A patient is ordered 1 mg of diazepam. 2 mg tablets are available. How many tablets will you give?

$$\frac{1\ mg}{2\ mg} = 0.5\ tablets$$

Example B – A patient is ordered 200 mg of sodium valproate. 100 mg tablets are available. How many tablets will you give?

$$\frac{200\ mg}{100\ mg} = 2\ tablets$$

Example C – A patient is ordered 37.5 mg of clomipramine. 25 mg tablets are available. How many tablets will you give?

$$\frac{37.5\ mg}{25\ mg} = 1.5\ tablets$$

Example D – A patient is ordered 1.25 mg of clonazepam. 0.5 mg tablets are available. How many tablets will you give?

$$\frac{1.25\ mg}{0.5\ mg} = 2.5\ tablets$$

You will also need to know or check the recommended dose range for the drug and, when recalculating the drug dose, have a colleague recheck the dose. If you believe the dose is not correct or within therapeutic range then you must consult the treating doctor to discuss this before you proceed with administration.

4. Right time

All medications are given at a specific time to achieve and maintain therapeutic blood levels and to avoid toxicity. You may need to know the half-life of the drug and whether the absorption is affected by food. There are times when medications are withheld at the times they are prescribed; the reasons relate to specific diagnostic tests, laboratory tests, surgery or other clinical reasons (e.g. to clarify a possible adverse drug reaction).

5. Right route

   The right route of administration is necessary for the appropriate absorption of the drug. Commonly with psychoactive medications these are given PO (by mouth) and (IM) intramuscular (a parenteral route). Other routes of administration include:

   - SL (sublingual)
   - TP (topical)
   - parenteral (intradermal, subcutaneous and intravenous)
   - IH (inhalation)
   - buccal (between the gum and cheek)
   - rectal (between the cheeks).

   When administering psychotropic medications IM, you will need to know the areas on the body appropriate for IM medications and the appropriate size of the needles required, and use a sterile technique for the administration of the IM medication.

6. Right documentation

   As a legal requirement you must document the date and time the drug was given and your name or initials. The documentation for medications administered must be made immediately. If the patient/client refuses the medication or the medicines cannot be administered as scheduled, this must also be documented, along with the reasons. Importantly, if a medication error was made you must report the error immediately to your supervisor; document the error and consult the treating medical officer to ensure adequate follow-up care for the patient/client. These actions must be undertaken promptly.

CATHY'S STORY

Cathy is 33 years old with a diagnosis of bipolar affective disorder. Cathy has been prescribed Risperdal Consta®. She had not taken risperidone before so her doctor gave her a test dose of oral risperidone to ensure that Cathy could tolerate the drug. Since she tolerated the oral risperidone Cathy was given her first injection and kept taking the oral risperidone for a period of three weeks to give the injection a chance to start working (reaching therapeutic levels). Cathy now receives her injection every two weeks. Cathy was visiting her local mental health community clinic for her follow-up appointment with her psychiatrist and her regular depot injection.

You are a new staff member to the clinic and have been asked to administer injections to the regular community patients/clients who attend for injection. You don't know all the patients/clients yet and the waiting room is full. You call out Cathy's name. Cathy has gone to the toilet. You look around the waiting room and a client (Sarah) catches your eye. Sarah has a diagnosis of schizophrenia and has been experiencing command hallucinations that render her mute. You approach Sarah and ask, 'Are you Cathy?' Sarah nods. Sarah stands up and you begin to walk towards the injection room with her.

Ask yourself!

As a new health care worker who is in the situation described above:

1   Reflect on how you can ensure that the right medication is given to the right patient/client.

2   What steps should you go through before the administration of medication?

3   What steps can you take to ensure patient safety and reduce the potential for medication errors in a community setting where identification of patients/clients is complex and where patients/clients may not be able to communicate clearly with you?

Different schedules of drugs

All drugs have inherent potential for toxicity and can cause harm in some circumstances. Along with other factors, potential toxicity is a cornerstone in the process of scheduling. In Australia, there are separate schedules for drugs and poisons, and their allocation of a drug to a particular schedule is based on toxicity data, epidemiology of disease states, access to health providers, and sociological issues, all considered in balance. Scheduling may vary between jurisdictions, but Table 5.1 is a general description; it will be necessary to check with relevant state or territory regulations.

Table 5.1: Schedules of drugs

Schedule	Description
2	Pharmacy Medicine – should be available from a pharmacy or a licensed person.
3	Pharmacist Only Medicine – should be available to the public with direct involvement of a pharmacist (without a prescription).
4	Prescription Only Medicine, or Prescription Animal Remedy – the use or supply should be by or on the order of people permitted by state or territory legislation to prescribe and should be available from a pharmacy on prescription.
5	Caution – substance with a low potential for causing harm, the extent of which can be reduced through the use of appropriate packaging with simple warnings and safety directions on the label.
6	Poison – substance with a moderate potential for causing harm, the extent of which can be reduced through the use of distinctive packaging.
7	Dangerous Poison – substance with a high potential for causing harm at low exposure and which requires special precautions during manufacture, handling or use. These poisons should be available only to specialised or authorised users.
8	Controlled Drug – substance which should be available for use but requires restriction of manufacture, supply, distribution, possession and use to reduce abuse, misuse and dependence.
9	Prohibited Substance – substance which may be abused or misused, the manufacture, possession, sale or use of which should be prohibited by law except when required for medical or scientific research, or for analytical, teaching or training purposes with approval of Commonwealth and/or state or territory health authorities.

Source: Schedule 1 Standard for the Uniform Scheduling of Drugs and Poisons No. 23

Classification of medicines in New Zealand

The *Medicines Act 1981* (NZ) (administered by the NZ Ministry of Health) defines three classification categories for medicines:

1. Prescription Medicine

   Prescription medicines may be supplied only on the prescription of an authorised prescriber (as defined in the *Medicines Act 1981*). They may also be used by a registered member of another specified health profession when permitted in the First Schedule to the *Medicines Regulations 1984* or amendments.

2. Restricted Medicine (also referred to as Pharmacist Only Medicine)
   Restricted medicines may be sold without a prescription, but the sale must be made by a registered pharmacist, in a pharmacy, and details of the sale must be recorded.

3. Pharmacy-Only Medicine (also referred to as Pharmacy Medicine)
   Pharmacy-only medicines may be sold only in a community or hospital pharmacy, or a shop in an isolated area that is licensed to sell that particular medicine. The sale may be made by any salesperson.

Medicines in each of these classification categories are listed in the First Schedule to the *Medicines Regulations 1984* and amendments. Medicines not listed in the classification schedules are deemed to be unclassified, and are referred to as General Sale Medicines. These medicines may be sold from any outlet.

An update to the First Schedule to the *Medicines Regulations 1984* came into effect on 1 August 2011. *Medicines Amendment Regulations 2011* is a consolidation of new classifications and classification changes. The classification of medicines database can be used to check the classification of medicines (including general sale medicines and controlled drugs used as medicines) and can be accessed from Medsafe webpage (<www.medsafe.govt.nz/profs/class/classintro.asp>).

Recording dangerous drugs

No person can administer a dangerous drug to a patient except with written instruction of a medical practitioner. The person responsible for the storage of dangerous drugs must keep the drugs in an approved and locked receptacle and the key in their personal possession. The person responsible for the possession of dangerous drugs has a legal responsibility of maintaining accurate records:

1. The place where the dangerous drugs are stored must be recorded (at a central point in wards, pharmacies, operating theatres) and the person in charge must keep a single book to record all transactions with the dangerous drugs.

2. The description, quantity, and class of each dangerous drug must be recorded.

3. The date of issue with a description of the quantity and each class of dangerous drug purchased or obtained, including the designated wards it was issued to, must be recorded.

4. A single book must be used to record all transactions of dangerous drugs issued to a ward, operating theatre and department.

5. In addition to the description and quantity of the dangerous drug used and administered, the person responsible must supply the date and time of use, the name of the patient for whom the drug was used and a progressive balance of that class of dangerous drug remaining in stock.

6. Each page of the book must contain only entries relating to dangerous drugs of the same class.

7. Any doses lost, discarded or unused must also be recorded.

National inpatient medication chart

Patient harm caused by adverse medication events is of major concern for individuals, organisations and communities. It is believed at the governmental level in Australia that standardising communication about medications for the diverse disciplines which contribute to medication prescribing, dispensing, administering and reviewing can reduce potential harm to patients/clients. At the Australian Health Ministers conference in 2004, a National Inpatient Medication Chart (NIMC) (see Figure 5.1) was approved for use by all public hospitals and a majority of private hospitals in an effort to reduce medication errors and subsequently harm from errors. Modified and adapted versions are now in widespread use in aged and extended care facilities. The NIMC is available from the Australian Commission on Safety and Quality in Health Care. It provides a standard approach to prescribing, dispensing, administering and reviewing medications for inpatients. Table 5.2 outlines the key principles of the NIMC.

Figure 5.1: The National Inpatient Medication Chart (NIMC)

Medication Chart Page 1 of 4

AFFIX PATIENT IDENTIFICATION LABEL HERE AND OVERLEAF

URN:

Family name: NOT A VALID

Given names: PRESCRIPTION UNLESS

Address: IDENTIFIERS PRESENT

Date of birth: Sex: ☐ M ☐ F

First Prescriber to Print Patient Name and Check Label Correct: Weight (kg): _____ Height (cm): _____

ALLERGIES & ADVERSE DRUG REACTIONS (ADR)
☐ Nil known ☐ Unknown (tick appropriate box or complete details below)

Drug (or other)	Reaction/Type/Date	Initials

Sign _____ Print _____ Date _____

MEDICATION Chart No. _____ of _____

ADDITIONAL CHARTS
☐ IV Fluid ☐ BGL/Insulin ☐ Acute Pain ☐ Other
☐ Palliative care ☐ Chemotherapy ☐ IV Heparin

Facility/Service: _____ Ward/Unit: _____

ONCE ONLY, PRE-MEDICATION & NURSE INITIATED MEDICINES

Date Prescribed	Medication (Print Generic Name)	Route	Dose	Date/Time of Dose	Prescriber/Nurse Initiator (NI) Signature Print Your Name	Given By	Time Given	Pharmacy

TELEPHONE ORDERS (To be signed within 24 hours of order)

Date Time	Medication (Print Generic Name)	Route	Dose	Frequency	Nurse Initiate NR1/NR2	Dr Name	Dr Sign.	Date	RECORD OF ADMINISTRATION Time/ Given by	Time/ Given by	Time/ Given by	Time/ Given by

Medicines Taken Prior to Presentation to Hospital

(Prescribed, over the counter, complementary)   Own medications brought in? ☐ Y ☐ N   Administration Aid (specify).................

Medication	Dose & frequency	Duration	Medication	Dose & frequency	Duration

GP: Community Pharmacy:

Documented by: (Sign)   (Date)   Medicines usually administered by:

(Continued)

Figure 5.1: The National Inpatient Medication Chart (NIMC) (*Continued*)

Medication Chart Page 2 of 4

AFFIX PATIENT IDENTIFICATION LABEL HERE

Allergies and adverse drug reactions See page 1 for details	URN: Family name: Given names: Address: — NOT A VALID PRESCRIPTION UNLESS IDENTIFIERS PRESENT

Tick if, Slow Release | SR- Sustained, modified or controlled release formulation. If scored tablet, then half can be given. Does must be swallowed without crushing

Date of birth: Sex: ☐ M ☐ F

First Prescriber to Print Patient Name and Check Label Correct: _____

REASON FOR NURSE NOT ADMINISTERING
codes MUST be circled

(A)	Absent	(L)	On leave
(F)	Fasting	(F)	Not available – obtain supply or contact Dr
(R)	Refused – notify Dr	(R)	Withheld – enter reason in clinical record
(V)	Vomiting	(V)	Self Administered

RECOMMENDED ADMINISTRATION TIMES
GUIDELINES ONLY

Morning	Mane	0900			
Night	Nocte			1800 or 2000	
Twice a day	BD	0800		2000	
Three times a day	TDS	0800	1400	2000	
Regular 6 hourly	6 hrly	0600	1200	1800	2400
Regular 8 hourly	8 hrly	0600	1400	2200	
Four times a day	QID	0600	1200	1800	2200

WARFARIN EDUCATION RECORD
Patient Educated by:...............
Sign: ....
Date:.....................................
Given Warfarin Book: ....
Sign: ....
Date:.....................................

REGULAR MEDICATIONS

YEAR 20_____   DATE & MONTH ⟶

VARIABLE DOSE MEDICATION

Date	Medication (Print Generic Name)		Drug level
Route	Frequency		Time level taken
	Prescriber to enter dose times and individual dose		**Dose**
			Prescriber
Indication	Pharmacy		Time to be given: ....
Prescriber Signature	Print Your Name	Contact	Time given

Date	**WARFARIN** (Marevan/Coumadin) select brand	INR Result
Route	Prescriber to enter individual doses	Target INR Range	**Dose** mg mg mg mg mg mg mg mg mg mg mg
Indication	Pharmacy		Prescriber
Prescriber Signature	Print Your Name	Contact	1600 (Nurse 1)
			Nurse 2

DOCTORS MUST ENTER administration times

Date	Medication (Print Generic Name)	Tick if Slow Release
Route	Dose	Frequency & NOW Enter Times ⟶
Indication	Pharmacy	
Prescriber Signature	Print Your Name	Contact

Date	Medication (Print Generic Name)	Tick if Slow Release
Route	Dose	Frequency & NOW Enter Times ⟶
Indication	Pharmacy	
Prescriber Signature	Print Your Name	Contact

Date	Medication (Print Generic Name)	Tick if Slow Release
Route	Dose	Frequency & NOW Enter Times ⟶
Indication	Pharmacy	
Prescriber Signature	Print Your Name	Contact

Pharmaceutical Review:

Continue on discharge? Yes/No
Dispense? Yes/No   days Qty:
Duration:

Date: Pharmacist:

Print your name:

Prescriber's Signature:

◯ DO NOT WRITE IN THIS BINDING MARGIN ◯

Figure 5.1: The National Inpatient Medication Chart (NIMC) (*Continued*)

Medication Chart Page 3 of 4

AFFIX PATIENT IDENTIFICATION LABEL HERE

ALLERGIES & ADVERSE DRUG REACTION (ADR)
☐ Nil known ☐ Unknown (tick appropriate box or complete details below)

Drug (or other)	Reaction/Type/Date	Initials

Sign _____ Print _____ Date _____

URN:
Family name:
Given names:
Address:

Date of birth:

NOT A VALID
PRESCRIPTION UNLESS
IDENTIFIERS PRESENT

Sex: ☐ M ☐ F

First Prescriber to Print Patient
Name and Check Label Correct: _____

REGULAR MEDICATIONS

YEAR 20_____   DATE & MONTH ⟶

DOCTORS MUST ENTER administration times

Date	Medication (Print Generic Name)	Tick if Slow Release
Route	Dose	Frequency & NOW Enter Times ⟶
Indication		Pharmacy
Prescriber Signature	Print Your Name	Contact

(repeated blocks of the above for each regular medication)

Pharmaceutical Review:

Continue on discharge? Yes/No
Dispense? Yes/No
Duration: _____ days Qty: _____

Date:
Pharmacist:
Date:
Print your name:
Prescriber's Signature:

DO NOT WRITE IN THIS BINDING MARGIN

(Continued)

Figure 5.1: The National Inpatient Medication Chart (NIMC) (*Continued*)

AFFIX PATIENT IDENTIFICATION LABEL HERE

Medication Chart Page 4 of 4

Allergies and adverse drug reactions
See page 3 for details

AS REQUIRED "PRN" MEDICATIONS
YEAR: 20 _____

URN:
Family name:
Given names:
Address:

NOT A VALID PRESCRIPTION UNLESS IDENTIFIERS PRESENT

Date of birth: Sex: ☐ M ☐ F

First Prescriber to Print Patient Name and Check Label Correct: _____

Source: *Australian Council for Safety and Quality in Health Care National Inpatient Medication Chart Pilot Aggregate Data Report* (2012)

Table 5.2: Key principles of the NIMC

Patient's name always at the top of the chart

The medication chart should have a section for adverse drug reactions and that the area is clearly visible whenever prescriptions are written.

The chart should include a section for complementary medicines and those medicines taken by the patient prior to admission.

The chart should have a section for prn (when required) medications.

The chart should have space for pharmacy documentation of the medication supplied.

The chart should have space for the prescriber to clearly identify themselves and how they can be easily contacted (e.g. page number).

Source: *Australian Council for Safety and Quality in Health Care National Inpatient Medication Chart Pilot Aggregate Data Report* (2012)

Safe and unsafe abbreviations

One of the main causes of medication errors is related to abbreviations of medical terms and dose expressions. The common issues related to safe and unsafe abbreviations centre on a few factors:

✳ Language used for health care and the health care literature was historically derived from Latin, and today English is the predominant language used in the medical literature.

✳ Abbreviations can be misunderstood – what a prescriber uses may mean another thing for the person interpreting the prescription.

✳ Different health care workers with differing levels of training are now able to administer medications due to changes in policy. Recent training does not include Latin nor does each curriculum include comprehensive education in terms used for the administration of medicines.

Clear and unambiguous abbreviations and dose expressions must be used when **prescribing medications**. A set of recommended terms and error prone abbreviations, symbols and dose expressions is provided in Table 5.3.

Table 5.3: Recommended terms (intended meaning and acceptable abbreviations)

Intended meaning	Acceptable terms or abbreviations
Dose frequency or timing	
(in the) morning	morning, mane
(at) midday	midday
twice a day	bd
four times a day	qid
every 4 hours	every 4 hours, 4 hourly, 4 hrly
every 6 hours	every 6 hours, 6 hourly, 6 hrly
every 8 hours	every 8 hours, 8 hourly, 8 hrly
once a week	once a week and specify the day in full, e.g. once a week on Tuesdays
three times a week	three times a week *and* specify the exact days in full, e.g. three times a week on Mondays, Wednesdays and Saturdays
when required	prn
immediately	stat
before food	before food
after food	after food
with food	with food
Route of administration	
epidural	epidural
inhale, inhalation	inhale, inhalation
intra-articular	intra-articular
intramuscular	IM
intrathecal	intrathecal
intranasal	intranasal

(Continued)

Table 5.3: Recommended terms (intended meaning and acceptable abbreviations) (*Continued*)

intravenous	IV
irrigation	irrigation
left	left
nebulised	NEB
nasogastric	NG
oral	PO
percutaneous enteral gastrostomy	PEG
per vagina	PV
per rectum	PR
peripherally inserted central catheter	PICC
right	right
subcutaneous	subcut
sublingual	subling
topical	topical
Units of measure and concentration	
gram(s)	g
international unit(s)	international unit(s)
litre(s)	L
milligram(s)	mg
millilitre(s)	mL
microgram(s)	microgram, microg
percentage	%
millimole	mmol
Dose forms	
capsule	cap
cream	cream

Dose forms	
ear drops	ear drops
ear ointment	ear ointment
eye ointment	eye ointment
injection	inj
metered dose inhaler	metered dose inhaler, inhaler, MDI
mixture	mixture
ointment	ointment, oint
pessary	pess
powder	powder
suppository	suppository
tablet	tablet, tab
patient-controlled analgesia	PCA

Source: Australian Commission on Safety and Quality in Healthcare (2008), pp. 3–4

Some health care units have endorsed the use of Tall Man lettering (or Tallman lettering), where part of a drug's name is written in upper case letters to help distinguish sound-alike or look-alike drugs from one another. For example, in Tall Man lettering, 'quinine' and 'quinidine' might be written 'quinINE' and 'quinIDINE', respectively. In addition, the use of generic nomenclature (rather than brand names) in drug orders is also a good approach to minimising errors.

Labelling and packaging of medications

It is estimated that nearly a third of all medication errors occur due to labelling of the medicine and the package of the medication. A labelling and packaging review reference group has been convened by the Australian Government, Department of Health and Ageing, Therapeutic Goods Administration and as from April 2012 has been preparing recommendations for changes to medicine labels, names and packaging in a bid to reduce medication mistakes.

Patient's own medications

Patient's own medications (POMs) are the medication products brought into hospital at the time of admission, or brought in from an external source at a later time. These should include the current medications taken prior to the hospital visit and may include prescription medicines, over-the-counter medicines, clinical trials stock or complementary medicines.

Having these medications available helps health care professionals to establish an accurate medication history. Under some circumstances the availability of these medicines may allow the timely provision of essential treatment in emergency situations if a required medication is not immediately available in the hospital. POMs may only be used where it is safe and appropriate: sometimes the medicines brought into hospital are not readily identifiable or suitable for use, and it is important that any medications are appropriately assessed by qualified staff before use. Information about POMs should be documented according to individual institutional policy, and when returned to a patient this must also be documented. Where necessary they must be recorded on the relevant dangerous drugs register and stored in accordance with state legislation. POMs must also be stored in accordance with the manufacturer's recommended requirements (e.g. refrigeration).

The decision to allow the use of POMs during admission will need to be made by the individual hospital or health service. Like any other medication, they may be administered to patients/clients only if they have been written into the patient's medication plan by the treating medical practitioner.

Continuity of pharmaceutical care

The Australian Medication Management Plan (available at the Australian Commission on Safety and Quality in Health Care) is an initiative that provides nursing, medical, pharmacy and allied health staff with a standardised approach to recording and reconciling medication information upon admission and discharge. The Medication Management Plan provides the process to obtain, in collaboration with the patient, the best possible medication history – where the nurse, prescriber or pharmacist and other suitably qualified health care professional documents medicines taken prior to admission, including non-prescription and complementary medicines. The Medication Management Plan also involves doctor's plan section; confirmation that the information provided in the history is correct with a least two sources (e.g. GP, pharmacist, patient's own medicines); medication reconciliation (where the nurse or pharmacist compares medicines listed with the medication chart – this should occur as soon as possible after admission); medication issues; medication changes during admission; and a referral for a home medicines review.

Safe injection techniques

General safety principles

General safety principles includes hand hygiene, gloves where appropriate, other single-use personal protective equipment, skin preparation and disinfection. This chapter covers the following injections:

* intradermal, subcutaneous and intramuscular needle injections

* intravenous infusions and injections

* dental injections

* phlebotomy

* lancet procedures.

The World Health Organization defines a safe injection as:

> A safe injection, phlebotomy (drawing blood), lancet procedure or intravenous device insertion is one that: does not harm the recipient; does not expose the provider to any avoidable risk; does not result in any waste that is dangerous for other people. (World Health Organization, 2010, p. 1).

Injections are unsafe when given with unsterile or improper equipment or technique. Unsafe injections are those that lead to the transmission of bacteria, fungi, and pathogens. Unsafe injections can also cause adverse, non-infectious events such as abscesses (especially for those who receive regular injections).

Health care workers should wear non-sterile, well-fitting latex or latex-free gloves when coming into contact with blood or blood products, when performing venipuncture or venous access injections, if the health care worker's skin is *not* intact, and if the patient's skin is *not* intact. Personal protective equipment (PPE) is not indicated for injection procedures unless blood splashes are expected or the medication is considered toxic. PPE includes protective eyewear, mask, and gloves.

Skin preparation for the type of injection is also an important consideration. The two types of preparation are soap and water, and disinfection. According to WHO (2010) there is evidence for using disinfection for venous access, but there is insufficient evidence on the need to disinfect before an intramuscular injection. WHO recommends a soap and water cleanse for intradermal and subcutaneous injections. However, in practice most injection sites are swiped with an alcohol swab or cotton-wool ball dipped in 60–70% alcohol-based solution (isopropyl alcohol), wiping the area from the centre of the injection site working outwards, without going over the same area and allowing 30 seconds for the solution to dry before injecting.

When administering an injection:

* Check the drug chart or prescription for the medication and the corresponding patient's name and dosage.

* Perform hand hygiene.

* Wipe the top of the vial with 60–70% alcohol (isopropyl alcohol) using a swab or cotton-wool ball.

* Open the package in front of the patient to reassure them that the syringe and needle have not been used previously.

* Using a sterile syringe and needle, withdraw the medication from the ampoule or vial (World Health Organization, 2010, p. 11).

To ensure that waste is dealt with safely:

* Transport and store sharps containers in a secure area before final disposal.

* Close, seal and dispose of sharps containers when the containers are three-quarters full.

* Assign responsibility in written policy for monitoring the fill level of sharps containers and replacing them when they are three-quarters full.

* Discard waste that is not categorised as sharp or infectious in appropriate colour-coded bags.

* Ensure that infectious waste bags and sharps containers are closed before they are transported for treatment or disposal (World Health Organization, 2010, p. 12).

Sites for intramuscular Injections

The most common injection given in mental health services is the intramuscular injection (IMI). This applies to psychotropic medications such as Risperdal Consta®, haloperidol decanoate, and paliperidone palmitate. An IMI in the ventrogluteal site is suitable for adults. Patients/clients are usually comfortable lying on their side with a flexed knee or leaning on the examination table with knee flexed (on the side the injection is to be given). To administer the injection you place the heel of your hand on the patient's trochanter with your fingers towards the patient's head. The area for the injection is also known as the 'upper, outer quarter' (images A and B in Figure 5.2). With your index finger on the patient's anterior superior iliac spine, stretch your middle finger. If the patient prefers to have the IMI in the deltoid muscle the injection needs to be given beneath the acromion process and in the middle of the deltoid triangle. Image C in Figure 5.2 on the next page demonstrates IMI technique.

Figure 5.2: A   B

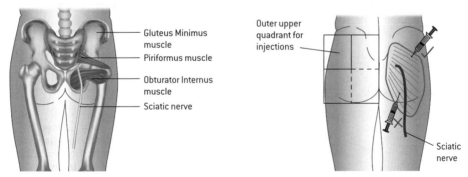

Monitoring drug efficacy and effects

Monitoring the efficacy of medication is an important role undertaken by health care professionals who administer medicines. These effects can be classified as desired (those you want to happen) and unwanted (those that you do not want to happen). Unwanted effects of medicines are sometimes serious, but generally they are manageable. Unwanted effects of medicines can occur with over-the-counter medicines, complementary medicines and/or prescribed

Figure 5.2: C

How to Give an Intramuscular Injection

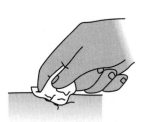

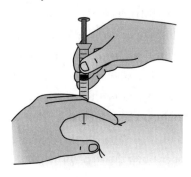

1. Use an alcohol swab to clean
   the skin where you will give
   yourself the shot.

2. Hold the muscle firmly and insert the needle into
   the muscle at a 90° angle (straight up and down)
   with an quick firm motion.

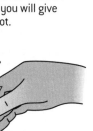

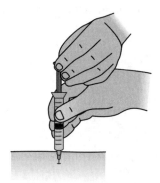

3. After you insert the needle
   completely, release your
   grasp of the muscle.

4. Gently pull back on the plunger of the syringe
   to check for blood. (If blood appears, withdraw
   the needle and gently press the alcohol swab
   on the injection site. Start over with a fresh
   needle.)

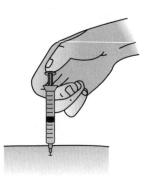

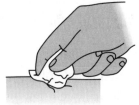

5. If no blood appears, inject all of
   the solution by gently and steadily
   pushing down on the plunger.

6. Withdraw the needle and syringe and press an
   alcohol swab on the spot where the shot was
   given.

medicines. Information related to the effects of medication can be presented in the product information leaflet that accompanies the medicine. As a prescriber, dispenser or an administrator of medicine it is your legal obligation to inform patients/clients about the medications they are prescribed. Unwanted effects are generally described as being common (1 in 10 people), uncommon (1 in 100), and rare (1 in 1000). Desired effects of medications will depend on the type of medicine prescribed (antipsychotic, anxiolytic, antiepileptic, etc.). Additionally, you must keep in mind that an unwanted effect in one person's situation may well be a desired effect for another.

For instance, chlorpromazine is a first-generation antipsychotic; it also has an affinity for histamine receptors (causing sedation) and has antiemetic and pain-relieving properties. Chlorpromazine as an antipsychotic can give rise to unwanted effects such as dry mouth, blurred vision, oversedation, **tardive dyskinesia** (in long-term use). Second-generation antipsychotics are preferred over first-generation antipsychotics since these are generally better tolerated by patients/clients in terms of effects. However, if a person presents to the emergency room with a migraine, chlorpromazine is one medicine that can be used with great effect.

Some adverse effects are quite serious and need to be reported. In Australia, the primary focus of adverse reaction reporting is to contribute to the early recognition of the harmful effects of drugs. Nurses, doctors, pharmacists, paramedics and other health care professionals, pharmaceutical companies and patients/clients can report any suspected adverse drug reaction to the Adverse Drug Reactions Advisory Committee. Reports undertaken by health care professionals may be submitted on a 'blue card' or online. Reports can also be made by email or letter to the Therapeutic Goods Administration.

In New Zealand adverse drug reactions are either reported online or in writing to the New Zealand Medical Assessor. The flow chart in Figure 5.3 may be helpful.

Ask yourself!

1   How could you keep up to date with the processes of reporting adverse reactions with medicines?

2   Why is it important to report the serious adverse events of medicines?

Figure 5.3: Action for adverse drug reactions (NZ)

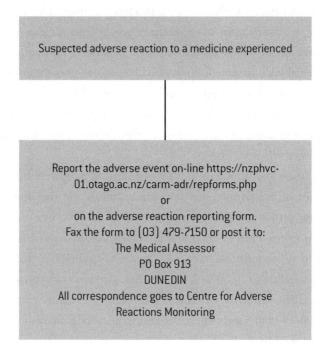

Suspected adverse reaction to a medicine experienced

Report the adverse event on-line https://nzphvc-01.otago.ac.nz/carm-adr/repforms.php
or
on the adverse reaction reporting form.
Fax the form to (03) 479-7150 or post it to:
The Medical Assessor
PO Box 913
DUNEDIN
All correspondence goes to Centre for Adverse Reactions Monitoring

Patient/client and carer education

Patient/client and carer education is an important consideration in medication administration. There are many reasons, not the least of which is the right of the patient to understand the medication they are taking and the possible wanted/desired and/or unwanted effects the medication may have on them. This is always conducted in agreement with the patient/client; however, the legal capacity of the person and the role of their carer are also taken into account. Medicine education can positively affect adherence to taking medicines – for instance, the patient/client may have fears or negative beliefs about the medication that can be demystified through education and the support that is provided through this therapeutic interaction. Education may also negatively affect the individual, such as creating fear of the medication, and therefore needs to be conducted in a way that allows time for people to ask clarifying questions of the health care worker. Additionally, medication education is to be understood as a dynamic and ongoing process, as medication regimens change over time and therefore education about medication regimens is not a single occurrence in the patient's/client's illness–health continuum.

Education related to medication needs to motivate and inform. This is in the context of a number of considerations such as duty of care, adherence behaviours, early warning signs planning (for symptoms or **adverse events**, etc.). The use of supplementary written information such as Consumer Medicines Information (CMI) may supplement verbal counselling, but it is important to note that CMI may not be appropriate where a drug is used 'off-label' in a mental health setting: for example, although anticonvulsants are widely used as mood stabilisers, CMI will generally make extensive reference to their use in relation to epilepsy.

In providing education the health care professional needs to look to the best available and most contemporary evidence. As the scope of medicines is constantly changing, reference to the evidence related to a particular class of drug and the various contexts in which that drug can be used is the imperative.

From the consumer's perspective – *How does this feel for me?*

There are quite a number of processes you need to go through when prescribing, dispensing or administering medicines to patients/clients. These processes require questioning the patient/client, and some of these questions may have been asked of them many times (especially in the case where they have experienced a protracted version of a mental disorder). Some patients/clients become irritated with many questions when they are with a health care worker, and may comment:

'Why are you asking me that question again? I told you last time.'

'You don't need to ask me those questions; my doctor covered it all with me at the appointment last week.'

'[To a nurse practitioner] You are not a doctor, so how can you prescribe me medication?'

Reflect on these statements and journal how you might respond to questions like these about medications. Keep in mind the goals of the person and the therapeutic goals of the treating team.

Summary

This chapter covered some key concepts and examples related to medication calculations and administration, including basic mathematical skills, medication administration, and your role in administering drugs for treatment, monitoring the efficacy of medicines, and patient and carer education relating to medication therapy. Importantly, the chapter highlights the fact that medication prescribing, dispensing and administration is a collaborative process and includes the patient, other health care team members and carers. Additionally, ensuring due diligence is paid to the processes involved in administration, recording and reporting matters related to medication therapy can positively affect patient/client outcomes and work towards the reduction of medication errors.

Discussion questions

1   *How* would you report a serious adverse event with medicines? Is this your responsibility?

2   *Who* can prescribe medicines in Australia?

3   *What* lessons can you take from Cathy's story?

Test yourself (answers at the back of the book)

1   A health care worker who prepares and administers medications will need to possess basic mathematical skills. Basic maths involves:

    A   addition, subtraction, multiplication and division

    B   addition, subtraction, division and decimals

    C   addition, multiplication, division and decimals

    D   all of the above

2   You will need to organise your drug calculations information using:

    A   desired dose; drug type; and the volume on hand

    B   drug type; concentration and the desired dose

    C   desired dose; concentration; and the volume on hand

    D   type of patient, desired dose and concentration

3   Schedule 3 drugs are:

    A   Pharmacy Medicine and should be available from a pharmacy or a licensed person

    B   Pharmacist Only Medicine and should be available to the public with direct involvement of a pharmacist (without a prescription)

C substances with a low potential for causing harm, the extent of which can be reduced through the use of appropriate packaging with simple warnings and safety directions on the label

D Prescription Only Medicine

4 The National Inpatient Medication Chart provides a standard approach to address issues related to:

A dispensing, administering and reviewing medications for inpatients

B prescribing, dispensing, administering and reviewing medications for inpatients

C prescribing, administering and reviewing medications for inpatients

D prescribing, dispensing, administering and reviewing medications for outpatients

5 A safe injection, phlebotomy (drawing blood), lancet procedure or intravenous device insertion is one that:

A does harm the recipient, does expose the provider to any avoidable risk, and does result in any waste that is dangerous for other people

B does not harm the recipient and does not expose the provider to any avoidable risk only

C does not harm the recipient, and does not result in any waste that is dangerous for other people

D does not harm the recipient, does not expose the provider to any avoidable risk, and does not result in any waste that is dangerous for other people

Useful websites

Australian Commission of Safety and Quality in Health Care available at <www.safetyandquality.gov.au>

National Medication Management Plan available at <www.safetyandquality.gov. au/our-work/medication-safety/medication-reconciliation/nmmp>

Therapeutic Goods Administration available at <www.tga.gov.au>

References

Australian Council for Safety and Quality in Health Care National Inpatient Medication Chart Pilot Aggregate Data Report (2012). Retrieved 2 May 2012, from <www.health.gov.au/internet/safety/publishing.nsf/content/national-inpatient-medication-chart>.

Australian Commission on Safety and Quality in Healthcare. (2008). *Recommendations for Terminology, Abbreviations and Symbols used in the Prescribing and Administration of Medicine.* Darlinghurst, NSW: Australian Commission on Safety and Quality in Health Care. Retrieved from <www.safetyandquality.gov.au>.

Schedule 1 Standard for the Uniform Scheduling of Drugs and Poisons No. 23. Barton ACT: Australian Government.

World Health Organization. (2010). *WHO Best Practices for Injections and Related Procedures Toolkit.* Geneva: World Health Organization.

Wright K. (2005). 'An exploration into the most effective way to teach drug calculation skills to nursing students' *Nurse Education Today* 25(6): 430–436.

Part 2

Context

Chapter 6

Mood Disorders

Chapter overview

This chapter covers the following topics:

* clinical features of important mood disorders

* discussion of the treatment of depression and bipolar affective disorder

* clinical pharmacology of antidepressants and mood stabilisers

* treatment of mood disorders in special populations

* approaches to management of treatment resistant mood disorders

Chapter learning objectives

After reading this chapter, you should be able to:

* describe the key features and differential diagnoses of major depression and bipolar affective disorder

* outline drug therapy options that are available for treatment of clinically important mood disorders

* discuss important adverse effects and drug interactions observed in association with the treatment of mood disorders

Key terms

Antidepressants
Bipolar I and bipolar II disorders
Electroconvulsive therapy (ECT)
Major depressive episode and major depressive disorder
Mood disorders
Mood stabilisers

Introduction

Mood disorder and affective disorder terminologies are sometimes used interchangeably, primarily because the terms 'mood' and 'affect' are closely related and describe similar but subtly different concepts. The term 'mood' is used to describe a person's predominant state of emotions/feelings, whereas 'affect' is more appropriately used to describe the external manifestation of internal emotional state. Put another way, mood is what is described by a patient/client, but affect is what is observed and documented by a clinician.

Mood disorders are certainly among the most common forms of mental disorders, with evidence from a range of sources suggesting that the lifetime prevalence rate for **major depressive disorder** among adults is probably in the order of 15–20% (higher for women than men). The incidence of bipolar disorder is much lower than that of major depression but, even so, the 12-month prevalence estimates for these forms of mood disorder among adults have been cited at 1.5–2%, and thus cannot be considered to be rare. Along with anxiety disorders, mood disorders have been referred to as 'high prevalence' disorders, distinguished from less common psychiatric illnesses such as schizophrenia. There are many circumstances where a person may experience mood alterations that do not satisfy criteria that are consistent with a diagnosable mood disorder – in the context of loss or disappointment it is normal to feel 'down, gloomy or flat'. It is important that appropriate precision is applied in diagnosis, as this can have important consequences for subsequent care coordination. Mood disorders can have devastating consequences for an individual and for those around them. For example, it is estimated that up to 15% of people with persistent major depression will eventually die by suicide, and the mortality rates associated with many major medical illnesses are definitively higher among those with major depression. Not all of the consequences of mood disturbance are reflected in physical morbidity or mortality: a person's actions during a manic episode may have enduring consequences such as financial repercussions, relationship breakdowns, work-related problems or failure to attend to important responsibilities (e.g. in caring for a child or grandchild).

The spectrum of mood disturbance

Conditions associated with depressed mood

Variability in mood is a normal part of life and certainly does not always connote the presence of an abnormal mental state or the presence of a mental illness. Transient mood alterations are often perfectly normal, and when a person uses terms such as 'feeling depressed' or 'on a high' in the vernacular context, this is often a way of verbalising feelings rather than describing important clinical features of a mood disorder. Daily life challenges, such as occupational or relationship problems or disappointment with the outcome of a process to which the individual attaches importance (e.g. exam results), may lead to a person feeling sad or disappointed. Another special situation to consider is bereavement, where the loss of a loved one or an important figure in a person's life is a natural source of sadness that will usually eventually abate in a well-recognised pattern (although not always, in which case a form of mood disorder *may* eventually be diagnosed). Conversely, very happy events and circumstances in a person's life may create an enhanced state of well-being, but this is not accompanied by other features that would be associated with a diagnosis of a mood disorder.

Major depressive disorder

In the context of a mood disorder, a person's mood and affect will usually be either depressed or elevated. When the mood is seriously depressed and other diagnostic criteria are present, a person is said to be affected by an episode of major depression (refer to Table 6.1). If a person experiences an episode of major depression in the absence of other plausible causes such as the effects of another mental illness (such as schizoaffective disorder), or a history of episodes of elevated mood (see later in this chapter), and the depressed mood cannot be attributed to the effects of a drug or substance or general medical condition, the person satisfies the diagnostic criteria for major depressive disorder. Under some circumstances, major depression can occur under specific circumstances, and may be referred to using specific terminology (e.g. postnatal or postpartum depression).

Table 6.1: Abridged description of diagnostic criteria for a major depressive episode, adapted from the *Diagnostic and Statistical Manual of Mental Disorders* (4th edn, Text Revision)

To satisfy the diagnostic criteria for an episode of major depression, a person must have five or more of the key symptoms described below, present during the same two-week period and representing a departure from their previous functioning or mental status.

At least one of the symptoms must be:

Depressed mood that is present for most of the day, nearly every day, either reported by the patient (they may describe feeling 'down', 'sad', 'hopeless' etc.), or observed objectively by others

or

Loss of interest or pleasure (sometimes called anhedonia), where there is markedly diminished interest or pleasure in most activities for most of the day, nearly every day

Depending on whether one or both of the key features (above) are present, at least three or four more of the following symptoms must also be present:

Significant weight loss/gain without dieting (> 5% of body per month), or altered appetite

Persistent insomnia or hypersomnia nearly every day

Psychomotor agitation or retardation nearly (objectively observable) every day

Fatigue or loss of energy nearly every day

Feelings of worthlessness or excessive or inappropriate guilt

Diminished ability to think or concentrate, or indecisiveness

Recurrent thoughts of death or suicidal ideation without a specific plan, or a suicide attempt or specific plan for committing suicide

In addition, to satisfy the diagnostic criteria, symptoms must not meet criteria for a mixed mood episode, must cause clinically significant distress or impairment in functioning, and must not be attributable to the effects of a substance/drug or medical condition. The criteria also state that symptoms should not be better accounted for by bereavement.

Source: American Psychiatric Association (2000)

Other clinical circumstances associated with depressed mood

Bereavement represents a special category of mood disturbance that is relevant in the context of the death of someone of special significance to the patient/ client. People experiencing bereavement commonly present for help in the primary care setting, and indeed it is quite common for some people to have symptoms that look very much like a **major depressive episode**. Although the person affected will often regard the symptoms they experience as being entirely normal, they may seek professional help for issues such as sleep disturbance or loss of appetite. Different cultural groups may regard different periods of mourning as being normal, but in general bereavement symptoms are usually not considered to be consistent with major depression until these have been present for a period of two months or more. Other symptoms may be present that can also point to the possibility of major depression – these might include survivor guilt, marked functional impairment or hallucinations.

Dysthymic disorder is another example of a mood disorder that is characterised by depressed mood. People with dysthymic disorder typically have chronically depressed mood present for most of the time over a period of two years or more. Other associated symptoms that are similar to those of a major depressive episode also need to be present (e.g. poor appetite, insomnia, low energy). People with dysthymic disorder often have low interest and self-criticism and may describe themselves as uninteresting or incapable, but are often not reported unless in response to a direct enquiry. The disorder is commonly associated with an insidious onset and a chronic course. Other examples of conditions where depressive symptoms are present but cannot be attributed to major depressive disorder include psychiatric illnesses where there is an association with *depressive features, substance-induced mood disorder* where prominent and persistent disturbance in mood is secondary to the direct physiological effects of illicit or medicinal drugs, and *mood disorder due to a general medical condition*, whereby mood disturbance is due to the direct physiological consequence of a general medical condition (refer to Table 6.2).

Table 6.2: Other causes of conditions associated with depressed mood

Effects of substances/drugs
Intoxication with or withdrawal from the use of alcohol, amphetamines, cocaine, opioids, sedative/hypnotics.
Various medicinal drugs are also associated with the development of mood disturbances, including some analgesics, anticholinergic agents, antiepileptic agents (including those used for psychiatric purposes), antihypertensives, oral contraceptives, antidepressants and corticosteroids.
General medical conditions
Parkinson's disease, cerebrovascular disease, thyroid disease, HIV infection, malignancies, and others.

Conditions associated with elevated mood

Discussion so far has centred upon the mood disorders associated exclusively with depressed mood, but there are several types of mental illness in which the important diagnostic features include other forms of affective disturbance. Bipolar I and **bipolar II disorders** and cyclothymia are associated with episodes where there is abnormally and persistently elevated, expansive or irritable mood. Depending on the nature, severity and duration of the symptoms involved, the mood episodes are described as being manic episodes, hypomanic episodes or mixed episodes. It is important to point out that episodes of abnormally elevated mood do not necessarily mean that the person affected is particularly happy or cheerful. Furthermore, the symptoms associated with this type of mood disturbance can actually present a significant danger to the patient/ client themselves, or to those around them – behaviour can become inattentive, erratic, overconfident, grandiose and unpredictable. In these circumstances, the potential for enduring adverse consequences from the actions of those affected can be profound, and it is quite common for patients/clients to be detained involuntarily for treatment in the interests of their own safety and that of the general public. Diagnostic details for affective episodes involving elevated mood states are outlined in Table 6.3.

Table 6.3: Diagnostic features for episodes of affective disturbance involving elevated mood

Manic episode

Distinct period of abnormally and persistently elevated/expansive/irritable mood, lasting for least one week (or any duration if hospitalisation is necessary)

During the period of mood disturbance (above), three (or more) of the following are persistently present:

- inflated self-esteem or grandiosity
- decreased need for sleep
- increased talkativeness
- flight of ideas or racing thoughts
- distractibility
- increased goal-directed activity or psychomotor agitation
- excessive involvement in pleasurable activities that have high potential for painful consequences

During the period of mood disturbance there is no evidence of a mixed episode (see below). The criteria also specify that there would be marked impairment in occupational or social functioning, and that symptoms should not be due to the direct physiological effects of substances or medications or a general medical condition. Elevated mood secondary to the effects of treatment for depression cannot be used as a basis for a diagnosis of bipolar disorder.

Hypomanic episode

Many elements of the diagnostic criteria for a hypomanic episode are identical to those for a manic episode (above). *The period of mood disturbance may be briefer* than for a manic episode (the diagnostic criteria state at least four days), and the episode must be consistent with an unequivocal change in functioning that is not typical of the person's usual state. The alteration in mood should be objectively observable by others, but not severe enough to cause marked impairment in social or occupational functioning, or require admission to hospital. Unlike a manic episode, *psychotic features are not present during a hypomanic episode.*

Mixed episode

The criteria for both a manic episode and a major depressive episode are met on nearly every day during a period of at least a week. Mood disturbance is severe enough to cause marked impairment in social or occupational functioning or to require hospital admission. Psychotic features may be present. Symptoms are not attributable to a substance or medication or general medical condition.

Source: American Psychiatric Association (2000)

Bipolar affective disorder

Bipolar I disorder

To satisfy the diagnostic criteria for **bipolar I disorder**, a person must have a longitudinal clinical course that is characterised by at least one manic episode or mixed episodes (refer to Table 6.3 above). It is common for people with bipolar I disorder to also have had one or more major depressive episodes (see Table 6.1). Mood disturbance secondary to the effects of a substance or medication, a general medical condition, or the effects of another psychiatric illness (e.g. a psychotic illness) cannot be used as a basis for a diagnosis of bipolar I disorder. Symptoms must cause clinically significant distress impairment in social or occupational functioning. Features of a manic episode can be represented using a simple mnemonic (see Figure 6.1).

Figure 6.1: The 'DIGFAST' mnemonic representing features of a manic episode

D	• Distractibility
I	• Indiscretion (pleasurable activities)
G	• Grandiosity
F	• Flight of ideas
A	• Activity increase
S	• Sleep deficit (decreased need)
T	• Talkativeness (pressured speech)

Bipolar II disorder

To be diagnosed with bipolar II disorder, a person must have a clinical course that involves one or more major depressive episodes as well as at least one hypomanic episode (refer to Table 6.3). *If a manic or mixed episode is present, the diagnosis of bipolar II disorder cannot be made.* Mood disturbance secondary to the effects of a substance or medication, a general medical condition, or the effects of another psychiatric illness (e.g. a psychotic illness) cannot be used as a basis for a diagnosis of bipolar II disorder. Symptoms must cause clinically significant distress impairment in social or occupational functioning. A person with bipolar II disorder may consider the effects of a hypomanic episode to be abnormal or even undesirable. Much of the perceived disability experienced by those with bipolar II disorder is related to the effects of recurrent episodes of major depression.

Non-pharmacological treatment of mood disorders

Psychological therapy

Psychotherapy and other non-pharmacological treatments are widely acknowledged as having a very important place in the management of mood disorders, in particular for the management of depression. Various cognitive treatments are useful in the treatment of depression, and include Cognitive behavioural therapy (CBT) and interpersonal therapy. These types of treatment are usually delivered by psychiatrists or psychologists, but can also be provided by mental health nurses or social workers with appropriate training and experience. In addition, psychoeducation for patients/clients, carers and families is also important to ensure that there is an accurate understanding of the illness, and the objectives and nature of treatment. Non-drug psychological treatment may be considered to be the treatment of first choice in some populations (e.g. children and adolescents, or when there might be contraindications to pharmacotherapy). In more severe cases of depression, psychological therapies are rarely used as the sole treatment approach, and are generally combined with pharmacotherapy or other non-drug biological approaches such as electroconvulsive therapy (see below). In contrast, psychological therapies appear to have considerably less utility in the management of bipolar affective disorder. Although helpful in some cases, non-drug treatments are rarely used as the sole modality of therapy for bipolar disorder, which is usually managed with targeted pharmacotherapy. More extensive discussion of psychological therapy techniques is provided elsewhere in this text (refer to Chapter 7 on anxiety disorders).

Electroconvulsive therapy and other biological treatments

Electroconvulsive therapy (ECT) is widely considered to be the most effective treatment for major depression and a range of other serious psychiatric conditions. Relatively rapid in onset, and often effective in refractory cases, ECT is widely used in hospital-based psychiatry, but does not have a significant role in the community setting. However, significant stigma is still associated with ECT and patients/clients and their families or carers can be resistant to its use because of fear about the nature of the treatment and its side effects. Mental health clinicians have a significant role to play in assisting through the provision of psychoeducation, which may be augmented by the use of high quality written materials or audiovisual products such as short films illustrating the main points. A patient may be less fearful if offered the opportunity view a film that shows the actual processes of the treatment, and the subject's perceptions and responses to it – many products of this type are available.

The mode of action of ECT remains unclear. A convulsion occurs if a large number of neurons discharge simultaneously. Changes in the extracellular resting potential of neurons spread seizure activity throughout the cortical structures of the brain and into deeper regions, eventually involving the whole brain in synchronous neuronal firing. Pulses of electrical current are applied to the scalp, thus causing seizures (see Figure 6.2). Sophisticated imaging techniques demonstrate that during seizures induced by ECT, cerebral blood flow and uptake of glucose and oxygen increase in the brain, and that after the convulsion blood flow and glucose metabolism decrease, correlating with therapeutic response. Many neurotransmitters are affected by ECT, and the treatment also produces other neurological changes that are similar to those observed during antidepressant pharmacotherapy. In fact, ECT is known to be an effective treatment for both major depression and also mania, and can also be used for the management of severe, acute psychotic symptoms. ECT is also recommended for use in the treatment of severe mood disorders that occur with some general medical conditions such as Parkinson's disease.

Figure 6.2: Application of electrodes to the scalp during ECT

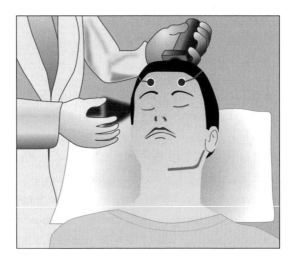

Some pre-existing conditions substantially increase the risk associated with ECT. Prior to the use of ECT, if a high-risk situation exists it is important that efforts are made to stabilise risk-related medical conditions. In the context of a recent myocardial infarction, there is a risk for reinfarction during ECT and most guidelines suggest that ECT should be avoided in the period spanning up to six weeks after a myocardial infarction. Uncompensated congestive cardiac failure and severe valvular heart disease are also thought to increase the risk of complications with ECT, as is any condition associated with increased intracranial pressure (e.g. space-occupying lesions, such as tumours), as the rise in intracranial pressure that accompanies ECT may cause brain herniation. ECT is not usually administered to a patient who has had a cerebrovascular accident. Given that ECT is administered with the assistance of a general anaesthetic, those patients/clients with severe cardiopulmonary disease or other illnesses that confer high anaesthetic risk are potentially at risk. Some medications may require modification or suspension during ECT: anticonvulsants and benzodiazepines may interfere with the achievement of an adequate seizure, and lithium may compound the risk of postictal confusion.

Some special populations require additional consideration. ECT can be used for older people, and evidence suggests that efficacy does not diminish with age. Concomitant medical conditions need to be accommodated and the approach to anaesthesia may require modification. The electrical stimulus intensity may actually need to be greater than that used for younger patients/clients, as the seizure threshold tends to increase with advanced age. Pre-existing cognitive impairment may be transiently exacerbated. ECT can be administered at any stage of pregnancy, but appropriate obstetric advice should be sought. In fact, the risk of teratogenesis associated with ECT is probably less than that associated with pharmacotherapy. ECT is a rarely used for children and adolescents, and specialist anaesthetic review will be required if there is an urgent need to do so.

ECT is usually administered in a timetable involving two or three treatments per week. Less frequent treatments may be helpful in the event that cognitive impairment or delirium develops. Typically, a course of 6–12 treatments is required, but in some cases more are necessary. Treatment continues until there is evidence that the therapeutic benefits realised through ECT have begun to plateau. The patient fasts from the night before the treatment, and an anaesthetist administers a general anaesthetic and muscle relaxant. A psychiatrist administers the electrical stimulus using a 'paddle', inducing the seizure. For a seizure to be effective it should last at least 25 seconds, and some ECT equipment actually includes an electroencephalogram monitor to allow precision in the measurement of the duration and intensity of the fit. Because of the very brief nature of the anaesthesia, intubation is not usually required, and the patient will awaken shortly after treatment. After being monitored in an appropriate environment for a short time, the person can usually return to the psychiatry unit soon after ECT.

Drugs used in ECT

ECT is always performed with general anaesthetic, which involves the use of drugs. The intravenous anaesthetic agents used may vary in accordance with local practices, or in accordance with the preferences of the anaesthetist involved. Many practices now use propofol to induce anaesthesia, but others may use barbiturate derivatives such as thiopentone or methohexitone. The anaesthesia is preceded by preoxygenation to optimise oxygen saturation, which facilitates the seizure and reduces the likelihood of desaturation after the procedure. Suxamethonium, a depolarising muscle relaxant, is always administered as a part of the anaesthesia. Suxamethonium binds acetylcholine receptors and in doing so the receptor is activated, causing depolarisation. The onset of action is rapid but the duration of action very short, because of rapid metabolic clearance by plasma cholinesterase. Side effects include fasciculations (small, rapid muscle contractions) and myalgia. The duration of effect is approximately five minutes, and because of this the usual approach does not involve intubation, but rather mechanical ventilation ('bagging'). A course of ECT usually involves general anaesthetic twice or three times weekly, and it is thought that this may contribute to the mild amnestic effect observed in some people undergoing ECT.

ECT is regarded as a very safe therapeutic intervention and is always performed under the supervision of a psychiatrist with the assistance of an anaesthetist and a nurse. Although many patients/clients and families are apprehensive about the possible side effects of ECT, with the exception of the potential to exacerbate medical conditions that should be picked up during pretreatment screening, adverse effects are usually mild and transient (and arguably are actually just as attributable to the effects of the general anaesthetic). Some patients/clients experience confusion and disorientation immediately after treatment, and others describe headache, nausea and muscle aches. A common unwanted effect of ECT is memory impairment, where some people experience difficulty with memory; however, this effect is generally transient and mild, improving with time. Patients/clients with poor dentition or those where the seizure has not been adequately modified with a muscle relaxant may sustain damage to the teeth.

Ask yourself!

1　Why might a patient become anxious about the prospect of having ECT?

2　What are the major risks associated with ECT and how might these be explained to a patient/client and their family with sensitivity?

3　Why are people who are treated with ECT usually hospitalised during their treatment?

Other non-drug biological treatments for depression are currently being developed and researched. Transcranial magnetic stimulation involves the application of a magnetic field over the surface of the head to depolarise superficial neurons. It uses a hand-held magnet to allow painless electrical stimulation across the scalp and cranium. As major depression may involve hypoactive cortical areas this approach appears to be promising as a means to alleviate symptoms of depression.

Vagal nerve stimulation is another technique for the treatment of depression that is currently under investigation – a stimulus is delivered via a programmable pulse generator implanted in the left chest wall through a bipolar lead. Exposure to bright light therapy can also be helpful in specific situations such as seasonal affective disorder, a condition that is uncommon in Australia because of relatively long days and abundant sunlight.

Pharmacotherapy for mood disorders

General principles of treatment for major depression

Although non-drug treatment options such as those outlined above are proven effective treatments for major depression, it is important to acknowledge that the majority of cases are managed in the community setting by primary care clinicians, and that drug therapy is by far the most commonly employed treatment modality in this setting. In severe cases of depression where the patient is suicidal and/or requires admission to hospital for the management of significant symptoms of depression, pharmacotherapy is almost invariably a major component of the treatment approach. Even where other treatment modalities are used (e.g. psychotherapy, ECT) it is common for these to be supplemented with pharmacotherapy – this may be with the aim of achieving response in refractory cases, or to enable treatment response to non-drug therapy to be sustained in the longer term.

The primary pharmacotherapy options that are used for the treatment of depression are collectively referred to as 'antidepressants' or antidepressant agents/drugs. Although this terminology accurately depicts their therapeutic utility for the management of depression, as outlined elsewhere in this text, these agents have therapeutic applications beyond the treatment of depression (e.g. for anxiety disorders, **eating disorders** and some general medical conditions). Also, some drugs are used in the adjuvant treatment of depression and are not strictly antidepressants, but are used in combination with antidepressants to augment their effectiveness.

Much has been written about the relative merits of the various antidepressant drugs that are currently available, and arguably a large proportion of the debate has been driven by claim and counterclaim in support of individual agents through the promotional activities of the pharmaceutical industry. In reality, a majority of contemporary opinion supports the view that, although there are certainly differences between individual agents in terms of adverse effect profile, potential for drug interactions, suitability for use in specific patient populations and toxicity in the context of overdose, in large part the overall safety, tolerability and effectiveness (as measured in overall response rates and time to onset of action) should be regarded as broadly similar. This means that there is a wide choice of agents that can be effectively regarded as first-line treatment options, and that the selection of a specific treatment for an individual patient/client needs to be based upon a broad consideration of a variety of more subtle considerations that are specific to the circumstances of each case. Additionally, as it is quite common for a patient/client to fail to gain a full therapeutic response from the first pharmacotherapy option tried (or for treatment to be withdrawn on the basis of a lack of tolerability), it is often the case that sequential trials of various medications may be needed before the most appropriate option is eventually employed. Many clinicians espouse the view that if a person has had a previous excellent response to treatment with a specific agent during a previous episode of depression, then this agent would logically be regarded as the treatment of first choice for subsequent episodes (unless other circumstances have changed). The most important principle of all is the primacy of the consumer's view in relation to the acceptability of treatment. Factors to consider include the consumer's capacity to pay for the medication (is it affordable or subsidised?) and ability to obtain the drug (can it be accessed through uncomplicated supply mechanisms?), and whether the person finds the therapeutic and adverse effects of the medication acceptable to the extent that adherence is likely to be adequate.

A range of considerations that influence antidepressant drug selection is represented in Figure 6.3. The presence of particular psychiatric comorbidities may lend weight to the selection of a drug with therapeutic efficacy across a spectrum of disorders (e.g. a person with comorbid major depression and obsessive-compulsive disorder may benefit from treatment with a selective serotonin reuptake inhibitor (SSRI), which can be helpful for both conditions). The presence of specific medical comorbidities may render a specific drug class less appropriate – for example, those with severe, unstable ischaemic heart disease should not usually be treated with tricyclic antidepressants (TCAs). In other situations, the pharmacological profile of an individual drug or drug class may confer benefit for a person with concurrent irritable bowel syndrome.

Figure 6.3: Treatment choice considerations when selecting an antidepressant

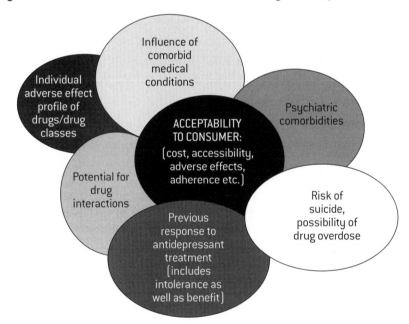

Drug interactions

The potential for drug interactions is an important consideration in the selection of an antidepressant medication in individual cases. Two different types of drug interactions can be relevant. With pharmacodynamic interactions the pharmacological effects of the antidepressant may add to those of another drug the patient/client is treated with, meaning that the effects will be cumulative. For example, when sedating TCAs are combined with other CNS suppressants such as opioids, benzodiazepines or antipsychotics, the extent of sedation and central respiratory depression can be significantly increased. On the other hand, the anticholinergic effect of TCAs may antagonise the therapeutic effect of cholinesterase inhibitors used for dementia. Another important manifestation of a pharmacodynamic drug interaction that is relevant to the use of antidepressant drugs is **serotonin syndrome**, sometimes referred to as serotonin toxicity. Serotonin syndrome is caused by a drug-induced excess of serotonergic activity, with clinical manifestations characterised by neuromuscular excitation, autonomic stimulation and mental status changes. Serotonin syndrome can actually happen as an adverse reaction to the normal therapeutic dose of an antidepressant, after a drug overdose or with drug interactions. The antidepressants that can cause serotonin syndrome include medications SSRIs, TCAs and monoamine oxidase inhibitors (MAOIs), as well as non-antidepressant agents such as pethidine, tramadol, the herbal supplement St John's wort, and illicit substances (e.g. MDMA or 'ecstasy'). Serotonin syndrome can be life-threatening and nearly all severe cases described to date have related to drug interactions. The clinical presentation of serotonin toxicity may be difficult to recognise because of the highly variable manifestations. Recognised diagnostic criteria for the serotonin syndrome are provided in Table 6.4.

Table 6.4: Diagnostic criteria for the serotonin syndrome

Coinciding with the commencement or increased dose of a known serotonergic agent, three or more of the following signs/symptoms should be present:

- cognitive-behavioural changes (agitation, confusion, hypomania)
- autonomic instability (diaphoresis, diarrhoea, hyperthermia, rigors, hypertension)
- neuromuscular changes (incoordination, hyperreflexia, myoclonus, tremor).

Other aetiologies should be ruled out, and a neuroleptic should not have been commenced or increased prior to the onset of symptoms.

Source: Sternbach (1991)

Antidepressants can also be involved in pharmacokinetic drug interactions, where the effects of one drug alter the clearance of another, as well as pharmacodynamic drug interactions. The anticonvulsant drugs carbamazepine and phenytoin lead to an increase in the rate of hepatic drug metabolism, which can compromise the effectiveness of many antidepressants. The SSRI antidepressants inhibit the hepatic metabolism of many other drugs, both psychotropics and those used for general medical conditions: the plasma levels of the second drug may rise, producing unintended toxicity. The types of drugs interacting will depend upon the doses of the drugs involved, the genetic phenotype of the patient/client (some have more extensive hepatic enzyme activity than others, and so are more prone to drug interactions), and the possibility of the involvement of alternative metabolic pathways (in which case drug interactions may be less clinically significant). The antidepressants most commonly implicated in this type of drug interaction are the SSRIs, and selected examples are illustrated in Table 6.5. An extensive exploration of antidepressants is beyond the scope of this discussion, and the reader should refer to a specialised reference text or consult a reliable drug information centre for further information if this is required in the context of the management of an individual case.

Table 6.5: Selected examples of drug interactions involving SSRI antidepressants

SSRIs + cytochrome 1A2 substrates
Most pronounced with fluvoxamine. Increased risk of toxicity or increased effects of various drugs metabolised by CY12A2 including caffeine, methadone, olanzapine, clozapine, donepezil, theophylline. Use with these combinations with extreme caution, if at all.
SSRIs + cytochrome 2D6 substrates
Most pronounced with paroxetine, fluoxetine, but can occur with any SSRI. Increased risk of toxicity or increased effects of various drugs metabolised by CYP2D6 including perhexiline, metoprolol, flecainide, haloperidol, risperidone, morphine and others. Use with these combinations with caution, if at all. Dosage adjustments of substrate drug will be required.
SSRIs + cytochrome 3A4 substrates
Most pronounced with fluoxetine, fluvoxamine and sertraline but can occur with any SSRI. Increased risk of toxicity or increased effects of various drugs metabolised by CYP3A4 including cyclosporine, tacrolimus, alprazolam, statins, zolpidem/zopiclone, carbamazepine and others. Use with these combinations with caution, if at all. Dosage adjustments of substrate drug will be required.

Antidepressants and overdose

Given the nature of the symptoms of major depression, suicidal intention and deliberate drug overdose are issues of serious concern. Although there is considerable discussion in the literature about the potential for a causal relationship between antidepressant treatment and suicide, the issue has not been resolved to an extent whereby 'confounding by diagnosis' can be excluded as a basis; this means that although suicidal ideation and suicide acts may be more common among those treated with antidepressants, it is not clear that this is caused by the drugs, or whether people with serious depression who are potentially suicidal are more likely to be treated with antidepressants. If the risk of suicide is considered to be high, and/or there is a history of past drug overdose, the drug with the safest profile in overdose should be used (e.g. SSRIs or moclobemide) and the amount of medication dispensed should be limited. Some medications such as TCAs and the older MAOI drugs (phenelzine and tranylcypromine) are highly lethal in overdose and should not usually be used for patients/clients at risk of suicide. Many other drugs (e.g. venlafaxine, mirtazapine, duloxetine) are associated with intermediate risk of toxicity in overdose – more dangerous than SSRIs and moclobemide, less dangerous than MAOIs and TCAs.

Choice of antidepressant

Current Australian best practice guidelines suggest that most of the currently available antidepressants can be regarded as potential first-line treatment (with the exception of TCAs, irreversible MAOIs and agomelatine, which on the basis of current data on safety and tolerability are regarded as legitimate second-line options). This being the case, the initial choice of antidepressant should be based on the general considerations outlined in Figure 6.3. A schematic representation of the differential properties of various antidepressants is provided in Figure 6.4.

The usual approach to the initiation of antidepressants involves use at the standard dose (refer to Table 6.6), for a period of approximately three to four weeks, after which there may be consideration of a dosage increase. In the event that there is little response after this time, or if there are intolerable unwanted effects, the usual approach would be to switch to a different drug. An alternative approach is the addition of an augmentation agent such as lithium, liothyronine, pindolol or an atypical antipsychotic. These agents are not antidepressants themselves, but may increase the efficacy of antidepressant drugs.

Figure 6.4: Schematic representation of the differential properties of various
antidepressants

SSRIs

Low toxicity:
relatively safe in
overdose

Extensive potential for drug–drug interactions involving a broad range of psychotropic
and medical drugs

Range of common side effects including nausea, diarrhoea,
tremor, headache, sexual dysfunction, possible bleeding
effects

Safety in comorbid medical illness good—well tolerated by those with
heart disease, little effect on seizure threshold. Dose adjustment usually
unnecessary for hepatic and renal dysfunction

Affordability and accessibility excellent – subsidised supply through pharmaceutical benefits
scheme. One daily dosing usual. Moderate potential for discontinuation syndrome upon
sudden discontinuation (except for fluoxetine – low potential)

TCAs

Very dangerous in overdose – risk of seizures, autonomic instability, cardiac arrhythmia.
Avoid for those at risk of suicide/overdose

Low – moderate potential for drug–drug interactions, mostly
pharmacodynamic interactions involving compounded risk for
sedation, hypotension etc.

Range of common side effects including dry mouth, blurred vision,
constipation, sexual dysfunction, confusion in the elderly

Safety in comorbid medical illness poor – not suitable for patients with heart
disease, destabilises seizure control

Affordability and accessibility excellent – subsidised supply through pharmaceutical benefits
scheme. One daily dosing, usually involving multiple tablets. Low–moderate potential for
discontinuation syndrome upon sudden discontinuation

(Continued)

Figure 6.4: Schematic representation of the differential properties of various antidepressants (*Continued*)

Irreversible MAOIs

Very dangerous in overdose – risk of seizures, autonomic instability, overdose difficult to manage. Avoid for those at risk of suicide/overdose

High potential for lethal drug–drug interactions, mostly hypertensive crisis after exposure to pressor amines in food (tyramine – "cheese effect") or interacting drugs such as cough/cold medications or sympathomimetics

Range of common side effects including dry mouth, blurred vision, constipation, sexual dysfunction, peripheral oedema

Safety in comorbid medical illness poor – not suitable for patients with heart disease, destabilises seizure control.

Affordability and accessibility adequate. Poor adherence because of need for dietary restrictions. Low–moderate potential for discontinuation syndrome upon sudden discontinuation

Moclobemide

Low toxicity: relatively safe in overdose

Almost no potential for drug interactions

Few serious side effects: nausea, headache, sexual dysfunction, peripheral oedema, transient anxiety

Safety in comorbid medical illness good–well tolerated by those with heart disease, little effect on seizure threshold. Dose adjustment usually unnecessary for hepatic and renal dysfunction

Affordability and accessibility excellent – subsidised supply through pharmaceutical benefits scheme. Twice daily dosing usual. Moderate potential for discontinuation syndrome upon sudden discontinuation. Seems less effective than other antidepressant for severe cases.

Figure 6.4: Schematic representation of the differential properties of various antidepressants (*Continued*)

Reboxetine

Moderate toxicity in overdose

Little potential for drug–drug interactions

Side effects include urinary retention, sexual dysfunction, sweating, increased blood pressure, headache

Safety in comorbid medical illness fair – use with caution for those with history of hypertension, little effect on seizure threshold. Dose adjustment required for renal dysfunction

Affordability and accessibility excellent – subsidised supply through pharmaceutical benefits scheme. Twice daily dosing usual. Moderate potential for discontinuation syndrome upon sudden discontinuation

Mirtazapine

Moderate toxicity in overdose – risk of seizures and autonomic instability

Low potential for drug–drug interactions

Side effects include sedation, peripheral oedema, significant potential for metabolic dysregulation, weight gain, hyperglycaemia, dyslipidaemia

Safety in comorbid medical illness fair – may exacerbate diabetes and hyperlipidaemia, significant effect on seizure threshold. Dose adjustment usually unnecessary for hepatic and renal dysfunction

Affordability and accessibility excellent – subsidised supply through pharmaceutical benefits scheme. One daily dosing usual. Moderate potential for discontinuation syndrome upon sudden discontinuation

(Continued)

Figure 6.4: Schematic representation of the differential properties of various antidepressants (*Continued*)

| Venlafaxine/Desvenlafaxine Duloxetine |

Moderate toxicity in overdose – risk of seizures and autonomic instability

Low potential for drug–drug interactions

Range of common side effects including nausea, diarrhoea, tremor, headache, sexual dysfunction, possible bleeding effects, dose-related hypertension

Safety in comorbid medical illness fair – may exacerbate hypertension, significant effect on seizure threshold. Dose adjustment required in renal dysfunction

Affordability and accessibility excellent – subsidised supply through pharmaceutical benefits scheme. One daily or twice dosing usual. Significant potential for discontinuation syndrome upon sudden discontinuation

| Bupropion |

Moderate toxicity in overdose – risk of seizures and autonomic instability

Low potential for drug–drug interactions

Side effects include insomnia, nightmares, potential for seizures, paranoia

Safety in comorbid medical illness fair – may lower seizure threshold. Dose adjustment usually unnecessary for hepatic dysfunction

Affordability and accessibility poor – not subsidised through pharmaceutical benefits scheme for depression (only for smoking cessation). Twice daily dosing usual. Low potential for discontinuation syndrome upon sudden discontinuation

| Agomelatine |

Toxicity in overdose appears low on the basis of limited data to hand

Low potential for drug–drug interactions

Adverse effects appear mild: headache; somnolence, fatigue; hyperhidrosis; raised LFTs

Safety in comorbid medical illness appears mostly good – may compound hepatic dysfunction

Affordability and accessibility poor – not subsidised through pharmaceutical benefits scheme for depression. Once daily dosing usual. Low potential for discontinuation syndrome upon sudden discontinuation

Table 6.6: Standard* daily doses for a range of antidepressant

	Starting dose (mg)	Maintenance (mg)	Maximum (mg)
SSRIs			
Citalopram	10	20	40
Escitalopram	5	10	20
Fluoxetine	10–20	20–30	60
Paroxetine	10–20	20–30	50
Sertraline	25–50	50–100	200
Fluvoxamine	50	50–100	200
TCAs			
Amitriptyline	25–50	50–150	300
Clomipramine	25–50	75–150	300
Dothiepin	25–50	75–150	300
Doxepin	25–50	75–150	300
Imipramine	25–50	75–150	300
Nortriptyline	25–50	75–150	150
Trimipramine	25–50	75–150	300
MAOIs			
Phenelzine**	15–30	30–60	90
Tranylcypromine**	10–20	20–40	60
Moclobemide**	300	600	600
Other			
Agomelatine	25	25–50	50
Bupropion	150	300**	300**
Desvenlafaxine	50	50–100	200
Duloxetine	30	30–60	90
Other			
Mirtazapine	15	30	45–60
Reboxetine**	8	10	12
Venlafaxine	75	75–225	375**

*May require adjustment for renal or hepatic impairment. More conservative doses used for children and the elderly. Caution is need in the presence of polypharmacy or multiple medical comorbidities
**Administered in divided doses

Considerations that should be taken into account when changing from one antidepressant to another are the 'washout' period that is required between stopping one drug and starting the next, and the possibility of a discontinuation syndrome. The washout period should be appropriate the plasma half-life and clearance of the first drug – the aim is to prevent adverse effects attributable to serotonin toxicity that occur because both drugs are present to a significant extent in the plasma. Some drugs require a long washout period because of a long half-life (e.g. fluoxetine) or an extended duration of action (e.g. phenelzine or tranylcypromine), whereas others have a very brief half-life and do not require a long washout (e.g. moclobemide venlafaxine). Note that drugs with a very short half-life are prone to be associated with a discontinuation syndrome. After stopping antidepressants such as venlafaxine, SSRIs and some others, discontinuation symptoms may include somatic features such as sleep disturbance, nausea, vertigo, sensory disturbances, and flu-like symptoms. The symptoms are usually mild and are not dangerous. Symptoms typically last for up to two weeks. The discontinuation syndrome is most likely after extended duration of treatment or with a high dose of the drug.

ELLEN'S STORY

Ellen is a 42-year-old married woman who presented to her local GP complaining of sleep disturbance and weight loss. She works part-time as an administration officer at a university and is the primary carer for her two teenage sons. On further enquiry Ellen describes a loss of appetite and grossly disturbed sleep – although she went to sleep at about midnight each night, she would consistently wake at about 3 am and find it almost impossible to get back to sleep. She found herself constantly exhausted and she described very little motivation to take on anything but the simplest of tasks. She has recently given up her gym membership, and said that she 'just didn't enjoy it anymore'. She said that she felt guilty about letting her family down, and that she had no interest in sex anymore. When asked about suicidal thoughts, she became very quiet and eventually said that she had thought about death a lot, but had not made any plans.

Her GP arranged for a series of blood tests and then prescribed paroxetine at a dose of 20 mg daily and asked her to come back in a fortnight to check on her progress. Two weeks later she presented again, looking tired and dishevelled. She looked upset and agitated and eventually burst into tears during the consultation.

She said she was feeling so awful that she had increased the dose of paroxetine to 40 mg of her own accord, but then stopped taking it altogether because of nausea and diarrhoea. Since stopping the medication she described feeling absolutely dreadful – agitated and dizzy, with constant headaches and strange sensations in her hands and feet. She was persuaded to try a different medication and was started on mirtazapine 15 mg at night, to be increased to 30 mg nightly after three days. She attended another appointment a week later and said that she felt 'better, but still not right'.

Ask yourself!

Thinking about Ellen's story:

1   What features of major depression were present at the time of her first presentation?
2   What happened to her after stopping the paroxetine?
3   How long will the medication take to work, and how long would she expect to need to be on treatment?
4   What care considerations would you include in Ellen's care plan related to her adherent/non-adherent behaviours?

From the consumer's perspective – *How does this feel for me?*

Depression can be all-consuming and can alter a person's perspective of their own life. Sometimes they are ashamed and may not reveal all of their symptoms.

Medications can cause side effects before they exert significant therapeutic effects – it is important to reinforce the need for good adherence.

'I'm struggling with life – I have a hard time just *existing*!'

'I feel so hopeless – nothing can help me, I need to pull myself together.'

'Sometimes I just want to go to sleep forever.'

Care Plan

The following is an example care plan for the patient/client presented in this chapter. The areas of daily living that are considered include bio-psycho-social factors and the plan is mapped out using the nursing process (Assessment; Planning; Implementation; Evaluation). Remember: the success is in the detail, so be specific about *who, when and what* in the collaborative plan; never include someone in the plan if they were not consulted in the planning process; and always work within a recovery-orientated framework (refer to Chapter 1).

Date: 30 July 2012

Name: Ellen

Case manager: GP

Areas of daily living	Assessment of current situation	Goal	Plan (undertaken with patient/client)	Implementation	Who is responsible? (Include only those who have been consulted in the planning process)	Evaluation/review date
Mental health	Depressed mood	Euthymia	Commence new antidepressant.	Fill prescription, follow-up appointment.	GP	6/8/12
Social	Married with two children	N/A	N/A	N/A	N/A	N/A
Biological	Non-adherent behaviour Discontinuation syndrome after cessation of SSRI	Facilitate effective pharmacotherapy and adherent behaviour.	Psychoeducation	Discuss motivation, beliefs and ambivalence for adhering or not adhering to medication/treatment.	GP and Ellen	6/8/12
	Monitor efficacy of medications	Minimise ADRs	Antidepressant side-effect checklist (Uher et al., 2009)	Weight gain Sedation Postural hypotension Other cardiovascular effects Hyperglycaemia	GP and Ellen	Progressive and ongoing

Environmental	Has recently given up gym membership due to anhedonia.	Re-engage with gym.	Speak with family about encouraging interests.	Family meeting	GP	TBA
Substance using behaviours	Nil detected	N/A	N/A	N/A	N/A	N/A
Risk behaviours	Suicidal ideation without plan	Minimise suicide risk.	Develop a suicide risk management plan.	Re-evaluate suicide risk at each appointment. Identify early warning signs, and strategy to address crisis. Refer to crisis assessment treatment team as appropriate.	GP and Ellen	6/8/12

General principles of treatment for bipolar disorder

Pharmacotherapy for bipolar disorder is complex and, unlike for major depression, the management of these conditions is rarely undertaken solely in the primary care setting: more often, pharmacotherapy is initiated by a specialist psychiatrist, although ongoing care may be continued by general practitioners. The treatment goals for bipolar illness may be divided into those which are appropriate for the acute management of episodes of mood disturbance, and those more relevant to ongoing prophylaxis against further episodes of depressed or elevated mood.

Management of mania or hypomania

Acute mania should be regarded as a psychiatric emergency and often requires timely admission to hospital. Mania affects about 1% of the population. The primary aim of treatment is the prompt control of symptoms. During a hospital stay it is common for the treating team to consider potential adjustments to prophylactic management, as well as appropriate supportive measures for the patient/client. A person with acute mania or hypomania may not necessarily be distressed, and in fact may actively resist therapeutic interventions.

After the safety of the patient/client and those around them have been addressed by the use of an appropriate treatment setting, the priorities for the management of acute mania are to address target symptoms such as psychosis and delusional thoughts (such as grandiose or persecutory delusions), as well as specific features of the affective disturbance such as hyperactivity, irritability and euphoria. Key measures that can be used to gauge the impact of treatment include the extent of sleep disturbance, pressure of speech, flight of ideas and hallucinations. The treatment aims are usually achieved through the introduction of one or more pharmacotherapies, with the choice of treatment usually predicated on the basis of the predominant symptoms at the time. At the outset of treatment it is important to check whether the person has been taking an antidepressant during the period prior to the presentation, as these medications are usually discontinued in the context of acute mood elevation.

Overall, antipsychotic drugs are more effective than mood stabilisers in treating acute mania. Risperidone, olanzapine, and haloperidol are among the best of the available options for the treatment of manic episodes

(Cipriani et al., 2011). Individual drugs that are commonly used for this purpose include olanzapine (up to 20 mg daily), quetiapine (up to 800 mg daily in divided doses), risperidone (up to 6 mg daily) or ziprasidone (80 mg twice daily). The threshold for the use of antipsychotic medication is usually regarded as lower if symptoms are severe or disruptive, or the elevated mood episode has occurred despite treatment with a mood stabiliser medication (see below). If there is prominent hyperactivity, or if the elevated mood appears to be refractory to antipsychotic drug therapy, a common strategy is to introduce concurrent treatment with a benzodiazepine medication. These agents potentiate the sedation that is achieved using the antipsychotic agents, and for this reason are sometimes referred to as antipsychotic-sparing agents. A long-acting benzodiazepine, commonly clonazepam, diazepam or lorazepam, is usually used for this purpose. As symptoms begin to subside, the dose of the benzodiazepine is reduced, and eventually changed to a regimen involving administration only when required for target symptoms that are clearly documented in the treatment plan.

Another routinely used approach to the management of mania is the introduction or adjustment of mood stabiliser medications. Several medications have proven mood stabiliser effects, and when used in the context of acute mood elevation these drugs can help to achieve a mood state close to **euthymia** (a mood state that is neither elevated nor depressed). For people not treated with mood stabilisers before the manic episode, or for those who had been treated but had not adhered to the treatment regimen, the introduction of a mood stabiliser alone can be sufficient as a management strategy, particularly if symptoms are not severe or refractory. On the other hand, it is quite common to combine mood stabiliser treatment with antipsychotics and benzodiazepines during an episode of acute mania, and to subsequently phase out treatment with these latter drugs after euthymia or near euthymia has been achieved. After initiation during the management of mania, mood stabiliser medications are usually left in place in the longer term as a part of the prophylactic approach to treatment.

The mood stabiliser drugs that are used in the management of acute mania are lithium, sodium valproate (also called valproic acid or divalproex sodium) and carbamazepine. Each of these drugs is administered orally, which may prove problematic with patients/clients refusing medications. The usual dose of lithium for healthy adults without renal impairment is initially in the order of 750–1000 mg per day, administered in divided doses – the objective should be to adjust the dosage in accordance with the trough serum concentration.

In acute mania some treatment guidelines advocate the use of slightly higher serum concentrations, in the order of 0.8–1.2 mmol/L, although at higher concentrations the side effects are more pronounced and the treatment is relatively poorly tolerated. Older people should usually be titrated to a slightly lower serum concentration. Later on, the serum concentrations used for maintenance treatment can be lower than those used for the management of acute mania, with many laboratories citing a reference range of 0.5–1.0 mmol/L. Sodium valproate is also used for the management of acute mania, and, although the reference range for use in psychiatric applications (as opposed to the original therapeutic application in the treatment of epilepsy) is less defined, most agree that the minimum effective serum concentration for this purpose is in the order of about 300 micromol/L (43 mg/L). Valproate treatment is usually introduced at a dose of 200–400 mg twice daily, with many people requiring a daily dose of up to 2000 mg to achieve therapeutic effects. Carbamazepine is the other option for use as a mood stabiliser during acute mania. Again, the dosage needs to be adjusted and most clinicians would aim for levels in the range of 20 to 50 micromol/L (5 to 12 mg/L). The starting dose for carbamazepine is usually 100 mg twice daily, and will require titration to achieve the appropriate therapeutic effect. Many people find that the rapid titration of carbamazepine required for the management of acute mania is associated with considerable side effects, most notably gastrointestinal and neurological in nature (nausea, dizziness, sedation). For this reason, carbamazepine is less frequently used for the management of mania than lithium or valproate.

Some people fail to respond to the standard treatments used for the management of acute mania. In these circumstances, it is important to establish that **compliance** has been adequate, and to optimise the serum concentrations of the drugs used. Combination treatment involving the simultaneous use of lithium, an anticonvulsant, an antipsychotic and a benzodiazepine may be required.

Management of depression in bipolar disorder

People with bipolar disorder will have episodes of major depression as a part of their illness, and these episodes are generally predominant for those who have bipolar II disorder. Particularly after an episode of mania/hypomania during which elation/euphoria has been present, the symptoms of a depressive episode are often experienced as particularly severe, and there is a substantial risk of self-harm (up to 15% of people with bipolar disorders die by suicide). During these times it is very important that the person is treated vigorously in a safe environment. The management of major depression in the context of bipolar disorder is the same as that for major depressive disorder, and the standard treatment approaches include antidepressant pharmacotherapy, ECT +/− psychological treatments such as CBT. There is emerging evidence to suggest that the newest mood stabiliser medication, lamotrigine, may be superior to others in both the management and prevention (see below) of recurrent major depressive episodes in people with bipolar disorder. Lamotrigine has the drawback of an association with potentially severe dermatological reactions, including life-threatening exfoliative reactions such as Stevens-Johnson syndrome and other dermatological toxicities. Serious skin reactions are more common with lamotrigine if the starting dose is up-titrated quickly, or if lamotrigine is used in combination with valproate. Currently available evidence suggests that maintenance treatment with antidepressants does not necessarily reduce the likelihood, severity, refractoriness or duration of depressive episodes among those with bipolar disorder. Another consideration that must be taken into account is the phenomenon of treatment-emergent affective switch (sometimes referred to as 'manic switch'), where the addition of ECT or an antidepressant may cause a patient to switch from depression to mania, hypomania, or a mixed episode. If this does happen, the antidepressant treatment should be stopped and the standard approaches to the management of elevated mood considered. There is no compelling evidence to suggest that any specific antidepressant medication is more likely to cause treatment-emergent affective switch than others.

Maintenance mood stabiliser treatment in bipolar affective disorder

Given the potentially catastrophic outcomes that can follow episodes of mood disturbance in the context of bipolar affective disorder, an important element of ongoing treatment is the use of prophylactic mood stabiliser treatment that is intended to reduce the frequency, duration and severity of episodes of mania and depressions. Lithium, valproate, carbamazepine, lamotrigine, olanzapine and quetiapine are all effective for this purpose. Lithium is generally regarded as the treatment of choice for this purpose, although not all patients/clients can tolerate this medication. The adverse **metabolic impacts** of the atypical antipsychotic agents mean that these drugs are generally reserved for circumstances where the other agents are not practical or effective. Lamotrigine may be preferred for those with treatment-resistant illness or where episodes of major depression are the predominant feature. The combination of lithium with valproate or lamotrigine may be used for those with refractory illness.

Ongoing mood stabiliser pharmacotherapy should be combined with an appropriate range of supportive strategies aimed at minimising comorbid **substance abuse** and maintaining physical health (e.g. dietary and exercise advice, monitoring blood pressure, body weight, blood glucose and lipids). It is also important to provide support for families and carers, and to offer appropriate psychological interventions and psychoeducation. Mood stabiliser treatment is associated with a range of adverse effects and it is critical that, in addition to periodic monitoring of serum concentrations, patients/clients should be reviewed regularly to check for signs of toxicities.

Lithium can cause serious toxicities if the serum concentration is not maintained within the reference range. Even at therapeutic concentrations, lithium can cause side effects including gastrointestinal symptoms such as nausea, vomiting and diarrhoea. Many people treated with lithium develop a fine tremor, which may actually become more coarse in nature at toxic serum concentrations. Skin reactions include activation or exacerbation of psoriasis or acne. Lithium can also cause thyroid dysfunction (most notably a reversible hypothyroidism) and hyperparathyroidism. As lithium is almost entirely cleared by the kidneys, regular assessment of renal function is critical to prevent toxicity.

Lithium toxicity can have potentially lethal consequences, and it is important that both clinicians and consumers are educated about and alert for the early signs of toxicity. Psychoeducation and the provision of written support materials are particularly important in this regard. Indications for measurement of the serum lithium concentration include the appearance of significant symptoms of toxicity, loss of control in prophylactic therapy, alterations in renal function, fluid restriction or poor oral intake, or intravenous fluid therapy, particularly in the perioperative period. Acute lithium toxicity (e.g. after overdose) is managed with dialysis. Chronic lithium toxicity is associated with poor outcomes, and it is important to ensure that patients/clients understand the signs and symptoms (refer to Table 6.7).

Anticonvulsant mood stabilisers also require ongoing monitoring to allow the detection of potentially serious side effects. Nausea and vomiting are common, as are dizziness, diplopia, ataxia (unsteady gait), and somnolence. Skin

Table 6.7: Features of lithium toxicity

Relatively mild (serum concentration < 1.2 mmol/L)	Fine tremor, nausea, vomiting, diarrhoea, muscle weakness, flu-like syndrome
Moderate (serum concentration 1.5–2.5 mmol/L)	Coarse tremor, severe gastrointestinal symptoms, dysarthria, sedation, hyper-reflexia
Severe (serum concentration > 2.5 mmol/L)	Stupor, coma, arrhythmias, seizures, cardiovascular collapse

rashes of various types are quite common, and may evolve to dangerous systemic hypersensitivity syndromes, particularly with lamotrigine and carbamazepine. Hepatoxicity and haematological adverse effects mean that regular monitoring of liver function and the complete blood picture is required. Elevation of the gamma–glutamyl transferase during treatment with carbamazepine may reflect hepatic enzyme induction which can compromise the effectiveness of other medications; this can be clinically important.

MICHELLE'S STORY

Michelle is 37-year-old single woman with a past psychiatric history of bipolar affective disorder, recently admitted to hospital for the treatment of an acute manic episode. Over the last two weeks her flatmate had noticed that she had become increasingly talkative, loud and intrusive. She told staff that she had increased energy and appetite. She had recently used her entire savings account to buy a second-hand prestige car. She said that while she has feeling 'up' she had lots of boyfriends, although she was not in a lasting relationship with anyone. She mentioned that she had recently stopped taking all of her prescribed medications except her venlafaxine. On examination she was agitated and restless, and answered questions in an overly expansive fashion. She made over-familiar gestures towards the medical and nursing staff. She was started on olanzapine 10 mg twice daily, clonazepam 2 mg twice daily + 0.5 mg extra when needed, and lithium 500 mg twice daily.

Care Plan

The following is an example care plan for the patient/client presented in this chapter. The areas of daily living that are considered include bio-psycho-social factors and the plan is mapped out using the nursing process (Assessment; Planning; Implementation; Evaluation). Remember: the success is in the detail, so be specific about *who, when and what* in the collaborative plan; never include someone in the plan if they were not consulted in the planning process; and always work within a recovery-orientated framework (refer to Chapter 1).

Date: 1 August 2012

Name: Michelle   Case manager: M. Mania

Areas of daily living	Assessment of current situation	Goal	Plan (undertaken with patient/client)	Implementation	Who is responsible? (Include only those who have been consulted in the planning process)	Evaluation/ review date
Mental health	Diagnosis of bipolar affective disorder.	Review current treatment regimen. Euthymia	Pathology examinations Physical examination Review mental state.	Mental state examination. Blood test for TFT, full blood examination, etc. Obtain baseline data – blood pressure, waist measurements, weight, temperature, pulse rate, respirations, serum LiCO3 etc.	Psychiatrist and M. Mania	3/8/12
Social	Single	N/A	N/A	N/A	N/A	N/A
Biological	Has ceased all medications except venlafaxine. History of non-adherence to medication/ treatment.	Recommence medications. Improve adherent behaviour.	Manage care in the least restrictive manner Discuss motivation, beliefs and ambivalence for adhering or not adhering to medication/treatment.	Monitor at home with CATT visits 3 times per day. When symptoms of hypomania abate, engage Michelle in discussions related to non-adherent behaviours.	CATT and M. Mania M. Mania and Michelle	Daily review. Regular fortnightly appointments.

Environmental	Lives with friend	N/A	N/A	N/A	N/A	N/A	N/A
Substance-using behaviours	N/A	N/A	N/A	N/A	N/A	N/A	N/A
Risk behaviours	Impaired judgment with spending savings. Previous disinhibition, possible unsafe sex.	Limit impact of behaviours experienced during mood elevation.	Provide education, refer to social worker.	N/A	Regular appointments with case manager provide opportunities for psychoeducation. Make appointment with social worker in local area for financial counselling and support.	M. Mania and Michelle	15/8/12 and fortnightly thereafter.

Ask yourself!

Thinking about Michelle's story.

1   Do you think it would be safe for Michelle to be treated for acute mania at home?

2   What factors might have contributed to this episode of mood elevation?

3   What monitoring will Michelle need over the next 12 months?

From the consumer's perspective – *How does this feel for me?*

People with bipolar disorder don't always have good insights into their symptoms. Treatment for acute mania may require involuntary detention in hospital.

> 'I can get so much done when I feel really energetic.'

> 'The tablets drag me down – I hate them.'

On the Horizon in Depression Pharmacotherapy

Although pharmacotherapy for depression is likely to continue as a major foundation approach, other treatments in the future may also involve new non-pharmacological treatments. The vagal nerve is involved in the communication of impulses into the cortical region of the brain. Vagal nerve stimulation is under investigation as a potential management option for depression. A small implantable electrical device is used to deliver electrical stimulation of the vagus, and this process has been observed to influence serotonergic and noradrenergic neurotransmission (these are two neurotransmitters known to be crucial to the activity of conventional antidepressant drugs). In early research, the antidepressant effect of vagal nerve stimulation has demonstrated comparable efficacy to that of medications for the treatment of depression, including treatment-resistant depression. Transcranial magnetic stimulation (TMS) is another non-drug approach that can be used for depression. A wire coil is used to allow electrical current to generate a powerful magnetic pulse, which passes through the scalp, stimulating the brain.

The dissociative anaesthetic drug ketamine has also recently been assessed as a treatment for major depressive episodes. People with treatment-resistant depression have been assessed for response to a single, subanaesthetic, intravenous dose of the drug, with impressive early response rates observed. Conventional antidepressants are thought to work by stimulating neurogenesis, eventually forming new synaptic connections over a period of weeks. Ketamine acts upon the glutamate system, increasing communication among existing neurons by creating new connections.

Other pharmacological advances in the treatment of depression are also expected. An antidepressant effect has been demonstrated with the cyclo-oxygenase inhibitor celecoxib, a drug conventionally used as an anti-inflammatory agent for people with arthritis. Celecoxib exerts inhibitory effects upon pro-inflammatory cytokines such as interleukin-6, with research confirming a link between reduction in serum IL-6 concentrations and decreased depression scores. Vilazodone is a recently approved antidepressant with a dual mechanism of action involving inhibition of serotonin transporters and partially agonist effects at serotonin-1a (5-HT1A) receptors. Another promising lead involves modulation of neuropeptides such as substance P and corticotrophin-releasing factor, and the intracellular messenger cyclic adenosine monophosphate (cAMP).

On the Horizon in Pharmacotherapy for Bipolar Affective Disorder

The development of new treatments for depression is likely to also be of benefit for the management of depressed mood in the context of bipolar disorder. Even so, a range of specific developments involving new applications of drugs already in use for other purposes show promise for application in various aspects of the bipolar disorder. Atypical antipsychotic drugs including olanzapine, quetiapine, risperidone, ziprasidone and others have now been investigated and demonstrated to be useful treatments for acute mania as well as effective mood stabilisers.

Modafinil is a drug originally used for management of excessive sleepiness due to narcolepsy or obstructive sleep apnoea. Recent research suggests that adjunctive modafinil may improve depressive symptoms in those with bipolar affective disorder. It is possible that glutamatergic abnormalities may contribute to the pathophysiology of bipolar disorder. Riluzole, a drug that modulates glutaminergic transmission, has benefits for people with bipolar depression, with early research suggesting that response to treatment may be rapid. The findings of a recent meta-analysis suggests that there is strong evidence to support the hypothesis that bipolar depression can respond to treatment with the adjunctive administration of omega-3 fatty acids, but there does not seem to be a role for use in attenuating mania.

There is a theoretical biochemical basis that suggests involvement of protein kinase C in the pathophysiology of bipolar affective disorder. Tamoxifen is a drug that has been used for the treatment of breast cancer and, because of its effects on protein kinase C, has been assessed as an adjunct to lithium for the treatment of acute mania. The combination of tamoxifen with lithium has been shown to be superior to lithium alone for the rapid reduction of manic symptoms.

Summary

Mood disorders cause severe symptoms for many who are affected, and pharmacotherapy is an important treatment modality in most cases. Both depression and mood elevation can cause significant morbidity and are associated with excess mortality. In each case it is critical that an appropriate treatment regimen should be carefully designed, initiated and monitored.

Discussion questions

1   What are the features of a major depressive episode?

2   What is the difference between a manic episode, a hypomanic episode and a mixed episode?

3   What are the standard pharmacotherapy options that are used as mood stabilisers?

Test yourself (answers at the back of the book)

1   In regard to the prevalence of mood disorders:

   A   the prevalence among men is higher than for women

   B   the prevalence among women is higher than for men

   C   the prevalence is not influenced by gender

   D   the prevalence of bipolar disorder is greater than that of major depression

2   Which of the following may contribute to the development of depressed mood?

   A   Thyroid disease

   B   Treatment with interferon

   C   Heavy use of alcohol

   D   All of the above

3   Which of the following is an example of a non-drug biological treatment used for management of mood disorders?

   A   Electroconvulsive therapy

   B   Anticonvulsant agents

   C   Cognitive behavioural therapy

   D   Psychoeducation

4   Which of the following drugs is metabolised by cytochrome P450 1A2?

   A   Risperidone

   B   Olanzapine

   C   Quetiapine

   D   Haloperidol

5   Which of the following drug classes would be regarded as least toxic in overdose?

   A   Tricyclic antidepressants

   B   Monoamine oxidase inhibitors

   C   Anticonvulsants

   D   Serotonin reuptake inhibitors

Useful websites

PubMed Health: *Major Depression* available at <www.ncbi.nlm.nih.gov/pubmedhealth/PMH0001941>

Sane Australia: *Bipolar Disorder* available at <www.sane.org/information/factsheets-podcasts/199-bipolar-disorder>

References

American Psychiatric Association. (2000). *Diagnostic and Statistical Manual of Mental Disorders*, 4th edn (DSM-IV). Washington, DC: American Psychiatric Association.

Cipriani A. et al. (2011). 'Comparative efficacy and acceptability of antimanic drugs in acute mania: a multiple-treatments meta-analysis' *Lancet* 378(9799): 1306–1315.

Rossi S. (2012). *Australian Medicines Handbook*. Chapter 18: Psychotropic drugs. Adelaide, South Australia: AMH Pty Ltd.

Sternbach H. (1991). 'The serotonin syndrome' *Am J Psychiatry* 148(6): 705–713.

Therapeutic Guidelines: Psychotropic – Version 6. Mood Disorders. Melbourne, Australia: Therapeutic Guidelines Limited, 2008.

Uher R. et al. (2009). 'Adverse reactions to antidepressants' *British Journal of Psychiatry* 195(3): 202–210.

Chapter 7

Anxiety Disorders

Chapter overview

This chapter covers the following topics:

* clinical features of major anxiety disorders

* discussion of the treatment of selected anxiety disorders

* relative merits of different treatment approaches for anxiety disorders

* important psychiatric comorbidities observed with anxiety disorders.

Chapter learning objectives

After reading this chapter, you should be able to:

* describe the key features of generalised anxiety disorder, panic disorder, post-traumatic stress disorder and obsessive-compulsive disorder

* outline drug therapy options that are available for the treatment of selected anxiety disorders

* discuss important adverse effects and drug interactions characteristically observed in association with the treatment of anxiety disorders.

Key terms

Anxiety and anxiety disorders
Generalised anxiety disorder
Obsessive-compulsive disorder
Panic disorder
Post-traumatic stress disorder

Introduction

The anxiety disorders are collectively the most common form of clinically significant mental disorders in developed economies, if not worldwide. Recent evidence suggests that the 12-month prevalence rate for anxiety disorders in Australia probably exceeds 14% of the adult population. Along with depression and substance-use disorders, the anxiety disorders are sometimes referred to as 'high prevalence' disorders, distinguishing them from less common important forms of psychiatric illness such as schizophrenia. Associated with very considerable disability and social isolation, anxiety disorders are characteristically associated with a high rate of comorbid depression and substance misuse. In many instances, people with anxiety disorders may present to their local doctor or pharmacy or to a hospital emergency department with complaints of physical symptoms such as chest pain, palpitations, headache, gastrointestinal upset, muscle aches or insomnia. Although short-term symptom-based treatments such as analgesia or hypnosedatives may be requested, if an anxiety disorder is present the symptoms are unlikely to resolve without some form of intervention directed at the underlying mental illness. In this chapter you will begin to understand the aspects of anxiety including both negative and positive aspects. For instance, anxiety is considered a great motivating force (such as responding to anxiety to be on time for an appointment). The chapter presents information related to pharmacological and non-pharmacological interventions for anxiety disorders and considers different antianxiety medications and drug interactions.

Anxiety is part of life, not always an illness

Although anxiety disorders are common and in many cases can be severe and disabling, it is important to acknowledge from the outset that not all anxiety is indicative of psychopathology. In fact, it is common for nearly everyone to be affected by anxiety at some times, and indeed it can be argued that normal anxiety serves appropriate motivational and protective purposes in everyday life. For example, many students who feel anxious about impending exams may be motivated to study and prepare, and thus the anxiety may help them to achieve better results. People who experience anxiety about potentially dangerous situations may adopt behaviours that are protective; for example, if a person is anxious about walking in a poorly lit and potentially dangerous part of town at night, they may adopt the protective behaviour of finding an alternative way home; and the smoker who is made aware of the considerable health risks associated with tobacco use may seek to quit, again fulfilling a protective function.

However, not all anxiety is functional. In some cases, the intensity of anxiety experienced by a person with an anxiety disorder may be so great as to cause intense distress and suffering on a daily basis. As a consequence of anxiety symptoms, the person affected may adopt maladaptive patterns of behaviour, such as self-medicating with drugs or alcohol. Some people with anxiety disorders become grossly avoidant, evading certain activities or contact with other people, refraining from being in public places (e.g. shopping centres or a workplace) to an extent that everyday living skills are affected. In anxiety disorders, the symptom of anxiety can become disconnected from any cause identifiable by the person affected.

State anxiety is an unpleasant emotional arousal in face of threatening demands or dangers. A cognitive appraisal of the threat is a requirement for the experience of state anxiety (Lazarus, 1991). Trait anxiety, on the other hand, reflects the existence of stable personality differences in the tendency to respond with state anxiety in anticipation of threatening situations. In Canada, Barrett and Armony explored the interaction between emotion and cognition and investigated whether trait anxiety alters cognitive performance and autonomic activity during an anticipatory anxiety task. Their results revealed that when 'anticipatory anxiety is increased, trait anxiety appeared to play a role in how participants performed tasks' (Barrett & Armony, 2006, p. 217). Clearly this result points to a psychological effect on performance.

A range of clinically significant anxiety disorders has been described, and is summarised in Table 7.1. In addition to these, anxiety disorders may occur secondary to a general medical condition (such as thyroid dysfunction, pheochromocytoma, hypoglycaemia, arrhythmias, some respiratory conditions and others). Similarly, **substance-induced anxiety disorder** is characterised by prominent anxiety attributable to the direct effects of substance intoxication or withdrawal (this may relate to recreational drug use, medications, or exposure to an environmental toxin).

Table 7.1: Abridged descriptions of some clinically important anxiety disorders listed in the *Diagnostic and Statistical Manual of Mental Disorders* (4th edn, Text Revision)

Panic disorder (with or without agoraphobia) involves recurrent panic attacks accompanied by persistent concern about these. A panic attack is said to occur when there is/are defined periods characterised by sudden intense apprehension, fearfulness, or terror, often associated with feelings of impending doom, which can be accompanied by a range of distressing physical symptoms. Agoraphobia is anxiety about and/or avoidance of situations/places that might be difficult to leave without embarrassment or excessive inconvenience.

Specific phobia occurs where there is reproducible and significant anxiety caused by exposure to a specific feared object or situation.

Social phobia is accompanied by significant anxiety provoked by exposure to certain types of social or performance situations.

Obsessive-compulsive disorder (OCD) is a mental illness where the affected individual may have obsessions (which cause marked anxiety or distress) and/or compulsions (which may relieve anxiety).

Post-traumatic stress disorder (PTSD) occurs after exposure to a traumatic event/s and may be characterised by reexperiencing of the event accompanied by symptoms of hyperarousal and/or avoidance of circumstances or cues that the affected individual associates with the event.

Generalised anxiety disorder (GAD) is characterised by at least six months of persistent and excessive anxiety and worry.

Anxiety can be a prominent feature associated with a range of other primary psychiatric disorders. For example, a person with a diagnosis of schizophrenia who experiences distressing delusions or command hallucinations may become anxious because of these. People with severe depression can develop ruminative anxiety or excessive worry about life events that may not have the same significance to them were they not affected by an affective illness. Some people with eating disorders become highly anxious in normal social situations where they are unable to restrict or modulate food consumption. In each case, the person affected has prominent anxiety as a feature of a mental illness, but is not necessarily affected by an anxiety disorder per se.

Non-pharmacological treatment of anxiety disorders

In addition to pharmacotherapy (which will be discussed in detail later), it is important to note that non-pharmacological treatments are very important strategies for the management of many anxiety disorders. Indeed, in some cases, non-drug treatment is regarded as the first-line approach for the management of anxiety disorders, and is used in preference to medications. Non-drug therapy has the advantage of being relatively free of the organically based side effects that are relatively commonly seen with medications. In addition, non-drug treatments for anxiety disorders (which are sometimes collectively referred to as 'psychological therapies') involve techniques that can be used by the individual on a recurrent basis, without necessarily being guided by a therapist during periods subsequent to the initial period of treatment. Usually delivered by a psychologist or psychiatrist or in some cases by specialised mental health nurses or social workers, this form of treatment can help a patient/client to develop a sense of self-mastery and a rewarding feeling that they themselves are making a substantial contribution to the treatment that results in the improvement of their overall well-being. In this way, learning effective psychological or behavioural techniques can help patients/ clients to increase self-esteem and diminish their perceived sense of reliance upon others for help. A range of non-pharmacological techniques can be used for this purpose, including the following:

✻ **Cognitive behavioural therapy (CBT)** can be used to alter the negative thoughts experienced by the patient/client, and is directed at influencing both behaviour and cognitions (the person's thoughts, perceptions and interpretations of their life experiences). Since excessive worrying is one of the main elements of anxiety, cognitive approaches can be very useful for the management of anxiety disorders. The first aim of CBT is to show the person how to modulate negative thoughts to allow them to gain insight into the ways in which thinking patterns contribute to their anxiety symptoms. The next steps focus upon strategies to allow the person with an anxiety disorder to change their thoughts and behaviours to lessen the frequency and severity of symptoms. CBT is particularly effective in reducing somatic complaints of people with anxiety disorders, and in doing so reducing headaches and muscular tension and lessening their subjective experience of distress.

* **Psychotherapy** can be employed to assist people with anxiety disorders to develop and maintain better coping mechanisms and to challenge and change unhelpful attitudes. Self-monitoring is advocated as the main component needed to allow this form of treatment to be effective. Patients/clients are helped to develop an awareness of situations that provoke anxiety, and to identify key overt behaviours, thoughts, images, emotions and physiological reactions associated with exacerbations of anxiety.

* **Psychoeducation** involves the skilled delivery of education about anxiety disorders and their treatment, and can be delivered by many different members of an interdisciplinary team. Providing patients/clients, partners and their families with education about the disorders themselves and the strategies that can be effective in their management can help to promote adherence to both psychological and pharmacological therapies. Other benefits can include a diminished experience of stigma, and promotion of general approaches that enhance the prospect of maintaining good mental health (e.g. healthy lifestyles, stress modulation, avoidance of substance abuse).

* Skilled practitioners deliver psychological treatment for people with anxiety disorder that is individually tailored to the person's unique circumstances, taking into account a wide range of factors such as severity and chronicity of symptoms, current life stressors, the individual's coping ability and style, barriers to processing information and learning new techniques. Individuals have differing specific personality traits, and variability in motivation to accept the challenges inherent in the use of these approaches, meaning that although general principles are helpful, an individual therapy technique should be designed and implemented for each person.

Conjecture continues about the relative merits of the combination of concurrent (or sequential) psychological and pharmacological treatment of anxiety disorders. At least superficially, the combination appears intuitively attractive, although the cases for and against this type of combined approach continue to be debated. Some proponents of psychological therapy argue that the influence of drugs may render psychological treatments less effective, perhaps by interfering with cognition and the ability of the person to receive, process and be motivated to act upon the elements of the sometimes complex information that is conveyed during psychological treatment. It has also been argued that some consumers are less likely to invest significant emotional energy and effort in learning skills for their own self-management if they are offered a simple solution in the form of medication to take. Sceptics point to the relatively modest margin of effects achieved by drugs relative to placebo, and to the high drop-out rates and incidence of adverse effects observed in clinical trials of pharmacotherapy for anxiety disorders, although these may reflect the somatic symptoms of the disorders that are being treated. On the other hand, proponents of drug treatment point out that pharmacotherapy may be quicker in onset, more effective in severe cases, and less involved and less expensive than an extended course of psychological treatment. Those who promote drug therapy also point out that placebo-controlled studies of pharmacological treatment are difficult, if not impossible, to achieve. Overall, the research results are mixed: some studies suggest benefit from combined psychological treatment and pharmacotherapy that is greater than that realised by either approach alone. Others suggest little or no synergism and, in fact, some research suggests that the use of one approach may even detract from the effectiveness of the other. This lack of clarity only serves to underscore the importance of individualising treatment to the unique requirements of each individual, and of being responsive to carefully obtained indicators of treatment efficacy in each case.

General principles of pharmacotherapy for anxiety disorders

Many of the same general principles that apply across all forms of pharmacotherapy apply equally in the context of the **pharmacological management** of anxiety disorders: the choice of drug and dosage should be judicious and should have regard to the individual characteristics of the patients/clients involved. Consideration of characteristics such as previous response to drug therapy, comorbid mental and medical disorders, and potentially interacting drugs already in the treatment regimen should be considered when planning and implementing treatment. Many of the drugs that are used in the pharmacotherapy of anxiety disorders will have other therapeutic applications in the management of other forms of mental and medical disorders, but it is important to bear in mind that the approach to dosage titration and duration of treatment may be specifically different in the context of anxiety disorders – this can create challenges with respect to adverse drug reactions and drug interactions. The acceptability of the proposed treatment to the consumer is very important, as this will critically influence adherence and consequently the overall likelihood of a successful treatment outcome. Where possible and within reason, it is important to accommodate the patient/client's preferences in this area, but at times it can be that the pharmacotherapy most sought by the patient/client may not necessarily be the most appropriate for long-term use.

One unique challenge in the pharmacotherapy of anxiety disorders is the high prevalence of associated comorbid substance disorders. People with serious anxiety disorders may in some cases use excessive alcohol, and may even inadvertently adopt a pattern of alcohol use as a form of self-treatment. This type of alcohol usage pattern may offer very temporary symptom relief but is never feasible as an enduring approach, and indeed the associated harm to physical and mental health can be considerable. With this in mind, it is often necessary to offer and coordinate psychological and pharmacological treatment for alcohol use disorders before or at the same time that specific drug treatment for anxiety disorders is implemented. As previously mentioned, anxiety disorders are frequently characterised by distressing somatic complaints including muscular tension, muscular skeletal pain, headache, gastrointestinal distress, tachycardia and insomnia or sleep difficulties. As the first point of contact with medical care for most patients/clients with anxiety disorders is in the primary care setting, it is imperative that effective communication between different health care sectors is emphasised to ensure that the treating clinicians involved are all aware of the previous investigations and treatments, and the intentions for future plans. Notwithstanding all of this, it is quite common for those with severe anxiety disorders to fall into patterns of strong analgesic and hypnosedative use that can be counterproductive, leading to potential for drug abuse, dependence and withdrawal. This pattern of drug use can be especially dangerous in the context of comorbid alcohol use.

Another problem to address in the management of anxiety disorders is the need for both clinicians and consumers to recognise and discern the relative place for different types of pharmacotherapy. The ready availability of drugs with potent antianxiety effects appears to offer benefits for those affected, but caution is required. The benzodiazepine class of drugs (e.g. diazepam, oxazepam, lorazepam, alprazolam) all commonly produce rapid, reliable and relatively safe anxiolytic effects, but these agents have potential drawbacks that need to be considered. All benzodiazepines have the potential for abuse, dependence, tolerance and withdrawal, and in each case these problems can have both physiological and psychological adverse effects. The unpleasant physical and psychological effects that are experienced by many people during benzodiazepine withdrawal can make it very difficult for a consumer to discontinue treatment, even if they express a strong desire to do so. In the most severe manifestations of withdrawal, serious medical complications (e.g. withdrawal seizures) can occur. Consumers may visit several prescribers to access supply ('doctor shopping') and may not necessarily accurately or completely report the extent, dosage or duration of usage to all clinicians involved in their care.

It is also important to point out that the benzodiazepines do nothing to address the underlying psychopathology of anxiety disorders, but rather they simply address some readily identifiable symptoms through temporary alleviation of anxious mood or insomnia.

When the effects of these drugs wear off, the symptoms return and more benzodiazepine is required. Furthermore, because of the phenomena of tolerance and tachyphylaxis (an increased need for greater doses to achieve the same effects as time goes by), it is common to observe dose escalation and the continuation of treatment with benzodiazepines for periods longer than was initially intended. It is important that if benzodiazepines are to be used for the temporary and short-term management of anxiety symptoms, all members of the treating team should clearly understand the predetermined objectives of treatment, and consistently communicate these to the consumer and other relevant people such as carers and family where appropriate. One way to communicate this message to patients/clients is to use an analogy based in another form of treatment: 'If you were in a car crash and broke your leg, we could give you morphine to kill the pain, but it wouldn't heal the bone fracture – you'd need surgery and a plaster cast for that.'

Long half-life agents such as clonazepam and diazepam have the potential to cause cumulative toxicity, especially in the elderly. On the other hand, short-acting, rapid-onset agents such as alprazolam can reinforce addictive behaviours (see below). The hazards of injudicious use of benzodiazepines for the symptomatic management of an anxiety disorder are illustrated in Figure 7.1.

Figure 7.1: Cycle of problems resulting from injudicious use of benzodiazepines

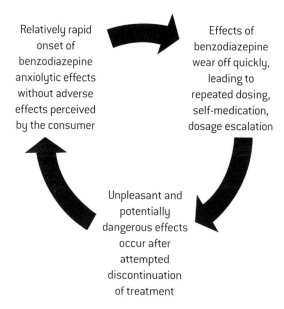

Relatively rapid onset of benzodiazepine anxiolytic effects without adverse effects perceived by the consumer

Effects of benzodiazepine wear off quickly, leading to repeated dosing, self-medication, dosage escalation

Unpleasant and potentially dangerous effects occur after attempted discontinuation of treatment

For the aforementioned reasons, treatment guidelines and psychiatric consensus have evolved to a point where extended symptom-based interventions for anxiety disorders using benzodiazepines are no longer routinely recommended. Management of the underlying disorder with targeted psychological and pharmacotherapy interventions is routinely used in contemporary practice.

On balance, a comprehensive and integrated approach to the diagnosis and management of anxiety disorders is now recommended, and needs to be tailored to the needs of the individual consumer. The important elements of this approach are outlined in Table 7.2.

Table 7.2: Principles of diagnosis and management of anxiety disorders

Accurate diagnosis and assessment

Accurate history to define nature, context, scope and duration of symptoms

Thorough physical work-up, laboratory investigations and imaging to exclude possible medical and/or comorbid psychiatric disorders that may account for symptoms

Comprehensive assessment and screening in relation to use of alcohol, tobacco, caffeine and recreation drugs

(Continued)

Table 7.2: Principles of diagnosis and management of anxiety disorders (*Continued*)

Specific medical interventions
Use of non-pharmacological interventions: cognitive behavioural therapy (CBT), psychotherapy
Psychoeducation
Reduction/cessation of tobacco and caffeine intake
Reduction/cessation of alcohol and other drug intake
Lifestyle and complementary interventions such as yoga, meditation, aromatherapy
Family/relationship/situational interventions
Pharmacotherapy: • brief use of symptomatic interventions to address key symptoms • targeted pharmacotherapy with appropriate drug selection and dosage tailored to individual underlying anxiety disorder
Address comorbid substance disorders and medical complications that may result from substance abuse or dependence.

Ask yourself!

1   What are the most commonly diagnosed anxiety disorders?

2   How does anxiety that is experienced as a symptom of an anxiety disorder differ from anxiety that is experienced commonly by many people as a part of their everyday lives?

3   Why is considerable caution needed when drugs such as benzodiazepines are used to treat anxiety?

Commonly encountered anxiety disorders and their treatment

In common with other forms of mental disorders, each of the major forms of anxiety disorder have discrete diagnostic criteria, regularly encountered comorbidities and specific pharmacotherapy approaches that have been supported by evidence from clinical trials.

Generalised anxiety disorder

Generalised anxiety disorder (GAD) is characterised by excessive anxiety or worrying that is present on more days than not, extending over a period of six months or more. People with GAD become excessively anxious about a range of specific events or activities, and find it difficult or impossible to control this. To satisfy the most commonly used diagnostic criteria, the anxiety needs to be accompanied by at least three of a group of additional symptoms: restlessness, easy fatigability, difficulty with concentration, irritability, muscle tension, or sleep disturbance. GAD can be diagnosed only if the anxiety is not attributable to the effects of another medical or psychiatric disorder, or the effects of a substance. People with GAD find their symptoms distressing, and will generally have resultant impairment in social or occupational functioning. In the experience of anxiety for people with GAD, the extent of anxiety is usually grossly disproportionate to the trigger event or circumstance.

Most guidelines and consensus statements will state that the first-line treatment options for the management of GAD should focus on non-pharmacological approaches such as psychoeducation, relaxation techniques and positive coping skills, supplemented with ongoing supportive psychotherapy or CBT.

During periods of severe or acute exacerbations the symptoms of GAD may become very distressing for the patient/client and indeed for those around them. One approach to the management of acute symptom exacerbations in GAD is to treat with a long-acting benzodiazepine such as diazepam, 5–15 mg daily in divided doses. Other benzodiazepines such as lorazepam, oxazepam or clonazepam could also be used for this purpose. In view of the high potential for dependence it is important to limit the use of benzodiazepines to a course of therapy, planned to continue for a period of no longer than two or three weeks followed by a downward titration of the dose with the aim of discontinuing treatment after about six weeks. Short-acting, rapid-onset drugs such as alprazolam should probably be avoided. The short-term use of benzodiazepine anxiolytics may prove to be helpful during the initial phase of implementation of other, long-term treatment strategies (see below).

Treatment for GAD

As benzodiazepine treatment is only useful for short-term management of severe symptoms, it is important that there should be consideration of a long-term treatment intervention for all patients/clients with GAD. These pharmacotherapies are generally used as supplements to non-drug treatments, and most commonly involve the use of medications that are generally referred to as antidepressants. In the context of anxiety disorders, including GAD, some antidepressants are used to address the underlying anxiety disorder and can produce a therapeutic benefit that is produced independently of a mood-elevating effect. Even so, many patients/clients are affected by comorbid anxiety and depression, and thus the antidepressant effects can be beneficial in their own right. The most commonly used antidepressant medications in the management of GAD are the selective serotonin reuptake inhibitors (SSRIs), serotonin/noradrenaline reuptake inhibitors (SNRIs) and some tricyclic antidepressants (TCAs). Another alternative to consider is the antidepressant anxiolytic agent, buspirone.

It is important to note that the anxiolytic onset of action of antidepressant medications in the treatment of GAD usually takes several days to become noticeable, and may not be completely developed until two to four weeks of treatment. In fact, during the initial treatment period, some patients/clients with GAD and other anxiety disorders actually experience a transient exacerbation of anxiety symptoms, meaning that short-term use of benzodiazepines may be helpful to address these symptoms during treatment initiation.

Further details of the clinical aspects of drug therapy for GAD are provided in Table 7.3.

Table 7.3: Clinical aspects of drug therapy for GAD

Benzodiazepines
Use long-acting agents at a modest dose for a defined period of time with a plan for the process of discontinuation – avoid alprazolam.
Be aware of potential for dependence, abuse and diversion.
May be helpful during the initiation of other treatments (below).
Do not address underlying psychopathology.
May increase risk of falls, fractures, injuries and incontinence, especially among the elderly.
Can impair ability to drive or operate machinery safely.

SSRI antidepressants

Commence at a modest dose, all drugs in this class probably equally effective for GAD:

- escitalopram – start at 5 mg daily, usually effective at 10 mg daily, max 20 mg daily
- citalopram – start at 10 mg daily, usually effective at 20 mg daily, max 40 mg daily
- paroxetine – start at 10 mg daily, usually effective at 20 mg daily, max 50 mg daily
- sertraline – start at 25 mg daily, usually effective at 50 mg daily, max 200 mg daily
- fluvoxamine – start at 50 mg daily, usually effective at 100 mg daily, max 200 mg daily.

May cause transient increase in anxiety symptoms initially.

Potential adverse effects may be misinterpreted as somatic complaints – gastrointestinal upset, headache, etc.

Potential for drug interactions (refer to discussion in section dealing with treatment of depression).

SNRI antidepressants

Commence at a modest dose, all drugs in this class probably equally effective for GAD:

- duloxetine – start at 30 mg daily, usually effective at 60 mg daily
- desvenlafaxine – start at 50 mg daily, max 100 mg daily
- venlafaxine – start at 75 mg daily, usually effective at 150 mg daily.

May cause transient increase in anxiety symptoms initially.

Potential adverse effects may be misinterpreted as somatic complaints – gastrointestinal upset, headache, etc.

Can cause elevation in systolic blood pressure, reduce dose in elderly or those with renal impairment.

Buspirone

Start at 5 mg twice to three times daily, usually effective at 30 mg daily, max 60 mg daily.

Not cross-reactive with benzodiazepines – will not prevent a benzodiazepine withdrawal syndrome.

Onset of optimal effect may take several weeks – no antidepressant properties.

Panic disorder

Panic disorder is a relatively common form of anxiety disorder, with a lifetime prevalence rate cited at up to 2%. Agoraphobia is often encountered among people with panic disorder: important clinical features of this disorder are summarised in Table 7.4.

Table 7.4: Clinical features of panic disorder

Panic disorder is characterised by recurrent panic attacks and persistent concern about further attacks and the implications of these.

Diagnostic features of a panic attack (adapted from the DSM-IV-TR)

A panic attack involves the development of symptoms where the person experiences a discrete period of intense fear or discomfort, with four or more of the following symptoms developing abruptly and peaking within 10 minutes:

- palpitations, pounding heart, or accelerated heart rate
- sweating
- trembling or shaking
- sensations of shortness of breath or smothering
- feeling of choking
- chest pain or discomfort
- nausea or abdominal distress
- feeling dizzy, unsteady, lightheaded, or faint
- derealisation (feelings of unreality) or depersonalisation (being detached from oneself)
- fear of losing control or going crazy
- fear of dying
- paresthesias (numbness or tingling sensations)
- chills or hot flushes.

Up to 80% of people with panic disorder will develop **agoraphobia,** involving anxiety about being in places or situations from which escape might be difficult (or embarrassing), or where help may not be available. This usually leads to avoidance of specific situations that cause apprehension. This avoidant behaviour may cause social or occupational disability, and may interfere with the routine activities of daily living.

Source: American Psychiatric Association (2000)

The key diagnostic feature of panic disorder is the finding of recurrent, unexpected panic attacks (refer to Table 7.4), accompanied by a period of at least one month of persistent apprehension about the possibility of further attacks, worrying about what the panic attacks might mean, and/or significant behavioural changes that arise directly from the attacks. To be able to diagnose panic disorder, other feasible explanations need to be excluded; these include the effects of a substance (including medicinal and illicit drugs), general medical conditions, or the effects of another psychiatric condition. The person experiencing the panic attacks does not necessarily identify a situational cue. Although the frequency of panic attacks can vary, many of those affected have attacks at least once a week, sometimes more. Those affected are generally apprehensive that the symptoms that they are experiencing actually signify the presence of a serious but undiagnosed illness. Indeed, some medical conditions such as hyperthyroidism, irritable bowel syndrome and mitral valve prolapse do appear to be more common among those with panic disorder.

Treatment for panic disorder

Cognitive behavioural therapy (CBT) is regarded as the treatment of first choice for panic disorder. One approach involves exposure to situations that are known to induce symptoms, paired with specific techniques for controlling symptoms and reattribution of symptoms to benign causes.

First-line drug therapy for panic disorder involves the use of SSRIs or venlafaxine, commencing at a modest dose and with slow upward titration in a fashion similar to that used for generalised anxiety disorder (refer Table 7.3). Short-term treatment with benzodiazepines during the initial period of other pharmacotherapy may assist in managing the periods of transiently increased anxiety symptoms that are commonly observed at the outset of pharmacotherapy, although caution is required because of the potential for dependence and abuse.

Alternative pharmacotherapy that might be considered if first-line approaches do not work include drugs such as tricyclic antidepressants (e.g. imipramine) or non-selective monoamine oxidase inhibitors (MAOIs) such as phenelzine. These agents are more frequently associated with adverse effects such as postural hypotension and anticholinergic effects such as dry mouth, blurred vision, cognitive impairment, constipation and tachycardia. In the case of the MAOIs, there is potential for serious drug interactions and these agents should be reserved for situations where other treatment options cannot be used. The selective MAOI moclobemide is a much safer alternative that can also be considered as a pharmacotherapy option of for panic disorder.

Drug treatment for panic disorder will usually need to continue for a period of up to a year. Treatment is usually combined with non-drug treatment approaches. Once a sustained response to pharmacotherapy has been achieved, drug treatment should be gradually withdrawn, with the dose reduced relatively slowly. If benzodiazepines have been prescribed for an extended period of time, it is important to gently decrease the dosage, if possible using a long half-life agent, so that the likelihood of a benzodiazepine withdrawal reaction can be minimised. Serious benzodiazepine reactions can be very dangerous, and carry a risk of withdrawal seizures (refer to Chapter 9 dealing with substance use disorders). In milder cases, benzodiazepine withdrawal is associated with increased anxiety symptoms, agitation and sleep disturbances. A characteristic discontinuation syndrome is also sometimes observed when SSRI treatment is withdrawn abruptly, particularly after extended treatment or with high doses. Although not dangerous, the syndrome can be very unpleasant and is often manifested through symptoms such as dizziness, nausea, paraesthesia, anxiety, agitation, tremor, sweating, confusion, electric shock–like sensations (sometimes referred to as Lhermitte's sign). Antidepressant discontinuation syndromes are most likely to be observed with drugs that have a relatively short half-life and/ or no active metabolites (e.g. paroxetine, venlafaxine).

JENNY'S STORY

Jenny, a 22-year-old woman, was assessed in an outpatient psychiatry clinic after referral by her local GP. A full-time university student in her second year of study towards an arts degree, she had visited her local doctor because she was becoming increasingly disabled by frequent 'hyperventilation attacks'. During the previous six months she found that she was constantly on edge and worrying about these episodes, to the extent that her previously good academic performance had deteriorated. She also reported that she had virtually stopped socialising with friends, and rarely left her flat except to go to university or to attend to errands such as shopping or banking. Throughout the initial interview, she repeatedly stated, 'I just want to know what's wrong with me'. On specific inquiry, she vividly described the distressing nature of the 'hyperventilation attacks' that were now occurring two or three times a week. During the attacks she would suffer from a choking sensation, and would begin to breathe rapidly. After a short time she would become increasingly breathless, dizzy and tremulous. She noticed that her 'heart was pounding rapidly in her chest', and that she felt nauseous. In addition to these physical symptoms, Jenny reported that she felt a sense of impending death, and was worried that she could 'stop breathing' or 'have a heart attack'.

Treatment with sertraline was commenced at a dose of 50 mg daily. On the instructions of her psychiatrist she increased the dose in a step-wise fashion over the next two weeks, attaining the target dose of 200 mg daily several days before her next review in the clinic. At this time she reported no benefit from treatment, claiming that, if anything, she now felt even more anxious and 'uptight'. Sertraline was discontinued that day, and her psychiatrist instructed her to wait for five days before commencing venlafaxine ER 75 mg daily.

Ask yourself!

If you were involved with caring for Jenny:

1   What factors might have contributed to the treatment failure with sertraline?
2   Would offering treatment with a benzodiazepine such as oxazepam have helped Jenny?
3   What other treatments should be offered to Jenny?

From the consumer's perspective – *How does this feel for me?*

Panic disorder can be a very frightening and distressing condition for those affected, and often the consumer will be worried about the possibility of a serious medical illness.

Consumers may need considerable coaching and advice to encourage them to accept non-drug treatment and to persist with pharmacotherapy.

'How long am I going to have to spend time talking about how I'm feeling?'

'The pills just make me more jittery.'

'If I have a few drinks I feel more relaxed and less worried about things.'

Post-traumatic stress disorder

Post-traumatic stress disorder (PTSD) is a serious anxiety disorder that develops after exposure to an extremely traumatic stressful event or circumstance. The type of trauma that might typically precede PTSD would involve actual or threatened death or serious injury, or witnessing a horrendous event that could involve death or injury (or the threat of these) for another person. To be consistent with the diagnostic criteria for PTSD, the person's response to the event must involve intense fear, helplessness, or horror. If exposure to this type of event does cause a person to develop PTSD, a characteristic suite of symptoms would be observed (refer to Table 7.5). Many types of traumatic events can give rise to PTSD, but common examples include warfare, combat, violent crime, torture and natural disasters such as bushfires or earthquakes. Childhood sexual abuse often forms the basis for PTSD reported in adulthood.

Table 7.5: Characteristic symptoms of PTSD

After exposure to a traumatic event a person with PTSD will experience characteristic symptoms.

The traumatic event is persistently re-experienced in one (or more) of several ways:

- recurrent and intrusive distressing recollections of the event (mental images, thoughts)
- recurrent distressing dreams of the event
- acting or feeling as though the event were recurring (may include hallucinations of flashbacks)
- intense psychological distress at exposure to cues that evoke an aspect of the traumatic event
- physiological reactions after exposure to cues that evoke the traumatic event.

People with PTSD often adopt behaviours that are consistent with persistent avoidance of stimuli that they associate with the traumatic event, and experience numbing of general responsiveness that was not present before the trauma. These features can include:

- efforts to avoid thoughts, feelings, or conversations associated with the trauma
- behaviours directed at avoiding activities, places, or people that cause recollections of the trauma
- inability to recall an important aspect of the trauma
- markedly diminished interest or participation in significant activities
- experiencing a feeling of detachment or estrangement from others
- restricted range of affect
- sense of a foreshortened future.

PTSD is also associated with persistent symptoms of increased hyperarousal, characterised by two or more of features such as:

- difficulty falling or staying asleep

- irritability and/or outbursts of anger

- difficulty with concentration

- markedly increased vigilance

- exaggerated startle response.

To satisfy diagnostic criteria, symptoms must be present for at least one month and must be associated with clinically significant distress or impairment in social, occupational or other key areas of functional capacity.

Source: Adapted from DSM-IV-TR, American Psychiatric Association (2000)

Symptoms of PTSD often very considerably affect the carers, partners and families of those affected. Comorbid substance abuse, including that involving alcohol, recreational drugs and prescribed medications, is very common. Difficulties with interpersonal relationships, occupational capacity and family dynamics are frequently encountered, and can compromise support systems that would otherwise be beneficial.

Treatment of PTSD

In common with many forms of anxiety disorder, current consensus suggests that the most appropriate first-line therapy should be non-pharmacological; specifically, the use of specialised CBT techniques including strategies such as graded exposure therapy involving desensitisation to the trauma is most commonly used. Despite this, many people with PTSD require adjunctive drug treatment. On the basis of currently available evidence and approvals from regulatory agencies such as the Australian Therapeutic Goods Administration (TGA) and the US Food and Drug Administration (FDA), the SSRIs are now accepted as first-line drug treatment for PTSD. Other antidepressants such as mirtazapine and venlafaxine have also been used with success as treatment for PTSD. In particular, mirtazapine appears to be effective for mitigating PTSD-related sleep disturbance, but this agent should be reserved for those not achieving an adequate response to SSRIs, as significant weight gain and metabolic disturbances including hyperglycaemia and hyperlipidaemia can be problematic.

For PTSD where anger, aggression, irritability, impulse control and mood instability are prominent features, the addition of an anticonvulsant mood stabiliser drug such as valproate or carbamazepine can prove helpful. A number of other drugs may also be of assistance where sleep disturbance and nightmares are prominent. Zopiclone can improve sleep quality but caution is needed because of the risk of dependency. Other treatments that have been shown to decrease nightmares and improve sleep include topiramate (which can also have the added benefit of reducing alcohol use and preventing weight gain secondary to other psychotropic drugs), prazosin, and propranolol. Atypical antipsychotics (e.g. quetiapine or olanzapine) have been used for the management of severe hyperarousal or agitation, particularly where intrusive symptoms have a delusory or hallucinatory nature. Long-term treatment with antipsychotics for PTSD should be avoided in view of the potential for side effects including weight gain, metabolic disturbances and movement disorders.

One area likely to become an increased focus of attention will be the use of medications in the period soon after exposure to trauma, with the aim of reducing the likelihood that those exposed will go on to develop PTSD. It is thought that future approaches will be designed to address biological changes that occur in the brain after exposure to trauma. The human response involves central and peripheral nervous systems, the endocrine system, and the immunological system.

During stress, corticotropin releasing factor is released and there are other neurochemical responses, but after the stress has passed, recovery of normal function is thought to be mediated through the effects of glucocorticoids, endogenous opioids and other hormonal factors. It is possible that future preventative drug therapy strategies will be based on corticotropin releasing factor antagonists, glucocorticoids, selective opioids agonists and other agents.

JEFF'S STORY

Jeff is a 63-year-old Vietnam veteran who was admitted to hospital for the assessment and management of symptoms of post-traumatic stress disorder (PTSD), which he has had for many years. Over the last month he had become increasingly irritable and aggressive. His usually heavy alcohol consumption had increased even more; he was sleeping poorly and he described escalating depression. The recipient of a full war-service pension, he had not been employed during the previous five years, but normally occupied himself with home-making duties. During his war service he had served as a forward scout in the infantry. His battalion had been involved in heavy fighting with extensive casualties, and several of his close friends had been severely injured. He had witnessed the death of one member of his company who was fatally injured after standing on a land mine. On many occasions he was exposed to the corpses of enemy soldiers and, in a number of instances, those of civilian villagers.

At the time of assessment he was tremulous and unkempt, and smelled strongly of alcohol. He was irritable and labile, crying openly at several points during the interview. He described frequent horrific nightmares with content relating to his war service, and reported a recent average of about four hours interrupted sleep each night. He had recently stopped shopping for the family's groceries, as he found that visiting the shopping centre was too intimidating. His exaggerated startle response was clearly demonstrated when a member of staff unexpectedly knocked on the door of the consultation room during the interview. He reported heavy use of cannabis and alcohol in the weeks leading up to his admission, drinking as much as a bottle of vodka daily during some weeks. In addition to this, he was smoking 50 cigarettes a day since his return from Vietnam. He was admitted as a voluntary patient and observed over the course of the next week. He went home for weekend leave after several days as an inpatient, but returned from leave clearly intoxicated, with facial injuries that he had sustained during a fight at the local hotel.

Ask yourself!

If you were caring for Jeff:

1 Which key features of PTSD are clearly present here?

2 What drugs would be the most likely to provide benefit for Jeff's PTSD symptoms?

3 What action is required with respect to Jeff's pattern of alcohol use?

Care Plan

The following is an example care plan for the patient/client presented in this chapter. The areas of daily living that are considered include bio-psycho-social factors and the plan is mapped out using the nursing process (Assessment; Planning; Implementation; Evaluation). Remember: the success is in the detail, so be specific about *who, when and what* in the collaborative plan; never include someone in the plan if they were not consulted in the planning process; and always work within a recovery-orientated framework (refer to Chapter 1).

Date: 5 August 2012

Client's name: Jeff

Case manager (TBA): Primary care nurse and treating doctor located at the hospital

Areas of daily living	Assessment of current situation	Goal	Plan (undertaken with patient/client)	Implementation	Who is responsible? (Include only those who have been consulted in the planning process)	Evaluation/ review date
Mental health	PTSD with labile mood.	Admitted for assessment and management of PTSD.	Pathology examinations Physical examination Review mental state	Mental state examination. Blood test for thyroid function test, full blood examination, etc. Obtain baseline data: blood pressure, waist measurements, weight, temperature, pulse rate, respirations, oral assessment to assess any oral health issues that may need attention, chest x-ray.	Primary care nurse and treating doctor.	8/8/12
Social	Unemployed, receives war pension.	No issues identified.	N/A	N/A	N/A	N/A
Biological	Poor sleep pattern due to nightmares.	Re-establish sleep pattern.	Refer to therapist to work with Jeff on PTSD symptoms such as re-experiencing, nightmares, hyper vigilance, etc.	Initiate medication to assist with sleeping problems. Engage Jeff in outpatient therapy. Explore possible enrolment in inpatient rehabilitation programs for war veterans.	Treating doctor Primary nurse and treating doctor and review with social worker.	8/8/12

Environmental	More isolated recently, avoids crowds. Stays home more.	Jeff would like to be able to shop for the family as he did before.	Discuss with Jeff his goals for accessing more support. Engage regular outpatient support for Jeff and his family.	Engage Jeff with a case manager/therapist to work with on an outpatient basis to address anxiety issues, to work with the family, and coordinate care.	Primary nurse and treating doctor.	8/8/12
Substance using behaviours	Recent heavy use of alcohol and cannabis. Smokes 50 cigarettes per day.	Reduce or eliminate substance use.	Identify in collaboration with Jeff physical and dental issues. Manage withdrawal symptoms. Engage Jeff in outpatient drug and alcohol rehabilitation.	Oral health assessment Physical examination (refer above) Review medications to assist with withdrawal symptoms. Review medications to assist with reduction or elimination of substance use. Work with Jeff regarding the option of nicotine patches with other smoking cessation interventions such as therapy (using motivational interviewing).	Primary nurse Primary nurse and treating doctor Primary nurse and treating doctor Primary nurse and treating doctor The ward team	8/8/12
Risk behaviours	In past month Jeff has become more aggressive and combative.	Harm minimisation	With Jeff, identify triggers for aggression.	Refer for psychotherapy in either group or one-to-one setting for veterans.	Primary nurse and treating doctor and allied health team located at the hospital	8/8/12

From the consumer's perspective – *How does this feel for me?*

People with PTSD often experience increased anger, irritability and frustration. Avoidant behaviour may interfere with a consumer's capacity to engage with treatment for PTSD.

'I'm sick of people telling me what is good for me – how would they know?'

'Sometimes I just feel like I'm going to explode.'

'I need something to help me sleep, to take the edge off.'

'Why bother with me? I'll be dead soon and they'll all be better off without me.'

Obsessive-compulsive disorder

Obsessive-compulsive disorder (OCD) is a major anxiety disorder that is characterised by the primary symptoms of recurrent obsessions or compulsions of sufficient severity to become time-consuming, or to cause marked distress or impairment (refer to Table 7.6). It is of interest that people with OCD recognise that the obsessions/compulsions are excessive or unreasonable. Furthermore, in keeping with other anxiety disorders, to diagnose OCD it is necessary to establish that the symptoms are not potentially attributable to the effects of a substance or comorbid medical condition.

Table 7.6: Features of OCD

People with OCD will have obsessions and compulsions.

Obsessions

- Persistent thoughts, impulses, or images that the person perceives to be intrusive/inappropriate
- Cause marked anxiety or distress
- Common obsessions include:
  - those centred on contamination themes (e.g. being unclean, dirty)
  - repeated doubts (e.g. is the door locked, are appliances turned off?)
  - a need to specifically order objects (e.g. a need for symmetrical arrangements).

In response to obsessions the person attempts to ignore or suppress such thoughts or impulses, or to neutralise them with a corresponding thought or action (i.e. a compulsion).

- Repetitive behaviours (e.g. hand-washing, ordering, checking)

- Repetitive mental acts (e.g. praying, counting, repeating words silently)

- Do not to provide pleasure or gratification

- By definition, clearly excessive or are not connected in a realistic way with what they are designed to neutralise or prevent

- Common examples include washing and cleaning, counting, checking, ordering objects

Source: Adapted from DSM-IV-TR, American Psychiatric Association (2000)

Treatment of OCD

Although non–drug therapy may be used for OCD, drug treatment is usually required. Pharmacotherapy for OCD is based on the use of SSRI antidepressant drugs. The recommended approach is to use standard starting doses that are similar to those used for other anxiety disorders, but it is common for the maintenance dose for OCD to be at the upper limit of the approved dosage range (e.g. 80 mg daily of fluoxetine, up to 300 mg daily of fluvoxamine). Alternatives to SSRIs include high-dose venlafaxine, or the tricyclic antidepressant clomipramine (again, maintenance doses of up to 250 mg daily may be required). At the high doses that are used for OCD, treatment tolerability is often poor, with pronounced adverse effects such as gastrointestinal upset and sexual dysfunction.

Ask yourself!

1   Some religions and personal belief systems involve ritualistic acts – how does this differ from OCD?

2   Why do many patients/clients fail to achieve a robust trial of pharmacotherapy for OCD?

JILL'S STORY

Jill, a 34-year-old woman, was referred by her GP for assessment and possible treatment by a consultant psychiatrist at a local hospital. The history of the presenting complaint included a visit from Jill and her spouse to the GP. During that consultation Jill's husband had complained that she was 'going mad' and 'needed to get help'.

During the initial consultation Jill admitted that she had begun to be disturbed by her thoughts and feelings during the last two years, since the birth of her first child. On specific inquiry, she reported that she worried constantly about the state of cleanliness of her home, and spends many hours each week washing and scrubbing floors, windows and other surfaces so that they would be clean enough. On any given day she would wash and disinfect the surface of floors up to five times, often recommencing less than an hour after completing the task previously. Although she could recognise that it was very unlikely that the floor would have become dirty during the short time since it was last washed, she reported that she 'just *had* to wash it again, just to be sure'. When asked what she thought might happen if she cleaned the house less often, she replied that she felt that her young son would probably catch an infectious disease and become very ill.

Her behaviour at home had now reached a point where there was considerable marital disharmony. She would devote so many hours each week to her cleaning rituals that other everyday tasks (e.g. shopping, food preparation) were often neglected. Social activities had all but ceased, and she had recently started staying up late at night to continue cleaning. During a recent weekend away, she had felt tense, anxious and upset that the house would be so dirty upon her return, and she spent most of her time worrying about the consequences that this might have for her family. The distress caused by her constant worrying had left her feeling miserable, and of recent times she had noticed a downturn in her appetite and sleep quality. She did say that she would like to have another baby 'if she felt well again'.

Ask yourself!

As a health care worker involved with caring for Jill:

1   What type of medication might be offered to Jill? Can you anticipate problematic side effects that might occur?

2   What will need to be considered if Jill were found to be pregnant again?

From the consumer's perspective – *How does this feel for me?*

Consumers with severe OCD can find that it completely takes over their life.

'I just don't have enough time in the day to do all the things I feel I need to.'

'The side effects of the medications are almost worse than the crazy thoughts.'

On the Horizon in Pharmacotherapy for Anxiety Disorders

Glutamate is an excitatory neurotransmitter in the central nervous system. One of the major glutamate receptors is the N-methyl-D-aspartate (NMDA) receptor group, which is a potential target for development of drug therapy for anxiety states. One compound that has attracted attention is D-cycloserine, which was originally developed as an antibiotic. D-cycloserine is a partial NMDA receptor agonist. The drug does not directly reduce anxiety, but seems to increase the effectiveness of non-pharmacological (psychological) treatments. D-cycloserine augmentation appears to show particular promise in the management of OCD and PTSD.

A variety of anticonvulsant drugs appear to show promise for some anxiety disorders. Gabapentin and pregabalin may eventually find clinical applications in the management of panic disorder and generalised anxiety disorder. PTSD appears to be responsive to the anticonvulsant drug topiramate, which has the added benefit of helping reduce alcohol consumption.

With respect to PTSD, one area likely to become important will be the use of targeted treatment in the period immediately after trauma, aiming to reduce the likelihood of PTSD developing or reducing severity of symptoms. The most important contributors to the stress response are the hypothalamic-pituitary-adrenocortical system and the locus coeruleus/norepinephrine-sympathetic system, both activated by corticotropin releasing factor. During stress, corticotropin releasing factor rapidly mobilises the hypothalamic-pituitary-adrenocortical system and locus coeruleus/norepinephrine-sympathetic mechanisms, but after the stress is past recovery of normal function is thought to be mediated through the effects of glucocorticoids and endogenous opioid-like compounds. Those most likely to develop PTSD are the people who produce the most intense hypothalamic-pituitary-adrenocortical system and/or locus coeruleus/norepinephrine-sympathetic activation, and it is possible that future preventative drug treatments will be based on corticotropin releasing factor antagonists, glucocorticoids, or opioid agonists. There is already some evidence to suggest that corticosteroids may exert a protective effect against the development of PTSD.

Summary

The anxiety disorders encompass a range of disabling mental illnesses that are often accompanied by comorbid depression and substance use disorders. Although medications are not necessarily regarded as first-line treatments for anxiety disorders, the refractory nature of symptoms means that it is quite common for drug therapy to be required. All clinicians involved with the management of people with anxiety disorders need to understand the target symptoms, and the relative merits of the different types of pharmacotherapy that can be used.

Discussion questions

1   What differentiates the normal life experience of anxiety from an anxiety disorder?

2   What are the potential drawbacks associated with the symptomatic management of anxiety with drugs such as benzodiazepines?

3   In what ways might drug treatment interact with other forms of therapy for anxiety disorders?

Test yourself (answers at the back of the book)

1   Which of the following anxiety disorders often involves flashbacks and nightmares?

    A   Generalised anxiety disorder

    B   Panic disorder

    C   Post-traumatic stress disorder

    D   Social phobia

2   Which of the following statements are true with respect to the management of anxiety disorders?

    A   Drug treatment is never useful.

    B   Drug treatment is always regarded as the first-line option.

    C   Psychological treatments can be very helpful.

    D   Psychological treatments never work.

3   Which of the following agents is most likely to create a risk of drug dependence if used for treatment of generalised anxiety disorder?

    A   Fluoxetine

    B   Olanzapine

    C   Buspirone

    D   Alprazolam

4 Which of the following drugs could be regarded as a first-line treatment of PTSD?

   A Quetiapine

   B Sertraline

   C Clonazepam

   D Lithium

5 Which of the following drugs may be effective for the treatment of OCD?

   A Carbamazepine

   B Fluvoxamine

   C Risperidone

   D Oxazepam

Useful websites

American Psychiatric Association. (2000). *Diagnostic and Statistical Manual of Mental Disorders Text Revision* (4th edn). Washington, DC: American Psychiatric Publishing.

Beyond Blue: *Types of Anxiety Disorders* available at <www.beyondblue.org.au/index.aspx?link_id=90.615>

National Institute of Mental Health: *Anxiety Disorders* available at <www.nimh.nih.gov/health/topics/anxiety-disorders/index.shtml>

Bibliography

American Psychiatric Association. (2000). *Diagnostic and Statistical Manual of Mental Disorders*, 4th edn (DSM-IV). Washington, DC: American Psychiatric Association.

Barrett J. & Armony J. L. (2006). 'The influence of trait anxiety on autonomic response and cognitive performance during an anticipatory anxiety task' *Depression And Anxiety* 23(4): 210–219.

Lazarus R. (1991). *Emotion and Adaptation*. London: Oxford University Press.

Rossi S. (2012). *Australian Medicines Handbook*. Chapter 18: Psychotropic drugs. Adelaide, South Australia: AMH Pty Ltd.

Therapeutic Guidelines: Psychotropic – Version 6. Anxiety Disorders. Melbourne, Australia: Therapeutic Guidelines Limited, 2008.

Chapter 8

Schizophrenia and Other Psychoses

Chapter overview

This chapter covers the following topics:

* characteristics of schizophrenia and other psychoses
* discussion of the treatment of psychosis
* overview of important adverse effects of antipsychotic drugs
* consideration of challenges inherent to the treatment of psychosis.

Chapter learning objectives

After reading this chapter, you should be able to:

* describe the key features of schizophrenia and other psychoses
* outline drug therapy options that are available for treatment of psychosis
* discuss important adverse effects and drug interactions observed in association with the use of antipsychotic drugs
* understand special challenges that may be encountered in the management of psychosis in specific subgroups
* describe issues that may prove to compromise adherence for consumers treated for psychotic illness.

Key terms

Antipsychotic adherence
Antipsychotic drugs
Extrapyramidal side effects
Metabolic adverse effects

Psychosis
Schizophrenia
Substance-induced psychosis

Introduction

Schizophrenia and other forms of psychoses are among the most clinically and epidemiologically complex psychiatric illnesses encountered in modern day mental health care. Until the advent of the first antipsychotic drugs in the early 1950s there was relatively little that could be done to help those affected. The range of treatment options available has increased over the last 60 years, to the point where many different pharmacological approaches are now available as treatment options for patients/clients. Even so, the management of schizophrenia and other psychotic disorders with pharmacotherapy is frequently associated with drug-related problems, meaning that clinicians must be aware of strategies that can be used to maximise the likelihood of effective treatment outcomes and minimise the incidence and severity of adverse effects and other treatment-related issues. In this chapter you will explore the characteristics of schizophrenia and other psychoses, the general aspects of the treatment of schizophrenia, antipsychotic medications, the adverse effects of antipsychotic drugs, drug interactions with antipsychotics and adherence considerations with medications for people who experience schizophrenia and other psychotic disorders.

Psychosis – a set of symptoms, not a disease

'Psychosis' is a term that is used to describe a psychological and/or behavioural disorder characterised by the presence of one or more distinctive syndromes that cause a significant derangement of the capacity of the affected individual to be able to perceive and interpret their surroundings and existence. The extent to which this affects the individual concerned may vary, but in some cases can result in a gross disconnection from reality, meaning that in severe cases mental capacity is diminished to the extent that adequate self-care is not possible. The individual's ability to interpret reality, and to communicate and relate with others, can be impaired to the extent that even the minor aspects of the demands of everyday life can prove insurmountable.

In the *Diagnostic and Statistical Manual of Mental Disorders*, 4th edn (American Psychiatric Association, 2000), discussion of the syndrome of psychosis mentions various key features including delusions and hallucinations (refer to Table 8.1). These are certainly key features of psychosis, and may be accompanied by other symptoms such as disorganised speech or disorganised or catatonic behaviour.

Table 8.1: Important features of psychosis

Delusions are falsely held belief systems that are often characterised by misinterpretation of personal perceptions or experiences. The most common form of delusion is the persecutory delusion, where the affected individual may believe they are being monitored or spied upon, or where there is a belief that others seek to exploit the person or deliberately create disadvantage for them. Ideas of reference may be observed whereby the person believes that certain aspects of their surroundings or experiences carry special meanings for them (e.g. they may interpret news or media to have a particular specific meaning for them alone). In the context of strongly held cultural or religious philosophies, it can be difficult to differentiate delusions from belief systems that may not be shared by some elements of society.

Hallucinations are falsely perceived sensory input that may be auditory, visual, olfactory, gustatory or tactile in nature. Auditory hallucinations are the most commonly observed, and most often take the form of hearing voices.

Disorganised thinking is also referred to as formal thought disorder, and may often be reflected in disorganised speech.

Grossly disorganised behaviour may result in serious agitation or even dangerous personal conduct. One severe manifestation is catatonia, where the affected individual adopts a rigid posture and resists attempts to move them.

Different forms of psychoses are sometimes subclassified according to their likely origins. Some are known to occur in association with organic brain syndromes (such as those related to the effects of substance intoxication), whereas others appear to have origins in genetic predisposition and structural brain abnormalities (e.g. schizophrenia). Psychosis can be a feature observed in the context of many psychiatric illnesses – common examples include substance use disorders (where psychosis may occur in the context of either intoxication or substance withdrawal), bipolar disorder (particularly during manic episodes), major depression ('psychotic depression'), and Korsakoff psychosis (a complication of thiamine deficiency associated with heavy and chronic misuse of alcohol). Importantly, psychosis can arise in association with a range of general medical conditions including neoplasms, cerebrovascular disease, Huntington's disease, multiple sclerosis, some forms of epilepsy, thyroid dysfunction, electrolyte disturbances and systemic lupus erythematosis. There are also many drugs for which psychosis is a recognised adverse effect (see Table 8.2).

Table 8.2: Drugs that may cause psychosis

Drugs used for recreational/illicit purposes
Alcohol
Amphetamines
Cannabis
Cocaine
Hallucinogens
Inhalants
Phencyclidine and related substances
Drugs used for medicinal purposes
Some anaesthetic agents (e.g. ketamine)
Analgesics
Anticonvulsants
Drugs for Parkinson's disease
Corticosteroids
Tricyclic antidepressants

Schizophrenia

Schizophrenia is arguably the most important of all psychotic illnesses, a condition which is devastatingly disabling for those affected, and with significant effects upon the families and carers as well. Associated with considerable morbidity and also increased mortality, schizophrenia creates a societal impact that is reflected in the considerable costs associated with hospital care and lifelong pharmacotherapy that usually is required for the effective palliation of symptoms. Although the reported prevalence rate for schizophrenia has varied in different epidemiological research, a commonly cited figure in international literature is

0.5% to 1.5%. Schizophrenia is characterised by the onset of psychotic symptoms (refer to Table 8.1) which most commonly first appear in the late teenage years or during the third decade of life. Most of those affected will also have some form of prodromal (early) phase associated with symptoms that are relatively less distinctive (e.g. social isolation; social, occupational or academic dysfunction; poor self-care; bizarre or unusual behaviours). There is considerable evidence to support a genetic predisposition, with first-degree relatives of affected probands being considerably more likely to develop schizophrenia than controls from the general population (see Figure 8.1).

The most widely accepted diagnostic criteria for schizophrenia essentially specify that two or more of a suite of critical symptoms need to be demonstrable for a significant proportion of a one-month period (less if successfully treated). These symptoms include delusions, hallucinations, disorganised speech and

Figure 8.1: Relative genetic predisposition for expression of schizophrenia

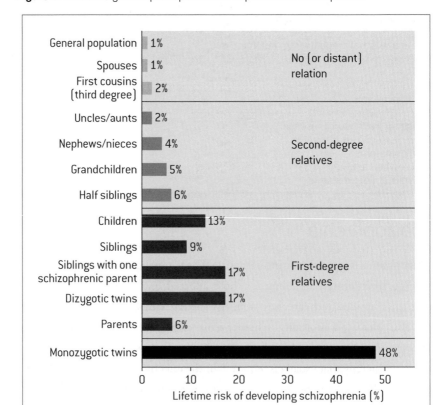

grossly disorganised behaviour. Collectively referred to as **positive symptoms**, these represent internally experienced aspects of reality that are added in the context of schizophrenia. A fifth, particularly important, category of symptoms comprises the so-called negative symptoms, which include disabling features like affective blunting (lack of emotional expression), alogia (difficulty in speaking attributable to a psychiatric disorder) and avolition (a general lack of drive or motivation to pursue meaningful goals). In reality, people with schizophrenia are often functionally impaired to a considerable extent, and this is reflected in compromised independent living skills, social functioning, and occupational and educational performance. These issues in turn contribute to broader problems such as homelessness, unemployment or under-employment, lack of meaningful interpersonal supports and relationships, and increased rates of substance misuse and suicide. As awareness of the impact of negative symptoms has grown, the importance of addressing these in the overall treatment approach has assumed equal (if not greater) priority to the management of positive symptoms. Additionally, there is evidence to suggest that some forms of pharmacotherapy used for schizophrenia may actually exacerbate negative symptoms, and this observation is one driver for change in the way this illness is treated in the contemporary practice setting.

One important issue that must be considered by any clinician involved in assessing the symptoms of schizophrenia (either for diagnostic purposes or when monitoring the effectiveness of therapeutic interventions) is that individual perceptions need to be viewed in an appropriate socio-economic and cultural context. It is not uncommon for ideas or behaviours that are considered to be relatively normal in one culture to be interpreted as evidence of psychosis in another (e.g. believing in magic or supernatural beings). In some religions, devotees may claim to converse directly with God or with deceased people. A lack of goal-directed activity may not necessarily represent motivational problems, and an inability to express feelings and thoughts may be appropriate where language or cultural barriers exist.

In addition to the genetic aspects of schizophrenia (see Figure 8.1), there is considerable interest in other biological aspects of this condition. The most widely held, if somewhat simplistic, biological theory for the underlying pathophysiology of schizophrenia is the so-called 'dopamine hypothesis', which is based on a theory that the illness results from overactivity in the dopamine systems of the brain. The indirect evidence for this paradigm is partly based in the observation that all of the effective medications that relieve the symptoms of schizophrenia are known to block dopaminergic receptors in the central nervous system, in particular the dopamine 2 (D2) subtype of receptors. Drugs such as amphetamines (which increase dopaminergic activity in the brain) can precipitate or exacerbate psychosis. Other neurotransmitters such as serotonin and glutamate are also now understood to be influential and this is reflected in the pharmacological profile of newer drugs that are effective for the treatment of schizophrenia.

Treatment of schizophrenia

When an disorder is as serious and as complex as schizophrenia, there are many considerations that need to be deliberated for incorporation into a holistic management approach. Although drug therapy is certainly an important aspect of the overall treatment that must be provided, many other issues need to be considered. The medications that are used for the treatment of schizophrenia are collectively referred to by many names (e.g. major tranquilisers, neuroleptics), but 'antipsychotic' has now become the most widely used term, reflecting the specific therapeutic utility of the drugs. Issues that need to be considered are outlined in Table 8.3, and the antipsychotics are discussed in detail later in this chapter.

Table 8.3: A holistic approach to the management of schizophrenia

Accurate diagnosis and assessment
Comprehensive and accurate longitudinal history from the patient/client and close relationships
Appropriate completion of imaging and pathology assessment, including substance misuse screening
Collateral history from other hospitals and health care providers

Psychosocial supports
Psychoeducation for consumers, families and carers
Housing assistance and support

Adherence support and education

Assistance in dealing with substance use/misuse issues

Access to advice and specialist services such as Home Medicines Review

Support and/or pastoral care for families and carers

Specific medical interventions

Use of non-pharmacological interventions:

- adjunctive psychotherapy
- specialised interventions where indicated (e.g. electroconvulsive treatment).

Pharmacotherapy:

- selection of the most appropriate drug therapy/therapies
- selection of optimal drug delivery approach:
  - monitoring for drug interactions, adverse effects
  - implementation of brief adjunctive pharmacotherapy where indicated
  - discontinuation of treatments that are no longer indicated or required
  - specialised screening before/after introduction of some medications.

Management of associated general medical issues:

- screening for metabolic complications of treatment, management of these
- management of important comorbid medical and psychiatric illnesses
- lifestyle interventions – smoking cessation, alcohol use modulation, exercise, diet.

Ask yourself!

1 If the incidence of schizophrenia in the wider community is about one in 100 people, why would it be that many health care workers have never met a person with the illness outside of their work environment?

2 Why do the family and carers of consumers with schizophrenia often require extensive practical psychosocial support from health services?

Antipsychotic medications

In October 1955, a group of eminent clinicians met in Washington, DC, in the United States to discuss the effects of new drugs that were at that time creating an enormous impact on patient care in psychiatric hospitals. These 'new drugs' were actually chlorpromazine and reserpine (reserpine is used to treat high blood pressure; it is also used to treat severe agitation in patients/clients with mental disorders), and their impact upon the care of people with psychotic illnesses at that time cannot be overstated. Interestingly, the meeting transcript suggests there was a general belief that the use of effective drug treatment with antipsychotic drugs would invariably be accompanied by side effects, with clinicians at the time noting that 'Parkinsonism … [might be used] as an index of the activity of the drug' (Duvall & Goldman, 2000). During the period of nearly 60 years that has followed, much experience has accumulated regarding the use of these first (conventional) antipsychotic drugs, also referred to as typical antipsychotics. More recently, the psychiatric community has watched the introduction of a new generation of antipsychotic medication, sometimes referred to as second-generation agents (i.e. atypical or novel antipsychotics). Despite this, in many parts of the developing world, conventional agents remain in widespread clinical use, in many cases as drugs of first choice.

First-generation antipsychotics (typical antipsychotics)

The earliest examples of the antipsychotic drugs included chlorpromazine and haloperidol, although the development of many others eventually followed, including agents such as thioridazine, trifluoperazine, zuclopenthixol, fluphenazine, perphenzine, pimozide and others. Many of these older antipsychotic drugs, collectively referred to as 'first-generation', 'conventional' or 'typical' antipsychotics, are still in widespread use now, particularly in developing countries where health funding may be limited. The first-generation antipsychotics share a range of common characteristics: all are effective in the management of psychosis, and in particular the positive symptoms of schizophrenia are responsive to the therapeutic effects of these drugs, whereas the negative symptoms of schizophrenia are often relatively refractory (and may even be worsened). Many of the first-generation antipsychotics are relatively sedating agents, although the extent of sedation when administered at effective antipsychotic dosage varies between drugs (refer to Table 8.4). In addition, these older agents exert potent alpha-adrenergic blockade, which in the peripheral vasculature is associated with a tendency to postural hypotension and orthostasis-related falls in the elderly. The anticholinergic effects of these drugs is responsible for a wide range of potentially serious adverse effects, including delirium, confusion, constipation, urinary hesitancy, dry mouth, blurred vision and tachycardia. Conversely, the extent of intrinsic anticholinergic effects associated with each drug is inversely related to the likelihood of parkinsonian side effects. The relative nature of the clinical effects of a range of first-generation antipsychotics is outlined in Table 8.4.

Table 8.4: Relative nature of the clinical effects of a range of first-generation antipsychotics

Relatively sedating drugs associated with a higher incidence of anticholinergic and hypotensive side effects but with a relatively low incidence of serious extrapyramidal side effects.
For example – chlorpromazine, pericyazine
Moderately sedating drugs with less potential for anticholinergic and hypotensive effects, but with a greater incidence of extrapyramidal side effects.
For example – trifluoperazine, fluphenazine
Drugs which produce little sedation, but have very little potential for causing anticholinergic effects or hypotension. These drugs are often associated with extrapyramidal side effects.
For example – haloperidol

As well as adverse effects attributable to the underlying receptor blockade pharmacology of the drugs, the first-generation drugs are associated with idiosyncratic side effects (e.g. photosensitivity with chlorpromazine and metabolic issues, covered later in this discussion). The potential for serious adverse effects and relative lack of efficacy against negative symptoms of schizophrenia have meant that the first-generation agents have been largely superseded in clinical practice, and the use of these agents has diminished markedly relative to newer drugs.

Atypical antipsychotics

A range of newer antipsychotics that include widely prescribed drugs such as olanzapine, risperidone and quetiapine, as well as amisulpride, aripiprazole, clozapine, paliperidone, quetiapine, asenapine, sertindole and ziprasidone, are collectively referred to as 'second-generation antipsychotics' or 'atypical antipsychotics'. These drugs are considerably more expensive than their predecessors, but notwithstanding this have become the basis for the usual standard of modern psychiatric care for schizophrenia.

The profile of receptor blockade in the central nervous system that is associated with the atypical antipsychotic drugs is more complex, and involves dopamine D2 receptor blockade but also additional blockade at different receptors including dopamine D1 and D4, and a subtype of serotonin receptor (serotonin 5HT2A). The 'gold standard' atypical antipsychotic in terms of efficacy is clozapine, regarded as having superior efficacy that is limited in clinical utility because of the potential for a range of life-threatening adverse effects: for this reason, clozapine is generally reserved for use in the management of treatment-resistant cases. Considered in terms of efficacy against the positive symptoms of schizophrenia, second-generation antipsychotics are all just as effective as the first-generation drugs, but are probably more effective for negative symptoms. An additional characteristic shared by most atypical agents is a lesser likelihood of extrapyramidal side effects.

Dosage and administration of antipsychotic drugs

All available antipsychotic drugs (including first-generation agents) are relatively effective in the management of positive symptoms of psychosis. Specific agents may have particular advantages and disadvantages in various practice settings: the relative merits of a particular therapy approach are largely based around dosage presentation, route of administration, specific adverse effect profiles, and drug interactions. These issues are addressed in detailed discussion elsewhere in this chapter, but in order to understand the potential benefits and disadvantages of individual treatment approaches it is important to have a clear understanding of the objective of treatment at each stage, schematically represented in Figure 8.2.

A range of antipsychotic formulations is currently available in Australia – selected prescribing considerations are outlined in Table 8.5.

Figure 8.2: Objectives and characteristics of antipsychotic treatment phases

Phase ONE

To attain medicated cooperation – treat psychotic agitation, reduce risk of harm to patient and staff. Provide significant sedation so that the patient is calmed and less distressed (and also so that the behaviours are less distressing and threatening to staff, visitors, carers etc.). Treatment often administered in short acting parenteral formulation or orally as liquid dose form or dissolving wafer. Calming effect and tranquilisation often achieved before significant impact upon positive or negative symptoms.

Phase TWO

Seeking to consolidate gains from phase one, and to have therapeutic impact upon positive symptoms. Adjust dosage and drug selection to avoid unnecessary sedation if this can be achieved. Therapeutic impact may be observed after a relatively short period of treatment, where hallucinations and delusions diminish, or the patient becomes relatively less concerned or distressed. Parenteral formulation may still be required but aim to transfer to oral dose form as soon as possible.

Phase THREE

Stabilisation phase – continue to adjust drug dosage and formulation, seeking to maintain benefits from phase two and to design a comprehensive treatment approach that has the potential to impact on negative symptoms also. Optimisation of pharmacotherapy should be supported with psychoeducation, strategies to support adherence and to minimise likelihood of substance misuse. Efforts are made to design a treatment regimen that accords with the preferences of the consumer. This phase often extends over a period of months and may involve a switch to a long-acting depot formulation.

Phase FOUR

This phase is directed at optimising quality of life and regaining significant functional capacity. Continue to adjust drug dosage and formulation, seeking to derive an effective and tolerable treatment approach that can underpin beneficial outcomes such as return to employment, stable relationships, safe housing etc.

Table 8.5: Selected prescribing considerations for various antipsychotic drugs

Drug	Dosage and formulations*	Clinical characteristics*
Amisulpride	Tablet, oral liquid: acute dose 200–400 mg twice daily, decrease for maintenance	Thought to be more likely than other atypical agents to cause parkinsonian side effects. Dosage adjustment required in renal impairment.

(Continued)

Table 8.5: Selected prescribing considerations for various antipsychotic drugs (*Continued*)

Drug	Dosage and formulations*	Clinical characteristics*
Aripiprazole	Tablet: 15–30 mg daily	Partial dopamine agonist. May have a higher incidence of akathisia than other atypical agents.
Asenapine	Wafer: 5–10 mg twice daily	Should not eat or drink for 10 minutes after administration.
Chlorpromazine	Tablet, oral liquid: variable, up to 1000 mg daily for acute psychosis Short-acting injection 25–50 mg every 6–8 hours by deep IM injection for management of acute psychiatric emergency	Associated with photosensitivity rash. Very sedating, significant anticholinergic effects, prominent orthostasis. Poorly tolerated by the elderly. IV injection can cause catastrophic hypotension; IM injection causes significant orthostasis and is associated with injection site pain and development of sterile abscess.
Clozapine	Tablet, oral liquid: slowly titrated to usual dose range of 200–600 mg daily, max 900 mg daily, response may correlate with serum concentrations	Significant adverse effects – although regarded as the most clinically effective antipsychotic, serious reactions such as agranulocytosis, myocarditis and seizures mean that this agent is not used for first-line treatment (reserved for severe/refractory causes and used with intensive monitoring). Weight gain and metabolic dysregulation with hyperglycaemia/diabetes/dyslipidaemia is frequently observed. Significant drug interactions including decrease in serum concentration with carbamazepine, increased serum concentration with fluvoxamine and also after smoking cessation.
Droperidol	Short-acting injection: IM/IV injection of 5–25 mg for extreme psychotic or manic agitation	Potential for Q-T prolongation and serious arrythmias. Avoid concurrent use with other agents that prolong the Q-T interval.
Flupenthixol	Long-acting depot injection: usual dose 20–40 mg every two weeks by deep IM injection	Delayed onset of action – not suitable for management of acute psychotic agitation.
Fluphenazine	Long-acting depot injection: usual dose 12.5–50 mg every two weeks by deep IM injection	Delayed onset of action – not suitable for management of acute psychotic agitation.

Drug	Dosage and formulations*	Clinical characteristics*
Haloperidol	Tablet, oral liquid: up to 30 mg daily in 2–3 divided doses Short-acting injection: 2–10 mg IM repeated as needed for psychotic agitation Long-acting depot injection: usual dose 50–100 mg every four weeks by deep IM injection	Prominently associated with parkinsonian side effects. High potential for tardive dyskinesia. Unlikely to cause orthostasis.
Olanzapine	Tablet, oral liquid: up to 20 mg daily in 2–3 divided doses Short-acting injection: 5–10 mg IM repeated as needed for psychotic agitation (max 30 mg/24 hours) Long-acting depot injection: usual dose 210–300 mg every two weeks by deep IM injection	Most sedating of the atypical agents. Weight gain and metabolic dysregulation with hyperglycaemia/diabetes/dyslipidaemia is frequently observed. Significant drug interactions including decrease in serum concentration with carbamazepine, and increased serum concentration with fluvoxamine and also after smoking cessation. Oral wafers may be used to enhance likelihood of adherence in acute psychosis. Monitor for postinjection delirium for three hours after injection of long-acting depot product.
Paliperidone	Slow release tablet: 3–12 mg daily Long-acting depot injection: titrate to maintenance dose of 25–150 mg monthly	Closely related to risperidone.
Pericyazine	Tablet: antipsychotic dose of 30 mg daily in divided doses	Often used at more moderate doses for sedative and anxiolytic effects.
Quetiapine	Tablet: 300–800 mg daily in divided doses	SR formulation may be administered once daily.
Risperidone	Tablet, wafer, oral liquid: titrate to 2–8 mg daily in divided doses Long-acting injection: 25–50 mg every two weeks	Associated with significant hyperprolactinaemia and metabolic disturbance. Long-acting injection must be stored in refrigeration.

(Continued)

Table 8.5: Selected prescribing considerations for various antipsychotic drugs (*Continued*)

Drug	Dosage and formulations*	Clinical characteristics*
Sertindole	Tablet: initially 4 mg once daily titrated as needed to maximum of 12–20 mg daily	Potential for Q-T prolongation and serious arrythmias. Avoid concurrent use with other agents that prolong the Q-T interval.
Trifluoperazine	Tablet, oral liquid: 2–15 mg twice daily	First-generation agent associated with high incidence of parkinsonism, tardive dyskinesia, metabolic disturbance/weight gain.
Ziprasidone	Capsule: 40 mg twice, titrated to maximum of 80 mg twice daily if needed Short-acting injection: 10–20 mg every four hours to a maximum of 40 mg daily, duration no greater than 2–3 days	Evidence suggests least likelihood of weight gain or metabolic dysregulation. Take capsules with food.
Zuclopenthixol	Tablet: 10–15 mg daily in divided doses Intermediate-acting injection: 50–150 mg every 2–3 days Long-acting injection: 200–400 mg every 2–4 weeks	Caution is required to ensure that the correct dosage form is selected.

*Not a comprehensive guide – refer to reference texts and manufacturer's information

Adverse effects of antipsychotic drugs
Extrapyramidal side effects

As the terminology implies, extrapyramidal side effects are mediated in the extrapyramidal tracts of the central nervous system. Although much less common with atypical antipsychotics than the first-generation predecessors, extrapyramidal side effects are still among the most important adverse effects to anticipate and closely monitor the patient/client for. These effects arise through dopaminergic blockade and are dose-related, and may be very distressing for the patient/client.

Extrapyramidal side effects are particularly frequent and severe with some specific first-generation agents such as haloperidol and trifluoperazine. There are various important manifestations of extrapyramidal side effects, discussed below.

Dystonic reactions (*dystonia*) may be described as muscle cramps, and are often characterised by muscular spasm in the face, neck, trunk and limbs. Dystonic reactions can have a rapid, acute onset. Typical examples of dystonic reactions include torticollis, retrocollis, carpopedal spasm, trismus and perioral spasm. The most serious manifestations include oculogyric crisis, laryngeal spasm and opisthotonos (a severe global spasm of the back muscles), which are medical emergencies requiring prompt treatment with parenteral anticholinergic agents (see below).

Akathisia is a subjective sensation of restlessness which may be very uncomfortable for the person. In some cases it can be difficult to differentiate between akathisia and psychotic agitation. Akathisia will usually improve with dose reduction and deteriorate when the dose is increased whereas psychotic agitation will usually improve if the antipsychotic dose is increased or deteriorate with a dose reduction. Akathisia is not usually responsive to anticholinergic drugs but refractory cases may respond to treatment with low doses of the beta adrenergic blocker propranolol (the only beta blocker that crosses the blood–brain barrier).

Parkinsonism (also referred to as *pseudoparkinsonism* or *parkinsonian side effects*) may manifest as a broad range of symptoms that have a resemblance to the clinical features of idiopathic Parkinson's disease. Commonly encountered features include tremor, rigidity or bradykinesia. Ideally, parkinsonism should be managed by a trial dose reduction of the antipsychotic, or in some cases a switch to a different agent. However, in some cases these approaches may result in a relapse or exacerbation of psychotic features. Under these circumstances the usual approach involves treatment with an anticholinergic drug such as benztropine or benzhexol.

Tardive dyskinesia is an abnormal involuntary movement syndrome that is most commonly observed to affect the face, mouth or tongue. In some cases there is more widespread involvement including the muscles of the head, neck, trunk or limbs. Most commonly tardive dyskinesia is observed after extended treatment with antipsychotic drugs for periods of months or years, and the syndrome appears to be more common with the older agents than with the atypical antipsychotics. Tardive dyskinesia may appear or become exacerbated after the dose of antipsychotic is decreased, or when the drug is ceased. Risk factors appear to be older age, female gender, cigarette smoking and diabetes mellitus. Very severe or refractory cases may respond to treatment with high dose vitamin E, or to tetrabenazine (which depletes presynaptic storage of dopamine in the central nervous system).

Neuroleptic malignant syndrome is a potentially fatal condition in which patients/clients develop fulminant symptoms including fever, marked muscle rigidity, altered consciousness and autonomic instability. An associated laboratory finding is elevation of plasma creatine kinase concentration (of skeletal muscle origin). Neuroleptic malignant syndrome is managed by ceasing the implicated antipsychotic agent and general, high-level supportive care (e.g. ventilation, dialysis, thromboprophylaxis), often in an intensive care unit. Anticholinergics or benzodiazepines may diminish muscular rigidity.

The extrapyramidal side effects are often amenable to management with anticholinergic drugs, although if possible it is best to avoid these agents for long-term use – a better approach might involve switching the antipsychotic or decreasing the dose of the antipsychotic. In some circumstances extrapyramidal side effects can be severe or may contribute to compromised treatment adherence, and under these circumstances an intervention with an anticholinergic agent is warranted. The most widely used anticholinergic agent in Australia is benztropine, administered orally at a dose of 1–2 mg twice daily, or by IM/IV injection at a dose of 1–2 mg for the management of acute or severe dystonias. Alternatives to benztropine include benzhexol, biperiden and orphenadrine. It is important to be cautious when using anticholinergic agents, particularly for elderly people, as serious unwanted effects such as angle closure glaucoma, urinary retention and delirium can occur. Other anticholinergic side effects to watch for include dry mouth, urinary hesitancy, constipation and tachycardia.

Metabolic side effects

Weight gain associated with antipsychotic drug treatment is very common, although the prevalence of this problem appears to be greater with some individual agents than with others. Atypical agents such as amisulpride, aripiprazole, asenapine, ziprasidone and the first-generation drug haloperidol are thought to have the lowest incidence of clinically significant weight gain. Clozapine and olanzapine are the drugs most likely to be associated with weight gain, and in some cases the extent and rate of increased body mass index can be extreme (15–20 kg over a six-month period has been recorded). The underlying mechanism appears to be multifactorial, and it has been postulated that histamine H1 receptor blockade, serotonin 5HT2C antagonism and effects of serum leptin contribute to alterations in food intake (both quantity and type of food) as well as diminished intentional and incidental physical activity. It is critical that the treatment plan for all people who are to receive ongoing treatment with any antipsychotic should include monitoring weight change, body mass index and waist circumference over time. Dietary advice and lifestyle assessment and assistance must be incorporated into an integrated approach aimed at maintaining physical health and well-being. Other aspects should include support and advice to facilitate smoking cessation and moderation of alcohol intake, and approaches designed to assist with maintaining physical activity and exercise.

All antipsychotic drugs increase the risk of hyperglycaemia and diabetes mellitus. Clozapine and olanzapine, and to a somewhat lesser extent risperidone and quetiapine, are prominently associated with abnormal glucose tolerance. Similarly, antipsychotic drug treatment confers additional risk of dyslipidaemia. The effects of impaired glucose tolerance, elevated lipids and obesity, combined with the effects of a sedentary lifestyle and smoking create very significant risk for cardiovascular disease and the significant consequences of cardiac ischaemia, stroke and other serious complications. The prevalence of diabetes is 10-fold higher in people who experience psychosis than in the general population. However, more evidence through research is needed to determine whether there is a direct causal effect between atypical antipsychotics and the development of diabetes. Importantly, these metabolic effects demonstrate a potential between drug-induced weight gain and increased risk of developing cardiovascular concerns and/or type 2 diabetes. Weight gain and diabetes caused by antipsychotic drug treatment continue to be clinical concerns (Edward, Rasmussen & Munro, 2010). All this emphasises the need to adopt an integrated monitoring and management for treatment of emergent adverse metabolic effects that should be used for all patients/clients undergoing extended treatment with antipsychotics.

Hyperprolactinaemia (abnormally high levels of prolactin in the blood) is another adverse endocrine/metabolic effect observed with antipsychotic drug treatment. Thought to be related to dopaminergic blockade in the tuberoinfundibular apparatus, hyperprolactinaemia is associated with a range of secondary complications such as gynaecomastia (abnormal development of large mammary glands in males resulting in breast enlargement), galactorrhoea (refers to milk secretion not due to breastfeeding), abnormal menses and anovulation, as well as various forms of sexual dysfunction which can affect either males or females. Longstanding hyperprolactinaemia may reduce bone mineral density and contribute to the development of osteopaenia or osteoporosis. Hyperprolactinaemia is most common with paliperidone and risperidone, and many of the first-generation antipsychotics. As well as contributing to adverse medical outcomes, hyperprolactinaemia can contribute to stigma and may have a substantial negative impact upon sustained adherence.

Ask yourself!

1   What barriers might exist that could interfere with open and frank discussion of metabolic adverse effects among those treated with schizophrenia? Do health care professionals and consumers always have aligned views about the relative importance of different adverse drug reactions?

2   If diabetes develops during treatment with an antipsychotic drug, how might this affect the treatment of schizophrenia? How might schizophrenia affect the management of diabetes?

Clozapine side effects

Clozapine is widely regarded as the most effective of all antipsychotic drugs; some research suggests that up to 50% of cases of treatment resistant schizophrenia may achieve a response (Lieberman et al., 1994). Considering this high rate of efficacy and the effectiveness against serious negative symptoms of schizophrenia, why then is clozapine not the most widely prescribed antipsychotic? Although highly efficacious, clozapine is associated with a range of very serious adverse effects, many of which occur at an incidence rate that precludes widespread or first-line use.

Blood dyscracias, in particular potentially fatal agranulocytosis or neutropaenia, occur at a rate of up to 4%. Although often reversible, clozapine-induced neutropaenia is a very serious complication and has necessitated the establishment of a structured approach to monitoring that is widely known as the Clozapine Patient Monitoring Service. Under the parameters of the Clozapine Patient Monitoring Service, patients must have regular and frequent complete blood examinations to ensure that the white blood cell count remains within safe limits. Initially, blood sampling is undertaken weekly, and the issue of each week's supply of medication is contingent upon a satisfactory blood test result. As the period of safe treatment extends, blood tests are relaxed to fortnightly and ultimately monthly, but in the event of an abnormal result, intensification of monitoring or cessation of treatment may be triggered. The invasive and intensive requirements for blood testing and the associated costs of this have been debated as potentially unacceptable limitations upon the suitability of the drug for routine use, with the effects of the monitoring regimen cited as a negative influence on quality of life and overall acceptability of the treatment to consumers.

The adverse effects of clozapine are not limited to haematological toxicities. Potentially fatal cardiac effects such as myocarditis and cardiomyopathy resulting in death or the need for cardiac transplantation are also known side effects of the drug. This in turn necessitates a complex regimen of cardiac screening and monitoring, involving tests including ECGs, echocardiograms and serial measurement of troponins – all contributing to diminished quality of life and potentially compromising adherence. Add to this the extensive metabolic impact of clozapine for many patients/clients (see above) and a known increase in the risk for other serious adverse effects such as seizures, pulmonary embolus and pancreatitis, and a clear picture emerges to explain why clozapine is reserved for very severe and refractory cases of schizophrenia. Even so, the remarkable results that can be achieved with this drug have ensured that it continues to merit a place among treatment options for difficult cases. The safety of treatment can be enhanced by the use of therapeutic drug monitoring and dosage adjustment based on measurement of clozapine serum concentrations.

Other significant side effects of antipsychotics

There is a range of other adverse effects associated with antipsychotics that necessitate careful history taking, monitoring, and a willingness to adjust dosage or switch agents if necessary. These include:

* Q-Tc segment prolongation on the ECG – thought to contribute to the increased incidence of sudden cardiac death among people treated for schizophrenia. Overall, the risk is believed to be higher for those treated with asenapine or sertindole, during treatment with other drugs known to contribute to Q-Tc prolongation (e.g. erythromycin, cisapride, methadone). Independent risk factors include electrolyte abnormalities (e.g. hypokalaemia, hypomagnesaemia, hypocalcaemia), or a history of anorexia nervosa or previous myocarditis. In the presence of these risk factors, judicious drug selection and intensified monitoring are needed. If during treatment the Q-Tc interval is over 440 ms for men or 470 ms for women, specialist advice

should be sought. If the Q-Tc interval exceeds 500 ms treatment should be suspended and a cardiology opinion obtained.

✱ Sexual dysfunction is relatively common, and may be a powerful motivator for non-adherence, particularly among younger patients/clients. A range of problems including erectile dysfunction, priapism and retrograde ejaculation or ejaculatory failure may affect men, whereas both genders may be affected by diminished libido and anorgasmia. These effects are complex to interpret in the context of illness-related psychosocial and interpersonal dysfunction, and those affected may be reluctant to discuss the issues, particularly where gender or cultural barriers exist.

✱ Antipsychotics are frequently sedating, and this is compounded by interactions with alcohol or other sedating drugs such as anticonvulsants (e.g. carbamazepine, valoproate, pregnable), hypnosedatives, opioid analgesics, and some antidepressants. As well as contributing to cognitive dulling, this may compromise the ability of the affected individual to drive a motor vehicle or operate heavy machinery safely. This in turn may mean that difficult decisions may be needed in relation to fitness to drive or the ability to remain in employment, and the implications of these factors may contribute to the patient/client withholding or minimising information given to the treatment team. Treatment with antipsychotic drugs need not mean that a person is not fit to drive – in fact, with adequate symptom relief, attentiveness and reaction time may actually improve, and thus expert assessment is often required to resolve these matters.

Drug interactions with antipsychotics

Drug interactions with antipsychotics may influence the safety and efficacy of antipsychotic treatment, or the stability of comorbid disease states. Comprehensive medication regimen review by a clinical pharmacist or reference to a reliable compendium of drug interaction information is advisable in the context of extensive medical comorbidity or **polypharmacy**. Although not a comprehensive list, a range of examples are provided here for illustrative purposes:

✱ The effects of other sedating medications such as benzodiazepines, opioid or anticonvulsants may profoundly accentuate sedation secondary to antipsychotics.

✳ Concurrent anticonvulsants such as phenytoin or carbamazepine may induce the metabolism and decrease the therapeutic effects of antipsychotics. Many antipsychotics are proconvulsant and may destabilise the control of epilepsy.

✳ The addition of an antipsychotic may destabilise glycaemic control and necessitate adjustment to the insulin or hypoglycaemic regimen for those with diabetes mellitus.

✳ Concurrent use of antipsychotic drugs with other drugs that can influence cardiac conduction may result in hazardous prolongation of the Q-Tc interval.

✳ Some SSRI antidepressants inhibit the hepatic metabolism of individual antipsychotics, leading to increased serum concentrations of the antipsychotic and enhanced adverse effects:

  - Fluvoxamine and fluoxetine increase the serum concentration of olanzapine and clozapine.

  - Paroxetine and fluoxetine increase the serum concentration of risperidone and haloperidol.

✳ Cigarette smoking induces the metabolism of olanzapine and clozapine and may decrease serum concentrations of these drugs to the extent that clinical efficacy is compromised.

✳ Conversely, if the patient/client stops smoking, the metabolism of olanzapine and clozapine will return to normal, meaning that without dosage adjustment the serum concentrations may increase causing toxicity. Note that this effect is produced by toxins in cigarette smoke itself, rather than nicotine. A smoker who stops smoking with the aid of nicotine replacement (e.g. gum, patches) may still experience antipsychotic drug toxicity.

Adherence and antipsychotic drug treatment

There are many complex issues to consider with respect to adherence to prescribed antipsychotic pharmacotherapy. Under some circumstances, the risk associated with suboptimal treatment of a psychotic illness creates an unacceptable level of risk for the patient/client, family or carer, staff or the broader community. Under these circumstances it may be necessary to utilise legislative provisions to mandate an involuntary admission to an approved hospital for treatment, or to create a community treatment order that compels a patient/client to receive treatment at an approved place. Oral treatment is rarely workable under these circumstances, and thus it is necessary to implement a regimen based on the long-acting depot formulation of drugs such as risperidone, paliperidone, haloperidol, fluphenazine, flupenthixol, olanzapine or zuclopenthixol. There is a limited place for directly observed therapy regimens of oral medication, where the patient/client must report for observation of a once-daily oral dose of medication under supervision.

The likelihood of attaining good voluntary adherence (and thus a better likelihood of good treatment outcomes) is increased by strategies such as adherence coaching and psychoeducation. Factors known to be predictive of better antipsychotic treatment adherence include:

* decreased exposure to illicit or recreational drugs such as cannabis or amphetamine

* experience of daily benefit – the patient/client can 'feel' the beneficial effects of the medication and can identify them

* a lack of side effects that are important to the patient/client themselves – to understand this requires an appreciation of the relative value/cost that an individual attaches to the medications they are taking or have taken in the past

* support from family, friends and carers – which may be enhanced by the provision of community-based support systems and planned 'time out' admissions.

Other strategies to enhance adherence include selection of a regimen based around once-daily self-administration of oral medications, or the periodic IM administration of a long-acting depot product (refer to Chapter 13 on adherence and concordance).

DAVE'S STORY

Dave is a 20-year-old Aboriginal man who was diagnosed with schizophrenia two years earlier. He lives alone in a small flat in a rural community and commutes to the nearest large urban setting for his assessment and to have prescriptions dispensed. He has been smoking 40 cigarettes daily and uses cannabis 'almost every day'.

He has not been employed since leaving school at the age of 15 years. His current treatment is limited to olanzapine 30 mg daily. He has recently presented with a severe exacerbation of his psychosis, having been found on the roof of his flat shouting obscenities at 'spirits in the air'. After the crisis team were called, he was detained for assessment and treatment in hospital. He volunteers little information to any of the female nursing or medical staff. His girlfriend tells the treating team that he has stopped taking his medication because he was worried about 'getting fat' and 'trouble in the bedroom'.

Ask yourself!

As a nurse involved with caring for Dave:

1   Why might Dave be reluctant to discuss his recent treatment and its effects?

2   Will the use of cannabis affect his schizophrenia?

3   What alternative treatments might be offered to enhance adherence and decrease the adverse effects important to Dave?

From the consumer's perspective – *How does this feel for me?*

Consumers may have impaired insight and judgment during an exacerbation of a psychotic illness such as schizophrenia.

Consumers may attach a different importance to aspects of their illness management than those chosen by the treating team.

'I'm not taking those tablets – you're trying to poison me!'

'I've never been as fat as this before – I hate it.'

'The needles hurt, I don't like having them.'

'I feel much better when I smoke a few cones.'

Care Plan

The following is an example care plan for the patient/client presented in this chapter. The areas of daily living that are considered include bio-psycho-social factors and the plan is mapped out using the nursing process (Assessment; Planning; Implementation; Evaluation). Remember: the success is in the detail, so be specific about *who, when and what* in the collaborative plan; never include someone in the plan if they were not consulted in the planning process; and always work within a recovery-orientated framework (refer to Chapter 1).

Date: 15/3/12

Client's name: Dave Client | Case manager: T. Player

Areas of daily living	Assessment of current situation	Goal	Plan (undertaken with patient/client)	Implementation	Who is responsible? (Include only those who have been consulted in the planning process)	Evaluation/ review date
Mental health	Diagnosis of schizophrenia, recent relapse of psychotic symptoms.	Minimise the adverse effects of psychotic symptoms.	Monitor early warning signs of psychosis, which are: • feeling more agitated and pacing more • poor sleep • poor concentration. Action – if early warning signs are present: • use distraction techniques • call T. Player to discuss and organise a possible review of medication.	Develop an early warning signs list and document this. Dave to keep a list of early warning signs with him and a copy to be attached to the fridge door.	Dave T. Player Dave	15/3/12 Ongoing

Social	Unemployed since leaving school.	Dave wants to get a job.	Dave to look for potential volunteer jobs as a starting point. Liaise with disability employment network groups for assistance.	Dave will attend an appointment at the disability employment network service. Appointment will be arranged by T. Player.	T. Player and Dave	19/4/12
	Some hesitancy with disclosure with female staff members.	Dave prefers to speak with male staff members.	Allocate male staff member to ensure gender-sensitive practice.	Ensure Dave has access (where possible) to male staff members when an appointment at the service is made.	T. Player	Ongoing
Biological	History of non-adherence to medication/ treatment due to sexual problems and weight gain associated with adverse effects of the medication.	Improve adherent behaviour.	Discuss motivation, beliefs and ambivalence for adhering or not adhering to medication/treatment.	Continue with regular appointments with T. Player.	T. Player and Dave	Every 2 weeks
	Prescribed 30 mg olanzapine daily.	Maintain therapeutic effect of olanzapine.	Maintain therapeutic effect of olanzapine.	Ensure regular appointments for Dave with psychiatrist related to positive effects of olanzapine.	T. Player	Every 12 weeks

(Continued)

Date: 15/3/12 (Continued)

Client's name: Dave Client | Case manager: T. Player

Areas of daily living	Assessment of current situation	Goal	Plan (undertaken with patient/client)	Implementation	Who is responsible? (Include only those who have been consulted in the planning process)	Evaluation/review date
		Monitor efficacy of medications.	Minimise ADRs.	Use PANSS (Positive and Negative Syndrome Scale). See also: • Brief Psychiatric Rating Scale (BPRS) • Scale for the Assessment of Positive Symptoms (SAPS) • Scale for the Assessment of Negative Symptoms (SANS). Positive and negative symptoms Weight gain Hyperprolactinaemia Sedation	T. Player	Every 12 weeks

			Extrapyramidal side effects Hyperlipidaemia Postural hypotension Other cardiovascular effects Hyperglycaemia		
Environmental	Lives in a rural community, possible isolation.	Minimise potential for isolation.	Explore membership to community groups related to Dave's interests. Develop a list of at least 2 interests of Dave.	Dave and T. Player	12/4/12
Substance using behaviours	Smokes 40 cigarettes per day.	Reduce the risks associated with cigarette smoking.	Explore Dave's motivations and beliefs related to cigarette smoking. Work together to discuss reduced smoking or smoking cessation.	T. Player and Dave	Each appointment
	Uses cannabis daily.	Reduce the risks associated with cannabis use.	Explore Dave's motivations and beliefs related to cannabis use. Work together to discuss reduced cannabis use or stopping cannabis use.	T. Player and Dave	Each appointment
Risk behaviours	Found on the roof of his flat shouting obscenities 'at spirits in the air'.		Develop strategies with Dave regarding being on the roof of his flat when he is distressed by symptoms. Work together to discuss alternatives to fear or stress induced by psychotic symptoms.	T. Player and Dave	Each appointment

On the Horizon in Schizophrenia Pharmacotherapy

Reduced dopaminergic activity in the prefrontal cortex probably contributes to negative symptoms of schizophrenia. Animal research suggests that drugs that exert alpha-2 adrenergic receptor antagonist activity in the brain increase dopaminergic activity in the frontal cortex when added to antipsychotic drug therapy. Drugs that can achieve this include clozapine, mianserin, mirtazapine and idazoxan. The effectiveness of clozapine against negative symptoms of schizophrenia is well known, and initial human research with this approach appears to suggest that these drugs may be promising adjuvant treatments in schizophrenia.

Novel drug delivery systems may assist in extending the range of options available for the management of symptoms of schizophrenia. One study found that inhaled loxapine reduced acute agitation compared with placebo, with onset of action as rapid as 10 minutes after the dose. Concerns do remain about the potential for respiratory adverse effects with this approach.

Schizophrenia may have a hormonal component in aetiology. Evidence suggests differences in the incidence and course of schizophrenia between genders and a possible protective role for oestrogen. Oestrogen has been demonstrated to influence CNS dopaminergic and serotonergic systems. One study has found that transdermal oestradiol augmentation was associated with significant improvements in symptoms of schizophrenia and also cognition, relative to the effects of antipsychotics alone. Raloxifene is an oestrogen receptor modulator and lacks the possible negative effects of oestrogen on breast and uterine tissue, and when used as adjunctive treatment for symptoms of schizophrenia in postmenopausal women was found to improve negative and positive symptoms in another study (Usall, Cobo & Serrano-Blanco, 2011). There is also evidence that oestrogen may be helpful for men with schizophrenia.

Pharmacogenetic approaches may help to elucidate why different people have different responses to the same antipsychotic drug therapy. Different metaboliser status may account in part for pharmacokinetic differences that influence response to treatment and the prevalence of serious adverse effects like metabolic dysregulation. Genetic influences upon neurotransmitter transport systems in the brain may also prove to be important. As more clinical trials include an element of DNA collection, additional information about these issues is likely to be revealed.

Summary

Psychosis, and in particular schizophrenia, is a complex condition that relies very heavily on pharmacotherapy for effective management. The medications that are used are only partially effective, and are heavily reliant upon consistent adherence to be able to achieve a response that will enable patients/clients to have good quality of life. The antipsychotic drugs are associated with a wide range of adverse effects and drug interactions, in some cases of considerable clinical significance. To ensure the maximum likelihood of good treatment outcomes a team approach is required with each clinician contributing in aspects where specialist expertise can make a real difference.

Discussion questions

1   What are the key features of a psychotic illness?

2   List several different types of adverse drug reaction that can have an impact upon the tolerability of antipsychotic drug treatment.

3   What factors are predictive of good adherence to a prescribed antipsychotic drug treatment regimen?

Test yourself (answers at the back of the book)

1   Which of the following is regarded as a diagnostic feature of schizophrenia?

   A   Nightmares and flashbacks

   B   Elevated energy and libido

   C   Hyperactivity and inattention

   D   Delusions and disorganised speech

2   Which of the following medicinal drugs is most likely to be associated with a drug-induced psychosis?

   A   Prednisolone

   B   Salbutamol

   C   Amoxycillin

   D   Bromhexine

3   Which of the following agents is an example of a first-generation antipsychotic agent?

   A   Citalopram

   B   Clozapine

   C   Carbamazepine

   D   Chlorpromazine

4   Blockade of which of the following receptors is regarded as critical to antipsychotic drug effects?

A   Histamine H1

B   Muscarinic M2

C   Dopamine D2

D   Dopamine D4

5   Which of the following drugs may administered by long-acting depot injection?

A   Clozapine

B   Paliperidone

C   Trifluoperazine

D   Quetiapine

Useful websites

Schizophrenia.com: *Daily Schizophrenia News* available at <www.schizophrenia.com>

Health Insite: *Schizophrenia* available at <www.healthinsite.gov.au/topics/schizophrenia>

Australian Psychological Society: *Schizophrenia* available at <www.psychology.org.au/community/schizophrenia>

References

American Psychiatric Association. (2000). *Diagnostic and Statistical Manual of Mental Disorders*, 4th edn (DSM-IV). Washington, DC: American Psychiatric Association.

Bazire S. (2012). *Psychotropic Drug Directory: The Professional's Pocket Handbook and Aide Memoire*. United Kingdom: Fivepin Publishing.

Edward K., Rasmussen B. & Munro I. (2010). 'Nursing care of clients treated with atypical antipsychotics who have a risk of developing metabolic instability and/or type 2 diabetes' *Archives of Psychiatric Nursing* 24(1): 46–53.

Duval A. M & Goldman D. (2000) 'The new drugs (chlorpromazine & reserpine): administrative aspects' *Psychiatr Serv* 51: 327–331.

Lieberman J. A., Safferman A.Z., Pollack S., et al. (1994) 'Clinical effects of clozapine in chronic schizophrenia: response to treatment and predictors of outcome' *Am J Psychiatry* 151: 1744–1752.

Taylor D., Paton C. & Kapur S. (2009) *The Maudsley Prescribing Guidelines*. 10th edn. UK: Informa Healthcare.

Rossi S. (2012). *Australian Medicines Handbook*. Chapter 18: Psychotropic drugs. Adelaide, South Australia: AMH Pty Ltd.

Usall, J., Cobo, J. & Serrano-Blanco, A. (2011) 'Raloxifene as an adjunctive treatment for postmenopausal women with schizophrenia: a double blind, randomised, placebo-controlled trial' *Journal of Clinical Psychiatry* accessed from www.pssjd.org/SiteCollectionDocuments/Article%20Judith%20Usall%20-%20sept.2011.pdf.

Chapter 9

Substance Use Disorders

Chapter overview

This chapter covers the following topics:

* dual diagnosis
* substance abuse
* substance dependence
* substance withdrawal.

Chapter learning objectives

After reading this chapter, you should be able to:

* recognise the two substance disorder categories and how they relate to mental illness
* have an overview of commonly used or abused substances including intervention and drug interactions.

Key terms

Dual diagnosis
Substance abuse
Substance dependence

Introduction

In this chapter you will explore substance use disorders and the effects of these upon people with comorbid mental illness, best practice for alcohol abuse or dependence intervention, issues relating to nicotine use and mental illness, cannabis and mental illness, the effects of 'ecstasy' and heroin upon mental illness, and care considerations for people with substance disorders.

What are substance disorders and how do they relate to those with mental illness?

A 'substance' can be described as anything ingested or taken into the body that results in alteration of affect, functioning or senses. The most commonly used substances in Australia are alcohol, nicotine, prescription drugs and other illicit drugs (heroin, 3,4-methylenedioxy-N-methylamphetamine (MDMA or 'ecstasy'), cocaine and marijuana). The *Diagnostic and Statistical Manual of Mental Disorders*, 4th edn (American Psychiatric Association, 2000) (DSM-IV) is used by most mental health clinicians to classify substance use disorders. In the section dedicated to Substance Disorders within the DSM-IV there are two categories: Substance Abuse and Substance Dependence. The categories relate to either the abuse of or dependence on any particular substance. Global epidemiological research confirms that co-occurring addictive and mental disorders are highly prevalent in Western communities (Kessler, Chiu, Demler & Walters, 2005; Kessler, Nelson, McGonagle, Edlund & Leaf, 1996; Teesson, Hall, Lynskey & Degenhardt, 2000); this is referred to as **dual diagnosis**.

Significantly, the prevalence of mental disorders and the resultant negative effects on role functioning are viewed to be generally higher than any other chronic conditions (World Health Organization, 2008). Notably people who have addictive and mental disorders are less likely to seek or engage in health care and this has implications when caring for this group of patients/clients.

Table 9.1: Diagnoses associated with class of substances

	Dependence	Abuse	Intoxication	Withdrawal	Intoxication delirium	Withdrawal delirium	Dementia	Amnestic disorder	Psychotic disorders	Mood disorders	Anxiety disorders	Sexual dysfunctions	Sleep Disorders
Alcohol	X	X	X	X	I	W	P	P	I/W	I/W	I/W	I	I/W
Amphetamines	X	X	X	X	I				I	I/W	I	I	I/W
Caffeine			X						–		I	–	I
Cannabis	X	X	X		I				I	–	I	–	–
Cocaine	X	X	X	X	I				I/W	I/W	I/W	I	I/W
Hallucinogens	X	X	X		I				I*	I	I	–	–
Inhalants	X	X	X		I		P		I	I	I	–	–
Nicotine	X			X					–	–	–	–	–
Opioids	X	X	X	X	I				I	I	–	I	I/W
Phencyclidine	X	X	X		I				I	I	I	–	–
Sedatives, hypnotics, or anxiolytics	X	X	X	X	I	W	P	P	I/W	I/W	W	I	I/W
Polysubstance	X								–	–	–	–	–
Other	X	X	X	X	I	W	P	P	I/W	I/W	I/W	I	I/W

*Also hallucinogen persisting perception disorder (flashbacks).

Note: S, I, W, I/W or P indicates that the category is recognised in DSM-IV. In addition, I indicates the specifier 'With Onset During Intoxication' may be noted for the category (except for Intoxication Delirium); W indicates the specifier 'With Onset During Withdrawal' may be noted for the category (except for Withdrawal Delirium); and I/W indicates that either 'With Onset During Intoxication' or 'With Onset During Withdrawal' may be noted for the category. P indicates that the disorder is Persisting. (American Psychiatric Association, 2000)

Alcohol

Alcohol is one of the most widely used substances globally, and has specific effects on the brain and behaviour. In many (but not all) societies, the use of alcohol is accepted as a social phenomenon and thus is easy to access due to this social acceptance and generally low cost.

What is a standard drink?

A standard drink contains 10 grams of alcohol, and the alcohol content of drinks is listed on labelling expressed as % w/v – the number of grams of alcohol that is found in 100 mL of the drink. For example, wine with an alcohol content of 12% will contain 12 grams of alcohol per 100 mL of wine – thus, a standard drink of this particular wine will be approximately 83 mL of wine. If the wine were a fortified wine of 20% alcohol, a standard drink would be just 50 mL. In this way, the alcohol content present in various wines, beers, spirits and liqueurs will vary very widely. It is important to note that drink serving sizes are often more than one standard drink. There are no common glass sizes used in Australia (Department of Health and Ageing, 2006). Note the following:

* For healthy men and women, drinking *no more than two standard drinks on any day* reduces your risk of harm from alcohol-related disease or injury over a lifetime. Guidelines also suggest that safe drinking patterns allow for alcohol-free days each week.

* Drinking *no more than four standard drinks on a single occasion* reduces the risk of alcohol-related injury arising from that occasion.

* Current guidelines in Australia and other jurisdictions suggest that no level of alcohol consumption during pregnancy can be designated as safe for the foetus.

When consumed, alcohol reaches peak concentrations within 30–90 minutes; however, there are metabolic differences due to body mass and gender. Alcohol interacts with many psychoactive medications and can also exacerbate existing mental health problems. With continued use, a degree of tolerance to the effects alcohol may develop, although this does not protect against end organ damage such as alcoholic liver disease or brain damage.

Based upon the latest available evidence (National Health and Medical Research Centre [NHMRC] level 1 [evidence obtained from a systematic review of all relevant randomised controlled trials] and evidence from the Joanna Briggs Institute [evidence category level A]), the Department of Health and Ageing in Australia recommends the interventions in Table 9.2 for alcohol abuse or dependence.

Table 9.2: Best practice for alcohol abuse or dependence intervention

Intervention Details	
Screening	Screening for risk levels of alcohol consumption and appropriate intervention systems should be widely implemented in general practice and emergency departments.
	AUDIT (Alcohol Use Disorders Identification Test) is the most sensitive of the currently available screening tools and is recommended for use in the general population.
	Indirect biological markers (liver function tests or carbohydrate-deficient transferrin) should only be used as an adjunct to other screening measures as they have lower sensitivity and specificity in detecting at-risk people than structured questionnaire approaches (such as AUDIT).
Assessment	A quantitative alcohol history should be recorded.
	Motivation to change should be assessed through direct questioning, although expressed motivation has only a moderate impact on treatment outcome.
	Patients/clients should be involved in goal setting and treatment planning.
Interventions	Brief interventions are effective in reducing alcohol use.
	Brief interventions are not recommended for people with more severe alcohol-related problems or alcohol dependence.
	Brief interventions may consist of the five components of the FLAGS acronym: feedback, listening, advice, goals, and strategies (or equivalent).
	Brief interventions should be implemented in general practice and other primary care centres and emergency departments.
Alcohol withdrawal: assessment, treatment and planning	Successful completion of alcohol withdrawal does not prevent recurrent alcohol consumption and additional interventions are needed to achieve long-term reduction in alcohol consumption.

Intervention	Details
Monitoring alcohol withdrawal	Alcohol withdrawal scales (CIWA-Ar, AWS) can be used to assess withdrawal severity, to guide treatment (such as symptom-triggered medication regimens) and to aid objective communication between clinicians, but should not be used as diagnostic tools.
Using benzodiazepines in alcohol withdrawal	Benzodiazepines are the recommended medication in managing alcohol withdrawal. In Australia, diazepam is recommended as 'gold standard' and as first-line treatment because of its rapid onset of action, long half-life and evidence for effectiveness. Loading with benzodiazepines (diazepam, lorazepam) and close monitoring for at least 24 hours is recommended after an alcohol withdrawal seizure.
Alternative and symptomatic medications in treatment of alcohol withdrawal	Carbamazepine is safe and effective as an alternative to benzodiazepines, although it is not effective in preventing further seizures in the same withdrawal episode. Antipsychotic medications should only be used as an adjunct to adequate benzodiazepine therapy for hallucinations or agitated delirium. They should not be used as stand-alone medication for withdrawal.
Pharmacotherapies for alcohol dependence	Pharmacotherapy should be considered for all alcohol-dependent patients/clients, in association with psychosocial supports. Naltrexone or acamprosate is recommended as relapse prevention for alcohol-dependent patients/clients. Disulfiram is no longer routinely recommended except in closely supervised patients/clients motivated for abstinence and with no contraindications.
Specific populations	Given the high prevalence of physical and mental comorbidities in the Indigenous population, clinicians should consider the possibility of physical and/or mental comorbidity in all presentations.
Managing co-occurring mental and alcohol-use disorders	Patients/clients with comorbid disorders of alcohol use and persisting mental health comorbidity should be offered treatment for both disorders. AUDIT is recommended for screening psychiatric populations.

Source: Department of Health and Ageing (2006)

Thiamine

Heavy alcohol drinkers are particularly prone to thiamine deficiency because of inadequate dietary intake, impaired gastrointestinal absorption, and impaired hepatic storage. Thiamine deficiency leads to a variety of serious neurological and cardiovascular signs. Early symptoms may be non-specific, and can include fatigue, irritability and abdominal discomfort. Severe deficiency can lead to the development of beriberi – cardiac, or 'wet' beriberi, is characterised by cardiac failure and oedema; 'dry' beriberi is characterised by peripheral neuropathy, muscle wasting and weakness, and paralysis. Wernicke-Korsakoff syndrome may also develop in severe cases of thiamine deficiency, often in association with chronic alcoholism. Wernicke's encephalopathy involves ocular abnormalities, gait ataxia and mental status changes, and can precede or occur concomitantly with Korsakoff's psychosis, a potentially permanent disorder of short-term memory loss that results in confabulation. Thiamine, given orally, intravenously or intramuscularly, is used in the treatment and also prevention of thiamine deficiency. The vitamin is available in Australia as thiamine hydrochloride 100 mg/mL ampoules and 100 mg tablets. Only small amounts of thiamine are absorbed from the gastrointestinal tract (the maximum amount absorbed after a single oral dose in healthy subjects is approximately 4.5 mg). Parenteral use is therefore usually recommended in severe deficiency to ensure adequate absorption. Adverse effects with thiamine are rare, but hypersensitivity reactions have occurred, primarily after parenteral doses. Thiamine is required for glucose metabolism; giving glucose in the presence of thiamine deficiency may potentially precipitate Wernicke's encephalopathy. Glucose and thiamine should therefore always be given at the same time to those at risk. At a dose of 100 mg orally each day, thiamine is an inexpensive and effective prophylactic measure that should be considered for all heavy alcohol users.

Ask yourself!

1   How could you incorporate regular alcohol and other substance screening into your routine practice?

2   What aspects of substance abuse or dependence relate to pharmacological considerations?

3   List three substances that mental health patients/clients may present with in terms of abuse or dependence. Include ideas related to how these substances may influence medication treatment (consider possible drug interactions with prescribed psychiatric medication).

Nicotine

Nicotine is a highly addictive and widely used drug, particularly by those who experience mental illness. Mental illness is associated with both higher rates of smoking and higher levels of smoking among smokers, with evidence from both the USA and Australia showing almost twice the rate of adults without mental disorders (Lawrence, Mitrou & Zubrick, 2009). Studies comparing smokers and non-smokers have shown that smokers have less grey matter density in the frontal brain area and larger amounts of nicotinic receptors. Research on the effects of smoking a cigarette confirms that smoking leads to the release of the neurotransmitter dopamine in brain reward areas and to nicotinic receptor binding (McClernon, 2009). Neurotransmitters are chemicals in the brain that allow the transmission of neural signals across synapses. Nicotine also mimics a common neurotransmitter in the brain called acetylcholine, which affects skeletal and heart muscle function.

The DSM-IV diagnostic criteria for drug dependency involves at least three of the following:

* The substance is often taken in larger amounts or over longer period than intended.

* There is a persistent desire or unsuccessful efforts to cut down or control use.

* A great deal of time is spent in activities necessary to obtain the substance, use the substance or recover from its effects.

* Important social, occupational or recreational activities are given up or reduced due to use of the substance.

* There is continued substance use despite knowledge of having a persistent or recurrent social, psychological or physical problem that is caused or exacerbated by the substance.

* Tolerance (the need for increased amounts to achieve effect) develops.

* Withdrawal symptoms occur.

The World Health Organization (International Classification of Diseases ICD-10) criteria for drug dependency relates to a cluster of behavioural, cognitive and physiological phenomena that develop after repeated use and that typically include:

* a strong desire to take the drug

* difficulty in controlling use

* a higher priority given to taking the drug than other activities or obligations

* persisting in use despite harmful consequences

* increased tolerance

* withdrawal symptoms.

The high rate of smoking translates to other complications such as cardiovascular risk; pulmonary disease can affect vision and cause stroke. There is also a gender-based debate emerging in the literature – the presence of schizophrenia spectrum disorder is a risk factor for tobacco use in men (Johnson, et al., 2010). This holds implications for using a gender-sensitive approach to smoking cessation programs. Importantly, increased nicotine metabolism in individuals using antiepileptic drugs (such as carbemazepine) has implications for increased smoking behaviour and exposure to more tobacco toxins (Williams, Gandhi & Benowitz, 2010). Given that some antiepileptics are used for their mood stabilisation effects, this has significant implications for people who experience mental illness.

One issue that may require attention in relation to the management of nicotine-dependent people is that policy decisions at state and local level may mean that while undergoing inpatient treatment, these people may not be able to use tobacco. For example, if a person is subject to a detention order in a non-smoking area, the lack of access to nicotine can precipitate significant withdrawal symptoms. These alone can contribute to increased agitation, anxiety, sleep disturbance and aggression, and there is evidence to suggest that nicotine withdrawal can contribute to the potential for violence and aggression, requiring drug and non-drug responses. To prevent or mitigate these problems, supplementary nicotine products such as gum, inhalers, patches or lozenges may be used to prevent or lessen symptoms of smoking withdrawal.

Tobacco smoking is known to influence the metabolism of other drugs, including caffeine, olanzapine, clozapine and donepezil. Cessation of smoking (even if using nicotine replacements such as patches) can reduce the clearance of these agents, meaning that caffeine intake should be reduced or the drug dosage decreased to prevent symptoms of toxicities.

It is clear that tobacco smoking contributes significantly to the increased morbidity and mortality associated with various psychiatric illnesses, and thus it is important to offer smokers assistance with smoking cessation. Cognitive approaches, combined with nicotine replacement therapy, can increase the likelihood of smoking cessation, although relapse rates remain high. Other specific pharmacotherapy such as bupropion and varenicline substantially increases quit rates relative to those achievable with nicotine replacement therapy or cognitive approaches alone, although caution is required, as these agents have themselves been associated with a range of adverse effects, including neuropsychiatric side effects.

Cannabis

In Australia, cannabis (marijuana) is an illicit drug that contains many psychoactive alkaloids, including the principal agent delta-9 tetra hydro-cannabinol (THC). Cannabis has an influence on mental health, where some experience distressing psychological effects (such as panic or extreme anxiety, confusion, and psychotic symptoms) when they use cannabis. These effects do not usually last after the effects of cannabis wear off, but for some the effects are more permanent. The longer term effects of cannabis use can relate to depression, suicidal ideation (in people with no prior history of a disorder), an increase in the risk of toxic psychosis (as mentioned), aggressiveness and memory impairment. A study undertaken in the 1980s supports the hypothesis that long-term cannabis use can lead to schizophrenia; it examined over 50 000 conscripts and followed them up for 15 years (Andréasson, Engström, Allebeck & Rydberg, 1987). This study found that the use of cannabis during adolescence increased the risk of schizophrenia. Similarly, a study that undertook a three-year follow-up of over 4000 people free from psychosis and about 60 with baseline psychotic disorder diagnosis demonstrated a strong relationship between cannabis and psychosis (Van Os, et al., 2002). In this study the length of cannabis exposure predicted the severity of the psychosis, and those who had a diagnosis of psychosis at baseline and used cannabis had a worse outcome (refer to Chapter 7 for more detail on psychoses). Cannabis use is also linked to a fourfold increase in depression and depressive symptoms (Bovasso, 2001) and an Australian study undertaken in 2002 reported a dose–effect association between cannabis, depression and anxiety (Patton et al., 2002). It is also clear that for people who already have a diagnosis of schizophrenia, use of cannabis destabilises symptom control and may contribute to non-adherence with prescribed antipsychotic treatment, compromising outcomes.

There is a high lifetime prevalence of cannabis use among people who experience severe mental illness, with rates of use higher in males in Western countries. Cannabis is believed to activate dopamine release in the brain and, unlike nicotine, alcohol and cocaine, it has been widely believed that cannabis was not addictive; however, this is not the case. It is believed that the dopamine release is part of the addictive propensity of cannabis (Copeland & Swift, 2009). There are reports that the antipsychotics quetiapine (Potvin, et al., 2006) and clozapine (Zimmet, Strous, Burgess, Kohnstamm & Green, 2000) can reduce cannabis use or craving.

Cocaine

Cocaine is an alkaloid found naturally occurring in the leaves of *Erythroxylon coca*, and was first isolated from the coca leaf in the mid 1800s. Towards the late 1800s cocaine was used as an anaesthetic and, towards the end of the 19th century, Sigmund Freud proposed cocaine for the treatment of mental disorders such as depression. An interesting piece of trivia related to cocaine is that in 1885 John Pemberton registered a drink in the USA that contained cocaine and the drink was later called Coca-Cola. (Modern Coca-Cola does not contain cocaine.)

Cocaine can be abused through inhalation, subcutaneous injection, intravenous injection and smoking. Due to poor absorption, cocaine is rarely ingested. There is a growing evidence base related to the risks of cocaine use for mental health and there are reports of high levels of comorbidity (dual diagnosis) among cocaine users who demonstrate a greater number of symptoms and higher levels of psychosis and depression (Gossop, Marsden, Stewart & Kidd, 2002; McKay, Alterman, Cacciola, Mulvaney & O'Brien, 2000). A study examining the brains of those who used cocaine found dopamine levels in cocaine users as compared to non-drug users was lower. The findings revealed more dopamine transporters in the brain as the brain's way of compensating for lowered dopamine levels, increasing the overall uptake of dopamine (Little et al., 2009). As is well known, excessive neurotransmission of dopamine is associated with schizophrenia and other forms of psychosis, and antipsychotics form a class of drug with a high affinity for dopamine receptors. The chemical structure of antipsychotics allows them to bind to dopamine receptors and block dopamine receptors without setting off an action potential, helping reduce the excess levels of dopamine and alleviating the positive symptoms of psychosis.

Ecstasy

3,4-methylenedioxy-N-methylamphetamine, or MDMA, is the chemical name for the drug 'ecstasy'. It was discovered in 1912 and originally intended for medicinal purposes (Freudenmann, Öxler & Bernschneider-Reif, 2006). There are many street names that ecstasy is known by: E, pills, doves, and Jack and Jills. Ecstasy is a stimulant, exciting the central nervous system and affecting the neurotransmitters dopamine, serotonin and noradrenaline. MDMA is ingested (usually by tablets or powder) and the effects last 3–6 hours.

The effects of ecstasy can include an increased feeling of well-being and increased self-confidence. The physiological effects of ecstasy include increased body temperature and pulse rate, sweating, nausea, anxiety and jaw clenching. High-dose ecstasy can produce distorted perception (hallucinations), aberrant behaviours, vomiting and convulsions, and long-term use can cause damage to the brain and liver. Mortality from ecstasy use is usually related to polydipsia (drinking too much), overheating and cardiac problems. Ecstasy can also produce a feeling of 'coming down' for individuals when the effects of the drug begin to wear off. Some of these effects include insomnia or excessive sleep, hunger, irritability and feelings of apathy. MDMA dependence is strongly associated with elevated psychopathology and interferes with psychoactive medications, in particular those that target dopamine and serotonin. A recent dangerous trend is the combined use of ecstasy with prescription antidepressant drugs such as SSRIs or moclobemide, with the intention being to intensify the serotonergic effects and decrease the likely 'coming down' effect. This in itself has not led to a street market for the antidepressants, but it is important to highlight that this practice is highly dangerous and may contribute to a substantially increased risk of serious toxicity, including the serotonin syndrome.

Heroin

Heroin is an opioid derivative discovered in the 1870s. Initially, heroin was marketed as a children's cough suppressant. Opium comes from the seed pods of poppy plants and includes compounds such as morphine and codeine. The effects of heroin may last 3–5 hours and include intense pleasure and a feeling of well-being, slurred speech, dry mouth, slowed breathing, affected coordination, pain relief and decreased blood pressure and heart rate. Heroin can also cause nausea and vomiting, a suppressed cough response and constricted pupils. Using greater quantities of heroin can cause poor concentration; nausea and vomiting is more likely to occur; sweating and itching can occur; and the user may fall asleep. If too much heroin is injected death can occur, usually by respiratory depression.

About 8–12 hours after the user's last heroin injection, a withdrawing individual will begin to experience flu-like symptoms: sneezing, weakness, muscle cramps, nausea, vomiting, diarrhoea. The symptoms increase in severity over two or three days, and within a week to 10 days the illness is over.

The ongoing use of injected heroin is associated with many adverse psychiatric, psychosocial and medical complications. Shared injecting equipment may contribute to the possibility of blood-borne diseases including viral hepatitis, human immunodeficiency virus (HIV) and others. The high costs involved may contribute to unlawful or dangerous behaviours such as theft or prostitution, to finance the purchase of drugs. Street heroin may be contaminated with impurities such as talc (a filler that increases profits for deals sold by weight). Dosages are not standardised, contributing to the risk of overdose. Many public health authorities advocate regulated supply of standardised heroin with clean injecting equipment as a means of harm minimisation.

Regulated opioid replacement using medications such as methadone or buprenorphine is widely used in Australia with the objective of harm minimisation. Patients/clients collect a daily dose of the medication from a registered and specified clinic or community pharmacy. The system of opioid replacement also operates extensively in corrective facilities such as prisons. Considerable caution is needed to avoid serious drug interactions with other CNS suppressant drugs such as benzodiazepines, which may increase the risk of death from respiratory depression. Some antidepressants such as fluvoxamine can increase methadone levels, leading to serious toxicities.

Crystal methamphetamine

Crystal methamphetamine, also referred to by the street name 'Ice', is a powerful form of amphetamine that has a rapid onset of action and longer duration of effect than other related drugs. The drug is usually is usually smoked using a pipe or injected, but may be inhaled or swallowed. Crystal methamphetamine causes effects such as euphoria, excitement and a sense of well-being, a sense of confidence, increased talkativeness, and increased libido. The agent causes many serious adverse psychiatric effects ranging from nervousness, anxiety, agitation and panic to serious paranoia, hallucinations, and uncontrollable hostility and aggression. Many heavy users experience psychosis, and may also develop serious withdrawal effects after discontinuation (e.g. restlessness, irritability, anxiety, paranoia, depression and increased sleep times). The use of this drug is associated with serious medical harm, affecting many organ systems. Like many illicit drugs, crystal methamphetamine can impair the ability to drive a motor vehicle, substantially increasing the risk of road accidents. The increasingly widespread use of this agent has contributed to increased presentations in Australian hospital emergency departments and the need to deal with violent and chaotic behaviours that are often observed during intoxication or withdrawal.

Prescribed medications

Although attention is often focused upon the effects of illicit drugs and social substance use (e.g. alcohol and tobacco), it is important to remember that prescribed medical drugs can also be implicated in substance use disorders. Drugs such as benzodiazepines and prescribed opioids may be used for legitimate purposes, but it is still common for a person to become dependent on these, or to use them in a pattern consistent with the diagnostic parameters for substance abuse. Abrupt discontinuation may result in severe withdrawal syndromes, and comorbid dependence upon illicit drugs or alcohol is also relatively common. Other prescribed medications are also subject to abuse potential, such as SSRIs in combination with MDMA, and antipsychotics such as olanzapine or quetiapine to mitigate the most severe aspects of crystal methamphetamine withdrawal. Oxycodone has rapidly become a substantial contributor to iatrogenic harm mediated through dependence or intoxication, with some research now suggesting that this prescription opioid may cause more presentations to emergency departments than heroin. An individual may not even be dependent upon these substances themselves, but may seek to gain supplies to on-sell for financial gain, or to finance a habit of illicit drug use.

IAN'S STORY

Ian is a 45-year old man with a 20-year history of alcohol dependency. He is divorced, and is living in a local hostel. He has three grown-up boys and has had several prison sentences in the past; offences range from shoplifting and drug dealing. He was recently caught stealing alcohol and was highly intoxicated at the time. He has a court case pending for this.

Ian has been known to the local mental health service for several years. He does not adhere to his treatment regimen at times and states he has 'really bad depression'. His diagnosis is alcohol dependence, psychosis and depression. He has been prescribed antidepressants and antipsychotics (olanzapine) by his GP.

Ian has had pathology tests ordered by his GP and test results have shown that his liver is badly affected by his drinking; he has been advised to reduce and/or stop drinking. Despite this, he is craving alcohol badly and finding this hard to cope with. Ian talks about drinking himself to death, is sleeping badly, and has been agitated and pacing around his accommodation most nights.

Ask yourself!

As Ian's health care worker:

1   What are your concerns about Ian?
2   When you develop a comprehensive care plan with Ian:
   • Indicate how you would engage Ian in developing the plan together. How would you engage Ian in treatment?
   • What is Ian's level of motivation to modify his lifestyle choices – drinking alcohol excessively – and how would you assess and then review this?
   • What services should be involved with Ian and what would their roles be within this care plan?
3   What risks should you consider when developing Ian's care plan?

Care considerations for people with substance use disorders

According to the United Nations Office on Drugs and Crime while a proportion of the world's population uses illicit drugs each year (about 5% between the ages of 15 and 64), only a small proportion of these are considered problem drug users (0.6%). An estimated 155 to 250 million people use street drugs each year globally (United Nations Office on Drugs and Crime, 2010). It has been reported in Australia that 40% of people with psychosis met the criteria for **substance dependence** or abuse, with this figure being similar in the United Kingdom and the United States of America (Croton, 2005).

An illustration of prevalence of dual diagnosis in those who experience mental illness can be drawn from United Kingdom research (Frisher et al., 2004), which suggests the prevalence of substance dependence and/or abuse disorder in patients/clients with a mental illness was especially high in people with a diagnosis of a psychotic disorder. In addition, other studies reveal substance use among people with first-episode psychosis was more common in men than women and was twice that of the general population (Addington & Addington, 2007; Barnett, et al., 2007; Farrelly et al., 2007), with the prevalence of substance use and early psychosis between 39% and 51% (Edward, Hearity & Felstead, 2011).

In Australia, historically, mental health and alcohol and drug services offered patients/clients treatment from two separate and different sets of specialist clinicians, resulting in the patient/client having to negotiate separate treatment pathways, with the risk of falling through the treatment service 'cracks' or gaps (Staiger, Long & Baker, 2010). To help people address mental health and substance misuse issues (Topp, 2007) current Health Department policy in Victoria, Australia requires clinicians from both sectors to develop expertise in each other's fields so that patients/clients are able to obtain treatment via entry points from both services. The initiative is labelled the 'No Wrong Door Policy'. In both the United States (Mojtabai, 2004) and United Kingdom (Wright, Smeeth & Heath, 2003) there has been a concentrated effort to develop guidelines for establishing expert practice and treatment programs for dually diagnosed persons.

From the consumer's perspective – *How does this feel for me?*

One dual diagnosis client said (Edward & Robins, 2012):

> Less than 2 months ago I was hospitalized, suicidal, psychotic, strung out …
> I stayed in the hospital for 2 weeks, got back on my meds, came home. I have
> tried to maintain my sanity, and function. Sure didn't take long to let myself
> down again. I still have my family fooled, but I'm unravelling as we speak …
> I'm exhausted, I'm alone, I need hope, I need so much …

Consider this quote and reflect on how you could maximise a client-centred
approach that assist the patient/client to well-being.

TOM'S STORY

Tom is a 39-year-old married man who lives with his wife and two children in a
metropolitan area. He has an eight-year history of psychosis and a comorbid
substance disorder. Tom is prescribed risperidone. Tom admits to drinking two
bottles of wine per day and he says he uses cannabis each day to relax. Tom is
currently unemployed.

Tom had never taken risperidone before, so to establish tolerability Tom was
prescribed with oral risperidone prior to initiating treatment with risperidone long-
acting injection.

Tom tolerated risperidone well and was later prescribed 25 mg every two weeks by
deltoid or deep IM gluteal injection. Oral risperidone was given with the first injection
and continued for three weeks to ensure adequate therapeutic plasma concentrations
are maintained prior to the main release phase of risperidone from the injection.

Although dose response for effectiveness has not been established for the
risperidone long-acting injection, some patients/clients not responding to 25 mg
may benefit from a higher dose of 37.5 mg or 50 mg. The maximum dose should not
exceed 50 mg every two weeks. Tom responded to the 25 mg dose.

Care Plan

The following is an example care plan for the patient/client presented in this chapter.
The areas of daily living that are considered include bio-psycho-social factors
and the plan is mapped out using the nursing process (Assessment; Planning;
Implementation; Evaluation). Remember: the success is in the detail, so be specific
about *who, when and what* in the collaborative plan; never include someone in the
plan if they were not consulted in the planning process; and always work within a
recovery-orientated framework (refer to Chapter 1).

Date: 15/8/12

Client's name: Tom   Case manager: DD Nurse   Present at meeting: Tom, Mrs Tom and DD Nurse

Areas of daily living	Assessment of current situation	Goal	Plan (undertaken with patient/client)	Implementation	Who is responsible? (Include only those who have been consulted in the planning process)	Evaluation/ Review date
Mental health	8-year history of psychosis and a comorbid substance disorder.	Minimise the adverse effects of psychotic symptoms.	Monitor early warning signs of psychosis, which are: • feeling more agitated • pacing more • poor sleep. Action: if early warning signs are present: • use distraction techniques • call DD Nurse to discuss and organise a possible review of medication.	Develop an early warning signs list with Tom and document this for Tom's record and DD Nurse record. Tom to keep a list of early warning signs with him and a copy to be attached to the fridge door.	Tom DD Nurse Tom	15/8/12 Ongoing

(Continued)

Date: 15/8/12 (Continued)

Clients name: Tom   Case manager: DD Nurse   Present at meeting: Tom, Mrs Tom and DD Nurse

Areas of daily living	Assessment of current situation	Goal	Plan (undertaken with patient/client)	Implementation	Who is responsible? (Include only those who have been consulted in the planning process)	Evaluation/ Review date
Social	Lives at home with wife and children. Marital stress related to budget concerns.	Review budget and reduce expenditure on substances.	Tom and his wife to review budget with a social worker.	DD Nurse to link Tom and his wife to social worker.	DD Nurse	15/8/12
Biological	History of non-adherence to medication/ treatment.	Improve adherent behaviour.	Discuss motivation, beliefs and ambivalence for adhering or not adhering to medication/treatment.	Continue with regular appointments with DD Nurse.	DD Nurse and Tom	Every 2 weeks
	Prescribed 25 mg resperidone IM.	Maintain therapeutic effect of resperidone.	Maintain therapeutic effect of resperidone.	Ensure regular appointments for Tom with psychiatrist related to positive effects of resperidone.	DD Nurse	Every 12 weeks

Environmental	Not working at the moment.	Would like to find work (including volunteer work).	Register with disability employment network group.	Tom to call disability employment network to register.	Tom and DD Nurse	12/9/12
Substance using behaviours	Consumes 2 bottles of wine a day.	Reduce the risks associated with risk drinking.	Explore Tom's motivations and beliefs related to drinking alcohol beyond what is recommended.	Work together to discuss reduced drinking or alcohol drinking cessation.	DD Nurse and Tom	Each appointment
	Smokes 8 joints of cannabis each day.	Reduce the risks associated with cannabis use.	Explore Tom's motivations and beliefs related to cannabis use.	Work together to discuss reduced cannabis use or stopping cannabis use.	DD Nurse and Tom	Each appointment

On the Horizon in Pharmacotherapy for Substance Abuse

The lack of meaningful recent progress towards the development of truly effective treatments for substance dependence has led to interest in alternative approaches that might address addiction at a fundamental molecular level. Anti-addiction vaccines are one approach that is currently being explored; this strategy relies upon agents that allow the production of antibodies to block the effects of drugs in the brain. Both passive and active immunisation approaches have been the subject of research into the treatment of dependence on cocaine, methamphetamine, nicotine, phencyclidine and heroin. It is thought that eventually it may be possible to develop antibodies that bind substances in circulation, preventing access and binding to sites in the CNS.

Topiramate is emerging as a promising treatment for alcoholism. It has been proven to be more effective than placebo, reduces the percentage of heavy drinking days, increases the number of days of abstinence, decreases the liver damage observed with heavy alcohol use, and enhances the quality of life and overall functionality of those treated. Some research also suggests that topiramate may in fact be more effective than naltrexone, a treatment that is already approved and in widespread use for this indication.

Although debate on the subject continues to polarise opinion among health care workers and the general public alike, the issue of supervised heroin injecting as a management strategy for opioid dependence appears to be worthy of further consideration. Some people who use heroin do not benefit from conventional treatments. Recent research has compared supervised injectable treatment with medicinal heroin supervised injectable methadone and optimised oral methadone for chronic heroin addiction (Strang et al., 2010). Those receiving injectable heroin were significantly more likely to have achieved the primary outcome (there is less laboratory evidence for the use of street heroin).

Summary

In this chapter you explored what substance disorders were including the two categories for substance disorders that are located in DSM-IV. From reading and working through this chapter you have discovered how substance disorders relate to people with mental illnesses, while considering their pharmacological implications for care; best practice for alcohol abuse or dependence intervention; nicotine and mental illness; cannabis and mental illness; ecstasy, heroin and mental illness; and care considerations for patients/clients with substance disorders.

Discussion questions

1 *How* would you negotiate dual services for those who experience dual diagnosis?

2 *Who* can provide care to people who are experiencing dual diagnosis?

3 *What* are the physiological implications for those with a mental illness and prescribed antipsychotic medications and are using cannabis?

4 *What* lessons can be learnt from a greater understanding of addictive behaviours?

Test yourself (answers at the back of the book)

1 Which of the following is regarded as a standard drink of alcohol?

   A 10 mL

   B 10 g

   C 20 mL

   D 20 g

2 Consideration of the administration of which of the following vitamins is most critical when dealing with the management of a patient/client with heavy or sustained alcohol intake?

   A Ascorbic acid

   B Riboflavin

   C Thiamine

   D Calcitriol

3 Which of the following drugs is an example of an agent used to assist with smoking cessation?

   A Citalopram

   B Bupropion

   C Moclobemide

   D Duloxetine

4   Metabolism of which of the following drugs may decrease markedly after smoking cessation?

   A   Sertraline

   B   Clozapine

   C   Alprazolam

   D   Lithium

5   If dealing with a person who has abruptly stopped drinking after heavy and sustained alcohol intake, which of the following drugs is helpful to reduce the likelihood of a significant withdrawal reaction?

   A   Diazepam

   B   Disulfiram

   C   Acamprosate

   D   Naltrexone

Useful websites

Alcohol Use Disorders Identification Test available at <http://whqlibdoc.who.int/hq/2001/who_msd_msb_01.6a.pdf>

Headspace available at <www.headspace.org.au/what-works/research-information/substance-use>

World Health Organization – *Psychoactive Substances* available at <www.who.int/substance_abuse/publications/psychoactives/en>

World Health Organization – *ATLAS 2010: First Global Report on Substance Use Disorders Launched*: <www.who.int/substance_abuse/publications/Media/en>

References

Addington J. & Addington, D. (2007). 'Patterns, predictors and impact of substance use in early psychosis: a longitudinal study' *Acta Psychiatrica Scandinavica* 115(4): 304–309.

American Psychiatric Association. (2000). *Diagnostic and Statistical Manual of Mental Disorders*, 4th edn, Text Revision (DSM-IV-TR). Washington DC: American Psychiatric Publishing, Inc.

Andréasson S., Engström A., Allebeck P. & Rydberg U. (1987). 'Cannabis and schizophrenia: a longitudinal study of Swedish conscripts' *Lancet* 330(8574): 1483–1486.

Barnett J. H. et al. (2007). 'Substance use in a population-based clinic sample of people with first-episode psychosis' *British Journal Of Psychiatry: The Journal Of Mental Science* 190: 515–520.

Bovasso, G. B. (2001). Cannabis abuse as a risk factor for depressive symptoms. *American Journal of Psychiatry* 158(12): 2033–2037.

Copeland, J. & Swift, W. (2009). 'Cannabis use disorder: epidemiology and management' *International Review of Psychiatry* 21(2): 96–103.

Croton, G. (2005). *Australian Treatment System's Recognition of and Response to Co-occurring Mental Health & Substance Use Disorders: Submission to the 2005 Senate Select Committee on Mental Health*. Retrieved 17 September 2007, from <www.dualdiagnosis.org.au/home/index.php?option=com_docman&task=doc_download&gid=4>.

Department of Health and Ageing. (2006). *National Alcohol Strategy 2006–2009: Towards Safer Drinking Cultures* (No. 3900). Canberra: Commonwealth of Australia.

Edward K., Hearity R. N. & Felstead B. (2012). 'Service integration for the dually diagnosed' *Australian Journal of Primary Care* 18: 17–22.

Edward, K. L. & Robins, A. (2012). 'Dual diagnosis, as described by those who experience the disorder: Using the Internet as a source of data' *International Journal of Mental Health Nursing* 21(6): 550–559. doi: 10.1111/j.1447-0349.2012.00833.x

Farrelly S., Harris M. G., Henry L. P. et al. (2007). 'Prevalence and correlates of comorbidity 8 years after a first psychotic episode' *Acta Psychiatrica Scandinavica* 116(1): 62–70.

Freudenmann R. W., Öxler F. & Bernschneider-Reif, S. (2006). 'The origin of MDMA (ecstasy) revisited: the true story reconstructed from the original documents' *Addiction* 101(9): 1241–1245.

Frisher M., Collins J., Millson D., Crome I., & Croft P. (2004). 'Prevalence of co-morbid psychiatric illness and substance abuse in primary care in England and Wales' *J Epidemiol Community Health* 58(12): 1036–1041.

Gossop M., Marsden J., Stewart D. & Kidd T. (2002). 'Changes in use of crack cocaine after drug misuse treatment: 4–5 year follow-up results from the National Treatment Outcome Research Study (NTORS)' *Drug and Alcohol Dependence* 66(1): 21–28.

Johnson J. et al. (2010). 'Gender-specific profiles of tobacco use among non-institutionalized people with serious mental illness' *BMC Psychiatry* 10(1): 101.

Kessler R., Nelson C., McGonagle K., Edlund R. & Leaf P. (1996). 'The epidemiology of co-occurring addictive and mental disorders: implications for prevention and service utilization' *American Journal of Orthopsychiatry* 66(1): 17–31.

Kessler R., Chiu W., Demler O. & Walters E. (2005). 'Prevalence, severity, and comorbidity of twelve-month DSM-IV disorders in the National Comorbidity Survey Replication (NCS-R)' *Archives of General Psychiatry* 62(6): 617–627.

Lawrence D., Mitrou F. & Zubrick S. (2009). 'Smoking and mental illness: results from population surveys in Australia and the United States' *BMC Public Health* 9(1): 285.

Little K. Y. et al. (2009). 'Decreased brain dopamine cell numbers in human cocaine users' *Psychiatry Research* 168(3): 173–180.

McClernon F. (2009). 'Neuroimaging of nicotine dependence: key findings and application to the study of smoking–mental illness co-morbidity' *Journal of Dual Diagnosis* 5(2): 168–178.

McKay J. R., Alterman A. I., Cacciola J. S., Mulvaney F. D. & O'Brien C. P. (2000). 'Prognostic significance of antisocial personality disorder in cocaine-dependent patients entering continuing care' *Journal of Nervous and Mental Disease* 188(5): 287.

Mojtabai, R. (2004). 'Which substance abuse treatment facilities offer dual diagnosis programs?' *American Journal of Drug and Alcohol Abuse* 30(3): 525–536.

Patton G. C. et al. (2002). 'Cannabis use and mental health in young people: cohort study' *BMJ* 325(7374): 1195–1198.

Potvin S. et al. (2006). Quetiapine in patients with comorbid schizophrenia-spectrum and substance use disorders: an open-label trial. *Current Medical Research and Opinion* 22(7), 1277–1285.

Staiger P. K., Long C. & Baker A. (2010). 'Health service systems and comorbidity: stepping up to the mark' *Mental Health and Substance Use: Dual Diagnosis* 3(2): 148–161.

Strang J., Metrebian N., Lintzeris N., Potts L., Carnwath T., Mayet S. et al. (2010) 'Supervised injectable heroin or injectable methadone versus optimised oral methadone as treatment for chronic heroin addicts in England after persistent failure in orthodox treatment (RIOTT): a randomised trial' *Lancet* 375: 1885–1895.

Teesson M., Hall W., Lynskey M. & Degenhardt L. (2000). 'Alcohol- and drug-use disorders in Australia: implications of the National Survey of Mental Health and Wellbeing' *Australian and New Zealand Journal of Psychiatry* 34(2): 206–213.

Topp, L. (2007). 'Comorbidity: a chance for change' *Of Substance* 5(1): 16–19.

United Nations Office on Drugs and Crime. (2010). *World Drug Report 2010.* New York: United Nations.

Van Os, J. et al (2002). Cannabis use and psychosis: a longitudinal population-based study. *American Journal of Epidemiology* 156(4): 319–327.

Williams J. M., Gandhi K. K. & Benowitz N. L. (2010). 'Carbamazepine but not valproate induces CYP2A6 activity in smokers with mental illness' *Cancer Epidemiology Biomarkers & Prevention* 19(10): 2582–2589.

Wright N., Smeeth L. & Heath, I. (2003). 'Moving beyond single and dual diagnosis in general practice' *BMJ* 326(7388): 512–514.

Zimmet S. V., Strous R. D., Burgess E. S., Kohnstamm S. & Green, A. I. (2000). 'Effects of clozapine on substance use in patients with schizophrenia and schizoaffective disorder: a retrospective survey' *Journal of Clinical Psychopharmacology* 20(1): 94.

Chapter 10

Mental Illness in Children and Adolescents

Chapter overview

This chapter covers the following topics:

* general considerations in child and adolescent psychiatry

* characteristics of attention deficit/hyperactivity disorder (ADHD)

* specific issues with psychotropic drug use in younger people.

Chapter learning objectives

After reading this chapter, you should be able to:

* describe the range of mental illnesses that may affect children or adolescents

* outline diagnostic and target symptoms of ADHD

* discuss the special considerations that must be taken into account when using psychotropic drugs for the treatment of children and adolescents.

Key terms

Attention deficit/hyperactivity disorder (ADHD)
Autism-spectrum disorders
Child and adolescent psychiatry
Tic disorders

Introduction

The manifestation of mental illness in childhood or adolescence presents many difficult dilemmas. Although some psychiatric conditions are most commonly or almost exclusively observed in childhood and adolescence, it is also evident that many mental disorders that are observed during adulthood may also affect children and teenagers. The parameters for the diagnosis and treatment of mental illness in **child and adolescent psychiatry** has at times created highly polarised debate in the general medical community, among paediatricians, within psychiatry and in the broader community. Special challenges exist for clinicians with respect to the diagnosis of mental illness in younger people, and also in the treatment of these conditions once diagnosed. In recent years, the emotive issue of suicide and suicidal behaviour in younger people treated with psychotropic drugs has been the subject of intense international discussion, with prominent clinicians promulgating strongly held viewpoints that are often conflicting in nature. This chapter will present issues related to child and adolescent psychiatry including ADHD, **autism spectrum disorders**, **tic disorders**, depression and other affective disorders in children and adolescents, and discussion throughout related to pharmacotherapy for patients/clients in this age bracket.

Special issues in child and adolescent psychiatry

The diagnosis and treatment of mental illness in children and adolescents present many specific challenges that are not necessarily important (or even relevant) in adult psychiatry. General issues that require special consideration in the context of child and adolescent psychiatry include:

✱ Self-description may not provide accurate or complete assessment. Children may find it difficult or impossible to express an accurate history and therefore clinicians seeking to obtain a mental state examination may find assessment difficult. This may be due to verbal skills which may not have developed to a point that allows reliable articulation of the symptoms or particular phenomenology the child experiences. Families and/or teachers may need to be accessed as sources of information, but even when these approaches are used, the full picture still may not be obtained. At times, if a clinician is perceived by the child as an authority figure, reporting of symptoms, thoughts or behaviours may be incomplete or misportrayed because of a fear of reprisals (which may not be revealed).

* Neurodevelopment is a complex process that evolves quite rapidly across the spectrum of childhood years and continues into early adulthood. As the central nervous system develops it is also subject to the effects of environmental influences, including the effects of individual parenting and educational style and a variety of cultural influences. There is great variability in the combined influences of genetic predisposition and environmental influences, meaning that the characteristics of mental illness in younger people may be highly disparate.

* The effects of gestational, perinatal and childhood brain damage may produce behavioural changes that position a child outside of traditional conduct norms, but this may not necessarily represent a diagnosable or treatable psychiatric disorder.

* Societal stigma related to mental illness, scepticism and disparate clinical views are particularly common in relation to paediatric psychiatry. There are still clinicians and others in the wider community who are sceptical about the existence of various mental illnesses that are diagnosed for children; for instance, the scientific validity of the diagnostic construct for conditions such as ADHD is still called into doubt by some. In some cases, there is a tendency to view abnormal behaviour among children as the result of character flaws or the direct effect of flawed parenting styles, even if the diagnostic entity has been long accepted in the medical and psychological arena.

* Child abuse or neglect is not a valid basis for the diagnosis of a mental illness among children or adolescents. In fact, in cases of significant child abuse or neglect, it would be expected that a child may have behaviours that differ from those of their peers. On the other hand, abnormal behaviours among children cannot be taken to imply that the child has been exposed to abuse or neglect.

* Children do not necessarily respond to the effects of psychotropic drugs in the same way as adults – pharmacokinetic and pharmacodynamic influences

can change the therapeutic effects of drugs and also the prevalence and nature of some adverse effects. Due to metabolic considerations, body mass and other factors, the dosage of the drugs will often require modification relative to that used for adults, and the monitoring regimen that is recommended may be different.

* Robust evidence from high quality clinical trials may not be available to inform the approach to paediatric pharmacotherapy in psychiatry. Children are less likely to be enrolled as subjects in clinical trials (often due to ethical considerations and implications), and there may be a lower threshold for withdrawing a child from a research study. This may mean that reliable guidance in relation to the dosage and administration of psychotropic drugs is lacking, and the use of these agents for younger people may be for 'off label' or 'non-approved indications'. It is important to remember under these circumstances that a lack of clear evidence to support a specific approach to management does not necessarily equate to clear evidence that an approach to clinical management is unsupportable. In real-life settings, clinicians are sometimes compelled to operate in an 'evidence vacuum'.

* Societal expectations engender a particularly conservative approach to the use of drugs for children. 'Black box' warnings and official statements issued by agencies such as the Australian Therapeutic Goods Administration (TGA) and the United States Food and Drug Administration (FDA) may have a profound impact upon prescribing practices for children.

* The nature of mental illness in the child or adolescent usually means that management is not regarded as routine practice for general health services/ generalist clinicians. Management of serious mental illness in a child is always included in routine practice for a paediatric mental health specialist. Access to such services may be limited or difficult in some settings.

Although many psychiatric syndromes seen in adults (e.g. major depression, mania, anxiety states and psychosis) are also sometimes diagnosed for children, there is a range of conditions that are most commonly encountered in children and adolescents (refer to Table 10.1).

Table 10.1: Examples of psychiatric syndromes observed in children and adolescents

Attention deficit and disruptive behaviour disorders: ADHD is associated with prominent inattention +/– hyperactivity and impulsivity. Other disorders in this classification include conduct disorder (a pattern of behaviour that violates the rights of others or major societal norms and rules), and oppositional defiant disorder (abnormally negative, hostile, and defiant behaviour).

Mental retardation: below-average intellectual functioning (IQ of 70 or below) with onset before the age of 18 years.

Learning disorders: below-expected academic performance relative to age, intelligence, and education. A well-known example is reading disorder, sometimes referred to as dyslexia.

Pervasive developmental disorders: impairment in reciprocal social interaction and communication; stereotyped behaviour, interests and activities. Examples include autistic disorder and Asperger's disorder.

Tic disorders: characterised by vocal and/or motor tics, e.g. Tourette's disorder.

Attention deficit/hyperactivity disorder

Probably the most well known of the psychiatric disorders affecting children and adolescents, **attention deficit/hyperactivity disorder** (ADHD) can also affect adults – in fact, in many cases where the condition is diagnosed in adulthood, a carefully compiled retrospective history can suggest the presence of diagnosable ADHD during childhood and which may have compromised potential academic achievement and normal childhood development. The prevalence of ADHD is estimated to be 3–7% among school-age children. The characteristic diagnostic features are inattention and/or hyperactivity and impulsivity symptoms that are seen with greater frequency or severity to that typically observed among peers. To be able to make a diagnosis, symptoms of ADHD causing impairment must have been present before the child's seventh birthday. Impairment relating to symptoms must be present in at least two contexts (such as at home and school) and would impair functional capacity relative to that which would otherwise be expected from developmentally equivalent peers. ADHD cannot be diagnosed if symptoms are attributable to another serious psychiatric illness such as a psychotic disorder, mood disorder or anxiety disorder. Symptoms of ADHD are outlined in Table 10.2.

Table 10.2: Diagnostic criteria for ADHD

To be diagnosed with ADHD, a child must have either:

- at least six of the key symptoms of inattention, present for six months or more, to an extent that is maladaptive and inconsistent with developmental level:

  - often fails to give close attention to detail, careless mistakes in schoolwork, etc.

  - often has difficulty sustaining attention in tasks

  - does not seem to listen when spoken to directly

  - often does not follow through on instructions and fails to finish tasks

  - has difficulty organising tasks and activities

  - avoids, dislikes, tries not to take on tasks requiring sustained mental effort

  - often loses things necessary for tasks or activities (e.g., schoolwork, pencils, books)

  - is easily distracted by extraneous stimuli

  - is often forgetful

or:

- at least six of the key symptoms of hyperactivity-impulsivity, present for six months or more, to an extent that is maladaptive and inconsistent with developmental level:

Hyperactivity:

- fidgets with hands or feet or squirms in seat

- often leaves seat in classroom or in other situations in which remaining seated is expected

- runs about or climbs excessively in situations where this would be inappropriate

- often has difficulty playing quietly

- is seen to be 'on the go' or often acts as if 'driven'

- often talks excessively

Impulsivity:

- shouts out answers before questions have finished

- has difficulty waiting their turn

- often interrupts or intrudes on others

Symptoms causing impairment need to have been present before seventh birthday, and impairment is present in two or more settings.

Source: American Psychiatric Association (2000)

Associated findings that may be seen can include low frustration tolerance, anger outbursts, stubbornness, mood lability, peer rejection and low self-esteem. Academic achievement is often diminished. Comorbid oppositional defiant disorder or conduct disorder are common.

Treatment of ADHD

Treatment of ADHD should not be considered until an appropriate evaluation has been undertaken by a properly qualified specialist (an experienced paediatrician or paediatric psychiatrist). Elements of the evaluation must include a full medical and developmental history, a mental state examination and a thorough physical examination. Collateral history about the child's behaviour should be obtained from parents and teachers, and this process should be repeated periodically to monitor the subsequent progress of treatment. Pharmacotherapy may not be required in mild to moderate cases, as behavioural therapy and education may prove to be sufficient.

The psychostimulant drugs are regarded as the first-line pharmacotherapy options for the treatment of ADHD, and produce benefits in reducing inattention and also hyperactivity and impulsivity. Both dexamphetamine and methylphenidate are equally effective treatments for ADHD, and if one agent is used without adequate response, a trial of the other should be considered. It is generally accepted that psychostimulants should not be prescribed for a child younger than four years. Careful monitoring is required to assess children treated with psychostimulants for possible adverse effects (refer to Table 10.3).

Table 10.3: Safety concerns with psychostimulant use in children

Common adverse effects include headaches, sleep disturbance, and gastrointestinal upset (including loss of appetite).
Psychostimulants may delay normal growth patterns in some cases, and weight and height should be monitored routinely. Drug holidays may be used to reduce this impact.
Psychostimulants are generally regarded as contraindicated for children with structural cardiac abnormalities or other cardiac disease that may be influenced by increased heart rate or blood pressure.
Tics are sometimes observed in predisposed children treated with psychostimulants. A range of psychiatric adverse effects has been observed, and include psychosis, mania and aggression.
Psychostimulants should not be prescribed where there is a history of psychosis or thought disorder.

Special care must be taken when using psychostimulants to ensure that all appropriate legal requirements for the prescribing of these restricted drugs are addressed. Some of the requirements are as follows.

Authorised prescribers include psychiatrists, specialist physicians or doctors and neurologists; they apply for an authorisation to prescribe dexamphetamine or methylphenidate under their respective criteria.

The potential for drug diversion should also be considered: given the abuse potential for these agents, there are circumstances where the drug may be used by a parent or sibling for illicit purposes, or on-sold for financial gain. It is important to check that the supply of medications is not being used before the timeline that would be expected has elapsed. Requests to replace 'lost' prescriptions or supplies of drugs should be considered carefully for these reasons.

For children four years of age or older, first-line psychostimulant treatment can be initiated with dexamphetamine 2.5 mg once to twice daily. The dose may be raised by 2.5–5 mg increments/day each week, until satisfactory clinical response is observed, or a ceiling dose of 0.5 mg/kg/day or 40 mg (whichever is less) in divided doses is attained. Alternatively, treatment may also be initiated with methylphenidate 5 mg once or twice daily, and gradually increased at weekly intervals to a maximum of 1 mg/kg/day or 60 mg (whichever is less), administered in divided doses. An alternative approach is to use long-acting modified-release preparations of methylphenidate. These products incorporate an immediate release phase in addition to a delayed release, and can be administered once daily. Notwithstanding the convenience and lower diversion potential of these products, treatment should be commenced with an immediate release product to allow effective dosage titration.

Atomoxetine is an alternative, non-stimulant agent that can be considered where psychostimulants are inappropriate, contraindicated or have proven to be ineffective or poorly tolerated. Adverse effects include decreased appetite, weight loss, gastrointestinal intolerance and mood swings. Like the psychostimulants, atomoxetine should be avoided for children with structural cardiac abnormalities. The dose of atomoxetine for children six years or older is suggested at 0.5 mg/kg (maximum 40 mg) orally, administered as a single daily dose each morning or in a divided dose (morning and late afternoon). After an initial period of seven days, the dose may be gradually up-titrated to the target dose of 1.2 mg/kg (maximum 80 mg). Other drugs that have been used for ADHD include clonidine and tricyclic antidepressants, but the routine use of these agents should be avoided because of adverse effects and lack of efficacy relative to the more established pharmacotherapy options.

Ask yourself!

1   What parameters might be monitored by using feedback from parents and teachers, to allow assessment of the efficacy of psychostimulants when used for the management of ADHD?

2   What problems might be anticipated and accommodated if it is necessary for a child to take psychostimulants during school hours?

ADHD is a recognised phenomenon, and up to 25% of those who had ADHD as children will still have symptoms by the age of 30 years. Treatment started in childhood should be continued in adulthood for those with symptoms that remain disabling.

Controversy in the treatment of ADHD

The diagnosis and management of ADHD continue to be controversial issues. There are some who assert that the disorder is overdiagnosed, and indeed there are even people who call the existence of the disorder into question. Stimulants used in the management of ADHD do have side effects, including the possibility of growth retardation and an association with serious psychiatric syndromes such as psychosis. Children cannot usually make their own decisions with respect to the treatment they receive, and thus the decision to use stimulants is usually made by a parent or guardian. The drugs themselves are subject to abuse and have a street value if sold for illicit use, creating the potential for diversion. There are complications relating to the need to manage these drugs in the school setting. Sceptics also suggest that the diagnosis and subsequent pharmacotherapy of ADHD is in part driven by the profit imperative of the pharmaceutical industry, which promotes the drug treatments heavily.

ZAC'S STORY

Zac is 10 years old, and lives with his mother Ella, who is 27 years old. Ella has been contacted by Zac's schoolteacher, who in a meeting describes a pattern of behaviour whereby he is frequently disruptive in class and is markedly behind his peers in the progress of his schoolwork. She produces some of his workbooks and shows the frequent mistakes that he makes in simple tasks, and asks if he has been doing work at home. Ella agrees that he seems to be constantly 'in a trance' and often forgets to take his school books and pencils with him in the morning. He fidgets constantly and has become unpopular with his classmates because he shouts over the top of them when they are speaking. Zac is later assessed by his GP, referred to a paediatrician and eventually is commenced on treatment with dexamphetamine. Despite eventual up-titration of his dose there appears to have been no therapeutic benefits that are reflected in his behaviour at school.

Ask yourself!

If you were involved in Zac's case:

1   What side effects might you be concerned about while Zac is being treated with a psychostimulant?
2   What are the possible reasons for the lack of response to treatment?
3   What alternative treatments could be explored for Zac?

From the consumer's perspective – *How does this feel for me?*

The use of psychostimulants by children during school hours can present special challenges for the child, the parents, the teachers and the school administration.

There is often considerable stigma for parent and child associated with the diagnosis of ADHD.

'People think I don't look after him properly, that he isn't disciplined.'

'I don't like the idea of my child taking "speed".'

'I worry about the side effects he might get.'

Care Plan

The following is an example care plan for the patient/client presented in this chapter. The areas of daily living that are considered include bio-psycho-social factors and the plan is mapped out using the nursing process (Assessment; Planning; Implementation; Evaluation). Remember: the success is in the detail, so be specific about *who, when and what* in the collaborative plan; never include someone in the plan if they were not consulted in the planning process; and always work within a recovery-orientated framework (refer to Chapter 1).

Date: 5 August 2012

Name: Zac   Case manager: General practitioner and/or mental health nurse in primary care

Areas of daily living	Assessment of current situation	Goal	Plan (undertaken with patient/client)	Implementation	Who is responsible? (Include only those who have been consulted in the planning process)	Evaluation/ review date
Mental health	GP assessment of ADHD and prescribed dexamphetamine with no improvement reported.	Assessment of mental state and cognitive function.	Review by child and adolescent psychiatrist.	Titrate down dose of dexamphetamine. Refer to child and adolescent psychiatrist for consultation and treatment.	Primary care team.	5/8/12
Social	Attends school in grade 4. Lives with mother.	Coordinate supports required for school.	Social worker referral	Liaise with Ella and school teacher.	Social worker.	5/8/12
Biological	Normal delivery, no physical illness reported.	Obtain baseline physical and mental assessment.	Assess physical and mental state.	Assess physical state including eyesight, vital signs, weight, hydration, etc.	Treating doctor and primary health team.	12/8/12

Environmental	Lives with mother Ella. Behind in school progress.	Support for Zac and Ella as appropriate.	Assess requirement for supports.	Assess supports required for Zac and Ella in terms of school and home.	Social worker or specialised mental health nurse.	12/8/12
Substance using behaviours	None identified	NA	NA	NA	NA	
Risk behaviours	None identified	NA	NA	NA	NA	

Autism spectrum disorders

Autism spectrum disorders are lifelong developmental disabilities. They are characterised by difficulties in communication, restricted and repetitive behaviours and impaired social interactions. Included in the autism spectrum is Asperger's syndrome and a variety of other less commonly encountered variants (such as Rett syndrome). In 2009, over 64 000 Australians were diagnosed as having autism (double the prevalence in 2003) (Australian Bureau of Statistics, 2011). The majority of people with autism (85%) are identified due to learning difficulties. The prevalence of autism is approximately 0.1%, while Asperger's disorder has a higher prevalence of up to 0.3%; the condition is more prevalent in boys than girls and the effects of an autism spectrum disorder can be minimised by facilitating an early diagnosis and timely and appropriate interventions. Features include difficult behaviours such as tantrums and aggression, marked difficulties with communication, disturbed sleep, picky eating, socially inappropriate behaviour and social isolation, often resulting in bullying. The diagnosis and pharmacological management of autism spectrum disorders are strictly the province of specialists. The word 'spectrum' is used to describe this type of mental disorder since the symptoms differ and the severity of the difficulties people with ASD experience are wide and varied.

A range of drugs including risperidone, psychostimulants and SSRIs has been used for the management of problem behaviours in these disorders. The choice of agent is usually based around the identification of the most pressing problem behaviours and the extent of associated impairment. For example, atypical antipsychotics such as risperidone are regarded as the first-line pharmacological treatment for children with autism spectrum disorders associated with prominent irritability. A suggested dosage regimen for dosing of risperidone for autism symptoms is a starting dose of 0.01 mg/kg/day, increasing gradually as needed to a maximum of 0.06 mg/kg/day. Some evidence suggests that melatonin may be helpful for sleep disturbance in children with autism. Benzodiazepines are not recommended for children with autism spectrum disorders.

Tic disorders

Transient tics can occur in up to 20% of all children, but Tourette's syndrome (persistent motor and vocal tics) has a prevalence of about 1%. Almost all children with tics will outgrow these by the time of adulthood. More common in boys than girls, tics may exacerbated by stress, inactivity and fatigue. Tics have been described as rapid, repetitive, non-rhythmic movements of sudden onset. Some presentations of simple childhood motor tics include blinking, shrugging and grimacing, whereas complex motor tics may be characterised by grooming, adoption of odd facial expressions or tapping. Common simple vocal tics include grunting and sniffing, whereas complex vocal tics include repeating words or phrases out of context, repeating others' words (echolalia) and using obscene language.

Tourette's syndrome is associated with both motor and vocal tics for at least a year and onset before the age of 18 years, with an incidence of about 0.05% in the general population. Tourette's syndrome is thought to be heritable and has a high association with comorbid obsessive-compulsive disorder. The onset of Tourette's syndrome is usually around the age of seven years, and symptoms are usually lifelong, but often become less severe in adolescence and adulthood. Tourette's syndrome may be responsive to behavioural interventions such as psychotherapy. Pharmacotherapy can be undertaken under specialist supervision, and may include the use of clonidine at a dose of 3–4 micrograms/kg/day. Haloperidol and risperidone are also effective, with the latter drug preferred on the basis of superior tolerability. Risperidone is now regarded as a more preferable approach than haloperidol because of a lower risk of serious complications such as tardive dyskinesia. For children older than five years of age, the staring dose of risperidone is 0.25 mg daily (for children weighing under 50 kg) or 0.5 mg (50 kg or over), increasing very gradually in weekly increments as required, up to a maximum of 0.05 mg/kg daily.

General psychiatry for children

As previously alluded to, children can be affected by many mental disorders that are more commonly observed among adults, such as affective disorders and psychosis.

Major depression in children and adolescents

Psychological interventions are regarded as the first-line treatments for depression in younger people. Pharmacotherapy may be needed in combination with psychological treatments in severe or refractory cases of depression. Cognitive behavioural therapy (CBT) and interpersonal psychotherapy are the psychological treatments most recommended for depression in children and adolescents.

At present, the antidepressant most widely to be considered as the drug of first choice in paediatric depression is the SSRI fluoxetine, which is used for children of seven years of age or older at a starting dose 0.25 mg/kg (maximum 10 mg) daily, increasing later to 0.5 mg/kg (maximum 20 mg) if needed. In the event of a lack of satisfactory response, the use of another SSRI under specialist supervision may be appropriate. There has been recent controversy about the risk of treatment-emergent agitation and suicidality relating to the use of antidepressants by children who are experiencing bipolar disorder, although opinions vary widely and the issue of 'confounding by diagnosis' and the distinction between suicidal behaviours (suicidal thoughts and acts as opposed to completed suicide) needs to be considered (refer to Figure 10.1).

Figure 10.1: Controversies in the use of antidepressants for children and adolescents

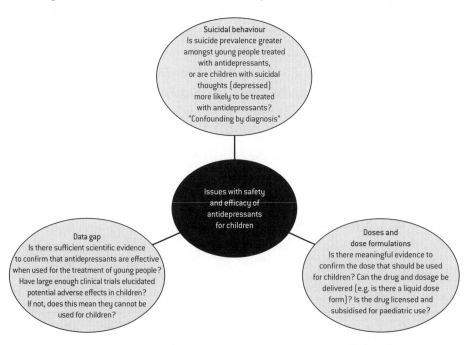

Up to a third of children and adolescents diagnosed with a major depressive episode will eventually be diagnosed with bipolar affective disorder. If symptoms

are suggestive of bipolar disorder emerging, treatment with mood stabilisers should be considered.

Bipolar affective disorder and psychosis

Bipolar disorder can be very difficult to diagnose in children and adolescents, largely because of the possibility that other mental illness may obscure the clinical picture (e.g. a diagnosis of ADHD may make the diagnosis of mania very challenging). If symptoms are clear and severe enough to allow a reliable diagnosis, current consensus suggests that pharmacotherapy should be based upon extrapolations from adult guidelines.

Antipsychotic drugs are regarded as the first-line treatments for manic episodes in children. Lithium and lamotrigine are mood stabilisers that are supported by some degree of clinical evidence for use in the pharmacotherapy of bipolar disorder in children and adolescents.

Prepubescent children almost never develop schizophrenia. Antipsychotic pharmacotherapy that is useful for adults with psychosis is also effective for children and adolescents, and can be administered in modified doses where appropriate. Adverse effects such as metabolic derangement and movement disorders are more common among younger people than for adults, and thus close monitoring is required.

On the Horizon in Paediatric Psychopharmacology

Extended-release guanfacine has recently been approved in the USA for use in the treatment of attention deficit/hyperactivity disorder (ADHD) in children and adolescents aged 6–17 years. Research suggests that this drug, which is a selective α-2A-adrenergic receptor agonist, can help children affected by the predominantly inattentive subtype of ADHD and combined type ADHD, but there is currently less evidence to support the use of the medication for those with predominantly hyperactive-impulsive ADHD.

Modafinil is a non-amphetamine stimulant agent that has been studied as a possible treatment for ADHD. Some research to date suggests that modafinil may well be at least as safe and as effective as standard stimulant treatment with drugs such as methylphenidate. Notwithstanding this, modafinil would not be regarded as a first-line treatment choice, and more extensive research is still required. Lisdexamgetamine is an amphetamine prodrug that requires metabolic activation by the liver to allow pharmacological activity. Although not expected to provide any advantage in therapeutic efficacy, this approach has been promoted on the basis of less potential for abuse and diversion.

Melatonin is synthesised in the brain from tryptophan, and is secreted by the pineal gland during periods of darkness (at night). Melatonin has been studied as a possible therapeutic strategy for use in autism spectrum disorders. A recent meta-analysis of melatonin-related research in this area suggests that this compound may be promising for improving sleep parameters.

Summary

The management of mental illness among children and adolescents is complex, difficult and should be undertaken by appropriately qualified specialists. The risk of suicide or suicidal behaviour during the early phases of psychoactive drug treatment for younger people is of significant concern, and may influence the setting in which the initial treatment is provided. Children and adolescents are particularly susceptible to the adverse effects of psychotropic drugs, and this should be acknowledged and incorporated into monitoring plans. If pharmacotherapy is to be used, it is important to set clear treatment goals, and to use close monitoring and feedback from parents and teachers to assist in the assessment of the effects of treatment.

Discussion questions

1 Which psychiatric disorders are seen among children and adolescents, and which of these are amenable to pharmacotherapy?

2 Describe the barriers that can interfere with the attainment of good therapeutic outcomes in the management of ADHD.

Test yourself (answers in the back of the book)

1 Which of the following statements is most accurate?

A Neurodevelopment concludes after the first trimester of pregnancy.

B Neurodevelopment continues until shortly after birth.

C Neurodevelopment continues until approximately five years of age.

D Neurodevelopment continues into early adulthood.

2   The management of depression in a child is most appropriately undertaken by:

   A   the usual GP

   B   a general paediatrician

   C   a general psychiatrist

   D   a specialist paediatric psychiatrist

3   Which of the following drugs would be regarded as a first-line agent for the pharmacotherapy of ADHD in children?

   A   Metamphetamine

   B   Moclobemide

   C   Methylphenidate

   D   Metoclopramide

4   Which of the flowing agents would be regarded as the most preferred option for use in the pharmacotherapy of tic disorders in children?

   A   Haloperidol

   B   Clozapine

   C   Risperidone

   D   Chlorpromazine

5   If pharmacotherapy for paediatric depression is required, which of the following would be regarded as the most suitable option?

   A   Clomipramine

   B   Phenelzine

   C   Bupropion

   D   Fluoxetine

Useful websites

American Academy of Child & Adolescent Psychiatry available at <www.aacap.org>

Attention Deficit/hyperactivity Disorder (ADHD) in Children available at <www.mayoclinic.com/health/adhd/DS00275>

The National Institute of Mental Health (NIMH): *Child and Adolescent Mental Health* available at <www.nimh.nih.gov/health/topics/child-and-adolescent-mental-health/index.shtml>

References

American Psychiatric Association. (2000). *Diagnostic and Statistical Manual of Mental Disorders*, 4th edn, Text Revision *(DSM-IV-TR)*. Washington DC: American Psychiatric Publishing, Inc.

Australian Bureau of Statistics. (2011). *Prevalence of Autism* available at <www.abs.gov.au/ausstats/abs@.nsf/Lookup/4428.0main+features42009>, retrieved 31 July 2012.

Rossi S. (2012). *Australian Medicines Handbook*. Chapter 18: Psychotropic drugs. Adelaide, South Australia: AMH Pty Ltd.

Taylor D., Paton C. & Kapur S. (2009) *The Maudsley Prescribing Guidelines*. 10th edn. UK: Informa Healthcare.

Chapter 11

Older People

Chapter overview

This chapter covers the following topics:

* the physical effects of ageing
* multiple comorbidities and the effects of prescribing and medicine taking
* polypharmacy in the older person.

Chapter learning objectives

After reading this chapter, you should be able to:

* describe the physical effects of ageing
* detail the care considerations in relation to polypharmacy in the older person
* describe the special considerations in prescribing in the older person.

Key terms

Ageing
Physical effects of ageing
Polypharmacy
Prescribing in the older person

Introduction

In this chapter you will explore issues related to prescribing and medication management for the older person. Throughout the chapter issues relating to the physical effects of **ageing**, polypharmacy, and special considerations in prescribing for older people will be discussed. A case scenario will also be presented to prompt you to think about the implications for your own practice and what the experience might be like for the person.

The physical effects of ageing

Declining organ system function

The liver and kidneys are the organs that are the most influential in the various processes that are responsible for the pharmacokinetic clearance of drugs. Most drugs or metabolites are eventually removed from the systemic circulation via filtration by the kidneys, but in some cases there may be some degree of reabsorption from the renal tubules. Many agents also require metabolism by the liver, where conversion to a more water-soluble compound (referred to as a metabolite) occurs, which can then be renally excreted. Drug absorption, distribution, metabolism and excretion are all processes that can profoundly influence a drug's serum concentration (and concentration at the site of action), and in turn can therefore influence the magnitude and nature of pharmacological effects. Accumulation of a drug because of altered pharmacokinetic parameters can lead to toxicity. The key principles of pharmacokinetics are discussed in detail in Chapter 3.

The normal processes associated with human ageing can have significant influences upon drug disposition and activity – it is important to understand that these changes (e.g. decreasing lean muscle mass, increasing body fat and water content, changes to the mucosal lining of the gastrointestinal system) happen in the absence of disease and are simply the consequences of growing older. Even so, the presence of pathological or disease states increases with age, and the influence of kidney disease, heart failure and hepatic impairment also leads to exaggerated clinical effects of medications. As a consequence the older person will often need a lower dose or modified administration regimen when compared to the younger person.

Brain and nervous system

As people age, the brain and the central nervous system become more sensitive to the effects of medicines. This is particularly the case for those with pre-existing neurological, cognitive or substance use disorders (e.g. alcohol abuse). Even when a diagnosis of a cognitive disorder (e.g. Alzheimer's disease) is not present, the memory of an older person can be influenced by the effects of age, and people may become forgetful and have trouble remembering how to take their medicines as directed. Various strategies can be employed by the treating team to help with memory deficits and medication regimens, such as dosage administration aids like Webster packs that are filled on a weekly basis by a pharmacist. Other strategies might include reminder charts or calendars and assertive outreach services as regular follow-up by aged care teams.

Eyesight

In the older person failing eyesight can cause problems with reading the small print medication labels and the medication information leaflets supplied with medications. It is important to consider these aspects of physical condition or deterioration in the assessments and ongoing evaluations of older people in order to accommodate for such impairments (e.g. larger print for those who need it).

Bones and joints

Bones and joints also deteriorate over time and this is a common concern in older people. A common condition to be aware of is arthritis. 'Arthritis' is often used as a generic term to describe these degenerative changes, when in reality there are a number of medical conditions affecting the musculoskeletal system and, more specifically, the joints. By far the most common specific disease state of this type is osteoarthritis, which causes inflammation, pain, stiffness and damage to cartilage, resulting in deformities of the joints, weakness and instability that can interfere with daily living (walking, driving a car, personal care, preparing food, dispensing medications from medication bottles, and so on). As the population ages, the number of people with arthritis is growing.

However, there is a commonly believed idea that arthritis is a consequence of age alone, but it is not a natural part of ageing. In fact 2.4 million of all people suffering from the disease are of working age (Arthritis Australia, 2007).

The other forms of arthritis include ankylosing spondylitis, rheumatoid arthritis and connective tissue diseases such as scleroderma and systemic lupus erythematosus (lupus).

Pharmacists can supply medicines in non-click lock containers (not child-resistant closures) upon request, but the older person will need to be reminded they must to keep non-click lock containers well out of the reach of children.

Multiple diseases – multiple medicines

Australia and New Zealand, like many other countries, has an ageing population. In 1996, 178 million prescriptions were written in Australia, with approximately 40% of those prescriptions being for people over the age of 65 (Roberts & Stokes, 1998). Old age is connected with many chronic diseases and associated disabilities, which often require multiple medications for management (in conjunction with other interventions). Multiple diseases (comorbidity) in the older person can include arthritis, hypertension, heart disease, stroke, depression, diabetes, and dementia (including Alzheimer's) as well as many other conditions. The term 'comorbidity' is used to describe the presence of two or more diseases at once. Due to the increase in longevity, the incidence of comorbidity is increasing as people age. According to the WHO the most prevalent chronic conditions are diabetes, asthma, heart disease and depression. Not only will chronic conditions be the leading cause of disability throughout the world by the year 2020; if not successfully managed, they will become the most expensive problems faced by our health care systems. In this respect, they pose a threat to all countries from a health and economic standpoint (WHO 2009).

Cognitive disorders (including dementia)

'Dementia' refers to symptoms due to changes in brain functioning (memory, behaviour and personality). In Australia in 2009 it was estimated that around a quarter of a million people Australia-wide had dementia (Alzheimer's Australia, 2010). Dementia is a significant burden in terms of health expenditure and is considered the fastest growing burden of disease. It is estimated that by 2050 over one million people in Australia will have dementia. It is important to be mindful that dementia is not a normal part of the ageing process, but after the age of 65 the likelihood of being diagnosed with dementia increases, with people who are 85 years or more having a one in four chance of developing dementia. Dementia is a word that includes different forms of brain diseases. It includes Alzheimer's disease, but also dementia with Lewy bodies, vascular dementia, frontotemporal dementia and dementia resulting from another condition (e.g. stroke).

The development of acetylcholinesterase (AChe) inhibitor drugs has followed the finding that cholinergic pathways in the cerebral cortex and basal forebrain are compromised in Alzheimer's disease. Cholinesterase inhibitors are prescribed to address the effects of dementia, and may assist in delaying the progression of features such as memory loss, impaired judgment, and impaired thinking and language. There is some evidence to suggest that cholinesterase inhibitors may also assist in lessening the severity and impact of behavioural and psychological symptoms of dementia, although where behavioural syndromes are refractory, severe or potentially dangerous it may be necessary to use a modest dose of a drug designed to address these issues (e.g. risperidone). There is considerable debate about the place of this type of approach, but most authorities agree that non-drug therapy should be the most important element of the management of such symptoms. People with Lewy body dementia are very sensitive to the effects of antipsychotic drugs, and may develop severe extrapyramidal side effects even when treated with low doses.

The commonly prescribed cholinesterase inhibitors are donepezil, rivastigmine and galantamine. Alzheimer's disease involves various pathological processes that compromise neuronal function related to the effects of the neurotransmitter acetylcholine. Cholinesterase inhibitors increase the synaptic concentration of acetylcholine by slowing down the breakdown of acetylcholine. Treatment is usually commenced on a low dose of cholinesterase inhibitors that is gradually increased over time, with dosage mostly dependent on how well treatment is tolerated.

The most frequently observed side effects are gastrointestinal in nature, commonly involving nausea, vomiting, diarrhoea, indigestion, abdominal pain and associated loss of appetite, and weight loss. Less common side effects include wakefulness, low energy and muscle cramps. Side effects tend to be mild and usually go away within a few weeks after treatment with the medicine is started. Another drug that is sometimes used is memantine, an agent that is an antagonist of the neurotransmitter N-methyl-D-aspartate (NMDA). Memantine may be used alone or in combination with cholinesterase inhibitors. Because of the extensive cost associated with the cholinesterase inhibitors and memantine, strict guidelines are applied as the basis for the supply of subsidised treatment. People who have dementia with a predominantly vascular origin may also respond to treatment with aspirin.

Delirium is another form of cognitive disorder which is different to dementia and is managed differently. Fundamentally, delirium is described as having transient and fluctuating and often reversible causes, often related to underlying organic aetiology. The 'DELIRIUM' mnemonic is sometimes used as a prompt to remember the various different underlying causes of the condition:

D – Degenerative neurological illness

E – Epilepsy (postictal confusion)

L – Liver failure

I – Intracranial pathology – injury, stroke, meningitis

R – Rheumatoid chorea

I – Infection

U – Uraemia

M – Metabolic (electrolyte imbalance)

The management of delirium involves short-term use of sedation, and addressing the underlying causes.

Other comorbidities

Other common chronic conditions in the older person include cardiovascular disease (CVD) and chronic obstructive pulmonary disease (COPD). Cardiovascular disease (CVD) increases dramatically as people age. CVD includes hypertension and heart disease and other cardiovascular disorders such as stroke and myocardial infarction. Heart disease is the current leading burden of disease worldwide, which in part is due to the ageing populations across the globe. CVD is the leading health and economic burden throughout the world, particularly in westernised, industrialised countries (American Heart Association, 2005). It has been predicted that CVD will become the main public health problem in the world by 2020 (Australian Institute of Health and Welfare, 2008; World Health Organization, 2009). Risk factors for stroke parallel those of CVD, namely hypertension, diabetes, low physical activity, hypercholesterolaemia, smoking and overweight (Australian Institute of Health and Welfare, 2008). Stroke is ranked second as cause of death, claiming 9% of all Australian deaths, or 12 300 lives a year (Australian Institute of Health and Welfare, 2002; Begg et al., 2007). Higher death rates are observed in regional and remote areas of Australia. Over the period 2004–06, 'regional areas had death rates that were 1.1 times as high as major cities, while death rates in very remote areas were 1.8 times as high' (Australian Institute of Health and Welfare, 2010, p. 243). In this context about one-third (32%) of Australians live in regional and remote areas (Australian Institute of Health and Welfare, 2008). Australians living in rural and remote areas generally have less contact with primary health care professionals (such as GPs), and this is a concern as there is an increased likelihood that they will develop certain diseases in the context of these geographical influences (Worrall-Carter, Edward & Page, 2012).

COPD in the older person is particularly dangerous as the older person may also be experiencing other chronic conditions (comorbidities) and these can exacerbate symptoms. COPD is almost always caused by smoking, and is also known as emphysema and chronic lung disease; it is treatable. The most common drugs used in the treatment of COPD are bronchodilators and corticosteroids. From time to time, antibiotics will be prescribed to treat lung infections caused by bacteria, and that could lead to pneumonia and death. Corticosteroids are used to reduce the inflammation in the bronchial tree, making breathing easier. Bronchodilators are used to reduce coughing, and make breathing easier. In end-stage COPD, the use of domiciliary oxygen may be needed.

On review of the evidence for this topic, only 3% of randomised, controlled trials and 1% of meta-analyses are published about prescribing for people over 65 years of age (Nair, 2002); this may be in part due to older people being infrequently recruited into clinical trials. The available literature for prescribing patterns for older people is disproportionate to the amount of prescribing that occurs in reality, and is relatively small (McLean & Le Couteur, 2004). The term 'polypharmacy' means 'many medications'. Polypharmacy is common in the older person; however, the body changes in composition with age, affecting the metabolism and distribution of drugs. As mentioned, this can led to toxicity in the older person, even when the dose is considered therapeutic for younger people. Alarmingly, some of the generic symptoms of an adverse effect of drugs (such as nausea, ataxia, sedation, oedema and changes in the gastrointestinal tract) can be mistaken for other illnesses, and additional medication may be added to the older person's medication regimen to treat these symptoms. It is important to remember that medications are not always necessary and that sometimes the older person's symptoms can be wrongly diagnosed. Additionally, older people may manifest the effects of social stressors that are generally common in older age, such as grief and bereavement though loss of a friend or partner, and feelings of isolation, loneliness and boredom (which may be misinterpreted as symptoms of depression). For a clinician working with older people, regular reviews of medication regimens should be commonplace. Additionally, assessment and regular evaluation of the bio-psycho-social context for the older person is also recommended so as to incorporate the whole clinical picture and potentially reduce the possibility of incorrectly medicating symptoms as management.

Ask yourself!

1   Describe what is considered polypharmacy.

2   Why is it important to conduct regular assessment or evaluation of medication regimens in the older patient/client?

3   What are the other care considerations to capture the 'whole clinical picture' for older patients/clients?

Increasing susceptibility to side effects of medicines

Table 11.1 shows how the body becomes more susceptible to the side effects of medicines as it ages.

Table 11.1: Medication implications and ageing organ systems

System	Ageing effects	Implications with medications
Cardiac system	Changes in cardiac musculature and blood vessels	Worsening circulation and less effective cardiac output, with diuretics and narcotics (morphine)
CNS (central nervous system)	Decline in neuroreceptors and pathways	Slower motor activity, so medications that affect motor function need to be monitored
	Increased sensitivity	Lower doses required as response to CNS agents is enhanced, i.e. opioids (fentanyl), barbiturates (diazepam)
Gastrointestinal (GI) system	Decrease in GI blood flow	Slower healing of drug precipitated bleeding
Respiratory system	Increased rigidity of chest wall	Compromised gas exchange with opioids
	Increased sensitivity	May have problems with sleep apnoea with barbiturates
Renal system	Decreased blood flow in kidneys	Influence drug levels of renally excreted drugs
Immune system	Greater susceptibility to infection due to reduced immunity to disease	Possible increase in use of antibiotics

Beers list (medication list)

The Beers Criteria for Potentially Inappropriate Medication Use in Older Adults is informally known as 'Beers list'. The Beers list is a reference source for health care professionals working towards safety when prescribing for older people, and is used widely in the clinical care of the older people, professional development and training, and health care policy development for the care of people 65 years and older. The list helps health care professionals working with older people to identify medications the harmful side effects of which may be life-threatening. First developed in 1991 (Beers et al., 1991) the list has been updated in 1997, 2003 and most recently in 2012.

The 2012 American Geriatric Society Beers Criteria was released in early 2012 via publication in the early online edition of the *Journal of the American Geriatrics Society* and is available at www.americangeriatrics.org. The 2012 Beers criteria differ from previous editions as, in addition to using a modified Delphi process for building consensus (a collaborative technique for estimating and forecasting among experts who interact autonomously discussing a particular topic, making comments and modifying opinions until mutual agreement is reached), all guideline developers additionally completed a systematic review of the evidence to inform their decisions.

Another significant change in the 2012 amended version is that each recommendation is rated for the quality of the evidence supporting the recommendation and the strength of the expert panel's recommendations. It is important to note that because medically complex older adults are often excluded from clinical trials, there is a shortage of evidence focused on this specific population.

Table 11.2: An abridged version of the AGS Beers Criteria for Potentially Inappropriate Medication Use in Older Adults (for the full version access the American Geriatrics Society at <www.americangeriatrics.org>)

Organ system or therapeutic category or drug	Rationale	Recom- mendation	Quality of evidence	Strength of recom- mendation
Anticholinergics	Highly anticholinergic; clearance reduced with advanced age, and tolerance develops when used as hypnotic; greater risk of confusion, dry mouth, constipation, and other anticholinergic effects and toxicity	Avoid	High– moderate	Strong

Organ system or therapeutic category or drug	Rationale	Recommendation	Quality of evidence	Strength of recommendation
Antiparkinson agents	Not recommended for prevention of extrapyramidal symptoms with antipsychotics; more effective agents available for treatment of Parkinson disease	Avoid	Moderate	Strong
Antispasmodics	Highly anticholinergic, uncertain effectiveness	Avoid (except in short-term palliative care)	Moderate	Strong
Antithrombotics: dipyridamole, oral, short-acting* (does not apply to extended release combination with aspirin)	May cause orthostatic hypotension; more effective alternatives available; intravenous form acceptable for use in cardiac stress testing	Avoid	Moderate	Strong
Anti-infective: nitrofurantoin	Potential for pulmonary toxicity	Avoid for long-term suppression	Moderate	Strong
Cardiovascular alpha1 blocker	High risk of orthostatic hypotension	Avoid use as an antihypertensive	Moderate	Strong
Antiarrhythmic drugs	Data suggest that rate control yields better balance of benefits and harms than rhythm control for most older adults.	Avoid antiarrhythmic drugs as first-line treatment of atrial fibrillation	High	Strong
Digoxin > 0.125 mg/day	In heart failure, higher dosages associated with no additional benefit and may increase risk of toxicity; slow renal clearance	Avoid	Moderate	Strong

(Continued)

Table 11.2: An abridged version of the AGS Beers Criteria for Potentially Inappropriate Medication Use in Older Adults (for the full version access the American Geriatrics Society at <www.americangeriatrics.org>) (*Continued*)

Organ system or therapeutic category or drug	Rationale	Recom-mendation	Quality of evidence	Strength of recom-mendation
Central nervous system:				
Tricyclic antidepressants	Highly anticholinergic, sedating, and cause orthostatic hypotension	Avoid	High	Strong
Antipsychotics, first (typical)and second (atypical) generation	Increased risk of cerebrovascular accident (stroke) and mortality in persons with dementia	Avoid	Moderate	Strong
Benzodiazepines	Older adults have increased sensitivity to benzodiazepines and slower metabolism of long-acting agents.	Avoid	High	Strong
Gastrointestinal system:				
Metoclopramide	Can cause extrapyramidal effects including tardive dyskinesia; risk may be even greater in frail older adults	Avoid	Moderate	Strong
Pain:				
Pethidine	Not an effective oral analgesic in dosages commonly used; may cause neurotoxicity	Avoid	High	Strong
Non-COX-selective NSAIDs, oral	Increases risk of GI bleeding and peptic ulcer disease. Upper GI ulcers, gross bleeding, or perforation caused by NSAIDs occur in approximately 1% of patients/clients treated for 3–6 months and in approximately 2–4% of patients/clients treated for 1 year. These trends continue with longer duration of use	Avoid	Moderate	Strong

Organ system or therapeutic category or drug	Rationale	Recom-mendation	Quality of evidence	Strength of recom-mendation
Skeletal muscle relaxants	Most muscle relaxants are poorly tolerated by older adults because of anticholinergic adverse effects, sedation, risk of fracture.	Avoid	Moderate	Strong

Source: Beers, et al. (1991)

Long-term effects of medication in the older person

Many medications have the potential to cause harm to or compromise the quality of life of elderly people, and yet there can be a reluctance to critically analyse drug therapy regimens with the objective of identifying the drugs that can be stopped without necessarily interfering with the achievement of specific therapeutic objectives. Many older people continue taking a medication for many years, simply because 'they've always been on that medicine'. In recent times there has been increasing focus on using a process to reduce the prescribing of potentially unnecessary or inappropriate medicines for older people; this approach is often referred to as 'deprescribing'. This process requires commitment from the prescriber and patient/client, and is underpinned by a collaborative partnership. To achieve deprescribing it is necessary to systematically review all current medications to assemble an accurate list of all drugs being taken, preferably involving the patient/client actually showing the prescriber or pharmacist the products they are using.

The indication and duration of treatment need to be determined and adherence assessed. Any potential adverse drug reactions should be identified, and the medications to be targeted as candidates for cessation established. Those not in current use should be discarded and repeat prescriptions destroyed. The drugs targeted can also be those used for conditions that have resolved, and medications used primarily to manage an adverse effect of another medication should be stopped when the offending drug is withdrawn. The deprescribing process should be carefully planned – it may be feasible to cease or reduce several drugs at the same time, but under other circumstances the preferred approach would be to achieve this in a sequential fashion. Drugs that have been identified as potential targets in deprescribing include benzodiazepines, antipsychotics used in the absence of psychosis, anticholinergic drugs, NSAIDs, digoxin and others. After deprescribing has been undertaken, it is important to arrange for regular review.

IAN'S STORY

Ian is an 80-year-old who lives alone, but near his son who looks in on him. He has a history of heart disease and hypertension, for which his cardiologist prescribes digoxin and an antihypertensive drug, respectively.

Eighteen months after his wife's death, Ian has become quite lonely with limited contact with his friends from the bowling club, he complains of feeling sad most of the time, he appears tired more often, and he complains that he cannot sleep at night due to constantly thinking about 'things'. His son becomes concerned and decides to take Ian to the general practitioner (GP). A benzodiazepine for insomnia and an antidepressant for his mood change are prescribed. The drugs initially improve Ian's mood, but soon he becomes confused, ataxic and forgetful. Ian's son once again takes Ian to the GP and his blood pressure is found to be low.

Upon review of Ian's medications, and in consultation with the nurse from the aged care team who is also involved in co-ordinating care for Ian, the GP finds the cardiologist who is treating Ian for his heart disease had increased the dosage of the antihypertensive medication to control Ian's rising blood pressure. The antidepressant, the insomnia medication and the hypertension medication collectively produced Ian's disorientation and vertigo. The nurse informs the GP that Ian also experiences allergies but it is not clear if he is taking anything for these.

Ask yourself!

If you were involved in Ian's care in the above scenario:

1   What other care considerations should you be thinking about for Ian?

2   Is it important to communicate with the cardiologist? How can you and the GP improve the communication between Ian's cardiologist and the rest of the treating team? What legal considerations do you need to think about when sharing medical information with a broader team?

3   What role does Ian's son have in the care planning?

4   What role does Ian have in the care planning?

5   What are the common side effects for antidepressants, benzodiazepines, and the hypertension medication?

6   Might Ian benefit from a HMR?

From the consumer's perspective – *How does this feel for me?*

Ian (as described above) is grieving for the loss of his wife to whom he was married for over 40 years. He is also from a generation where the 'doctor knows best'. Ian may become concerned if one doctor attempts to alter the treatment of another. Ian may think:

'Why do you need to speak to my cardiologist? He only looks after my heart condition?'

'Why is a nurse so concerned with my medications?'

'These antidepressants are making me feel tired so I might stop taking them.'

Drugs and falls in the older person

Falls are the most common type of reported patient adverse event, and a large percentage can cause minor injuries (Hitcho et al., 2004), such as bruises and soft tissue damage. Some falls can cause serious harm such as fractures, subdural haematoma and even death (Coussement et al., 2007). Most falls in older people are due to weakness, confusion, ataxia, the effects of some medications and the effects of polypharmacy. Medications are a major contributing factor to the incidence of falls in the older person. Older adults taking more than three or four medications are at increased risk of recurrent falls. The use of sedatives and hypnotics, antidepressants, and benzodiazepines have been demonstrated to have a significant association with falls in the elderly (Woolcott et al., 2009).

In terms of care considerations, health care professionals need to undertake a falls risk assessment (forms for this are often made available for recording falls risk at each health care facility). A falls risk assessment will provide the team with the necessary clinical information to provide appropriate interventions for individuals to help to prevent the probability of a fall. All interventions to reduce the incidence or probability of falls in older people involve a multidisciplinary approach and cross-disciplinary collaboration in assessment and interventions, strength building through exercise, a comprehensive clinical picture for each person related to comorbidities, medications and attention to any environmental hazards that may exist for individuals at home when considering discharge planning. For older people with a history of falls and osteoporosis, the use of hip protectors may confer additional protection.

One option that can be considered as a strategy to reduce the risk of medication-related morbidity in the elderly is to make arrangements for a Home Medicines Review (HMR), also referred to as a Domiciliary Medication Management Review (DMMR). Funded by the Commonwealth Department of Health and Ageing, the HMR process involves a referral from a general practitioner to an accredited pharmacist who visits the person in their home. The pharmacist reviews the patient/client and their medications and then prepares a report for the doctor, who discusses the information and recommendations with the patient at the time of next visit. The criteria for referral are at the discretion of the doctor, but some of the model criteria that have been suggested include:

* taking five or more medications

* more than 12 occasions of medication administration per day

* symptoms suggestive of an adverse drug reaction

* possible non-adherence

* treatment with a drug of low therapeutic index.

HMR has been proven to reduce drug-related harm and prevent hospitalisations in the elderly. Nurses can assist by prompting the person to seek a referral from their doctor, or by contacting the doctor directly to suggest a HMR. A similar form of review is also available for people living in aged and extended care facilities, and is referred to as Residential Medication Management Review (RMMR).

Ask yourself!

1   How could I incorporate a fall risk assessment in my routine practice?

2   If I am working in an inpatient environment, how can I facilitate a home assessment for potential environmental hazards that could increase the potential for falls for the older patient/client?

3   How does polypharmacy influence the potential for falls?

Table 11.3: Prescribing for older people and special considerations

Medicine	Potential concerns with treatment	Clinical considerations
Anticonvulsants (phenytoin, carbamazepine, valproate)	Can led to confusion, liver dysfunction, ataxia and vomiting	Monitor serum levels
Anticholinergics (benztropine, benzhexol)	Can lead to confusion, constipation, hypotension and urinary retention	Generally not appropriate for the older person
Mood stabiliser (lithium carbonate)	Can lead to oedema, central nervous system toxicity, weight gain and electrolyte imbalance	Important to monitor serum levels and use in low dose in the older person
Monoamine oxidase inhibitors (MAOIs)	Can lead to hypertensive crisis when taken in conjunction with certain foods; postural hypotension also can be a concern	May be difficult for the patient to adhere to food diet that is tyramine-free
Serotonin reuptake inhibitors (e.g. fluoxetine, sertraline)	Can lead to agitation, sleep disturbance, and anorexia	Not a first-line drug for older patients/clients

On the Horizon in Pharmacotherapy for Cognitive Disorders

With the rapid ageing of the world population and associated increased incidence of dementia, advances in the management of cognitive disorders are set to become increasingly important.

Cerebrolysin is a porcine brain-derived peptide that exhibits neurotrophic properties. Several randomised studies in Alzheimer's disease have demonstrated that cerebrolysin was better than placebo in improving global outcome measures and cognitive ability. Another large study that compared cerebrolysin, donepezil or combination therapy revealed benefits for all three treatment groups; it would appear that cerebrolysin may be a useful addition to the treatment options currently available for dementia.

Initial attempts at developing a vaccination to treat or prevent Alzheimer's disease proved to be unsuccessful. It has since become clear that targeting plaque amyloid alone is insufficient for improving clinical symptoms and signs, meaning that multiple targets may require attention. Another critical issue is to avoid autoimmune encephalitis and adverse inflammation observed with early attempts at this type of treatment. Polyclonal immunisation with activation of T helper type 2 T-cells appears promising.

Summary

As people age, their livers become less efficient at breaking down medicines and their kidneys become less efficient at excreting medicines. The prescriber for the older patient will need to take these ageing conditions into consideration and may need to prescribe a lower dose. Additionally, as people age the brain and the central nervous system become more sensitive to the effects of drugs. Also, failing eyesight can affect reading the small print on medication labels and the medication information leaflets supplied with medications. Prescribing medications is a significant contributing factor to the incidence of falls in the older person, where an older adult taking more than three or four medications at once is at increased risk of recurrent falls. Multiple diseases in older people can lead to polypharmacy and such diseases may include arthritis, hypertension, heart disease, stroke, depression, diabetes and dementia (including Alzheimer's). To augment practice in the context of medications, the Beers Criteria for Potentially Inappropriate Medication Use in Older Adults, informally known as Beers list, is a reference source related to the safety of prescribing for older people, and is used widely in clinical care.

Care Plan

The following is an example care plan for the patient/client presented in this chapter. The areas of daily living that are considered include bio-psycho-social factors and the plan is mapped out using the nursing process (Assessment; Planning; Implementation; Evaluation). Remember: the success is in the detail, so be specific about *who, when and what* in the collaborative plan; never include someone in the plan if they were not consulted in the planning process; and always work within a recovery-orientated framework (refer to Chapter 1).

Date: 1 August 2012

Client's name: Ian

Case manager: O. Aged

Areas of daily living	Assessment of current situation	Goal	Plan (undertaken with patient/client)	Implementation	Who is responsible? (Include only those who have been consulted in the planning process)	Evaluation/ review date
Mental health	Disoriented Depressed mood Ruminations Forgetfulness Confusion	Treat mood disorder and treat cognitive impairment.	Discuss with Ian the need to coordinate care with GP, psychiatrist and cardiologist.	Mental state examination. Cognitive assessment – referral back to aged care team.	Psychiatrist or mental health nurse on aged care team	4/8/12
				Secondary consultation with cardiologist regarding cardiac care plan and psychiatrist regarding review of antidepressant medication – case conference.	GP and case manager from aged care team to coordinate	8/8/12
Social	Son lives nearby and frequently visits. Limited contact recently with friends from bowling club.	Ian would like to get back to his bowls club activities.	Refer to aged care team.	Liaise with case manager and son and suggest referral for social worker assessment/involvement.	GP	1/8/12

(Continued)

Date: 1 August 2012 (Continued)

Client's name: Ian   Case manager: O. Aged

Areas of daily living	Assessment of current situation	Goal	Plan (undertaken with patient/client)	Implementation	Who is responsible? (Include only those who have been consulted in the planning process)	Evaluation/ review date
Biological	Allergies Insomnia Heart disease Hypertension, recently hypotension Vertigo	Stabilise physical state.	Stabilise physical state in consultation with cardiologist.	Assess physical signs including vital signs, weight, TFT, liver function test, full blood examination, etc. Secondary consultation with cardiologist regarding antihypertensive medication and cardiac condition Review medication with cardiologist and psychiatrist – case meeting.	GP and/or clinic nurse	1/8/12 8/8/12 8/8/12
Environmental	Lives alone	Supports for the home environment as appropriate	Refer to aged care team.	Liaise with case manager and suggest referral for social worker assessment/involvement.	GP	1/8/12
Substance using behaviours	Not identified	N/A	N/A	N/A	N/A	N/A
Risk behaviours	Risk of falls	Falls assessment	HMR DMMR	Home assessment Arrangements for a Home Medicines Review (HMR), also referred to as a Domiciliary Medication Management Review (DMMR)	GP and aged care team case manager	1/8/12

Discussion questions

1   *How* would I access the Beers list and how can I incorporate this list into the routine reference lists used in my area of work?

2   *What* aspects of an assessment of an older patient/client should comprise a falls risk assessment? How can you assess falls risk and should information about medication be included in this type of assessment?

3   *What* are the effects of ageing and how do these influence the effects of medications?

Test yourself (answers in the back of the book)

1   With respect to age-related changes in drug disposition, which of the following statements is most accurate?

A   Older people do not have significantly different drug disposition.

B   Renal elimination of drugs may be slower than for younger people.

C   Renal elimination of drugs may be faster than for younger people.

D   Hepatic elimination of drugs may be faster than for younger people.

2   Pharmacotherapy for dementia is generally based on the principle of:

A   reversing the extent of cognitive decline

B   arresting cognitive decline

C   slowing the progression of cognitive decline

D   preventing the onset of cognitive decline

3   People with Lewy body dementia are more likely to experience which of the following adverse effects when treated with antipsychotic drugs?

A   Hallucinations

B   Gait disturbance

C   Delirium

D   Blurred vision

4   The use of which of the following classes of agents is thought to increase the risk of falls among the elderly?

A   Antipsychotics

B   Benzodiazepines

C   Antidepressants

D   All of the above

5   Which of the following agents is used for the management of cognitive decline in people with Alzheimer's disease?

A   Lorazepam

B   Risperidone

C   Donepezil

D   Valproate

Useful websites

Medication for the Older Person (National Health and Medical Research Council) available at <www.nhmrc.gov.au/guidelines/publications/ac7>

AGS Beers criteria available at American Geriatrics Society available at <www.americangeriatrics.org>

References

Alzheimer's Australia. (2010). *Keeping Dementia Front of Mind: Incidence and Prevalence 2009–2050*. Retrieved 31 July 2012, from <www.fightdementia.org.au/new-south-wales/access-economics-reports-nsw.aspx>

Arthritis Australia. (2007). *Painful Realities: The Economic Impact of Arthritis in Australia in 2007*, pp. 1–88. Sydney, Australia: Arthritis Australia.

American Heart Association. (2005). *International CVD Statistics 2005*. Dallas Texas: The American Heart Association.

Australian Institute of Health and Welfare. (2002). *Trends in Death Data 1987–1998 with Updates to 2000*. Canberra: Australian Institute of Health and Welfare.

Australian Institute of Health and Welfare. (2008). *Australia's Health 2008*. Canberra: Australian Institute of Health and Welfare.

Australian Institute of Health and Welfare. (2010). *Australian Health – The Twelfth Biennial Health Report of the Australian Institute of Health and Welfare*. Canberra: Australian Institute of Health and Welfare.

Beers M. H., Ouslander J. G., Rollingher I., Reuben D. B., Brooks J. & Beck J. C. (1991). 'Explicit criteria for determining inappropriate medication use in nursing home residents' *Archives of Internal Medicine* 151(9): 1825.

Begg S., Vos T. B. B., Stevenson C., Stanley L. & Lopez A. (2007). *The Burden of Disease and Injury in Australia 2003*. Canberra: Australian Institute of Health and Welfare.

Coussement J., De Paepe L., Schwendimann R., Denhaerynck K., Dejaeger E. & Milisen K. (2007). 'Interventions for preventing falls in acute- and chronic-care hospitals: a systematic review and meta-analysis' *J Am Geriatr Soc* 56: 29–36.

Hitcho E. B., Krauss M. J., Birge S., Claiborne Dunagan W., Fischer I., Johnson S. et al. (2004). 'Characteristics and circumstances of falls in a hospital setting: a prospective analysis' *Journal of General Internal Medicine* 19: 732–739.

McLean, A. J. & Le Couteur, D. G. (2004). 'Aging biology and geriatric clinical pharmacology' *Pharmacological Reviews* 56(2): 163–184.

Nair B. R. (2002). 'Evidence based medicine for older people: available, accessible, acceptable, adaptable?' *Australasian Journal on Ageing* 21(2): 58–60.

Roberts M. S. & Stokes J. A. (1998). 'Prescriptions, practitioners and pharmacists' *Medical Journal of Australia* 168(7): 317–318.

World Health Organization. (2009). *Global Health Risks: Mortality and Burden of Disease Attributable to Selected Major Risks*. Geneva: World Health Organization.

Woolcott J. C., Richardson K. J., Wiens M. O. et al. (2009). 'Meta-analysis of the impact of 9 medication classes on falls in elderly persons' *Archives of Internal Medicine* 169(21): 1952.

Worrall-Carter L., Edward K. & Page K. (2012). 'Women and cardiovascular disease: At a social disadvantage?' *Collegian: Journal of the Royal College of Nursing Australia* 19(1): 33–37.

Chapter 12

Mental Illness in Special Populations

Chapter overview

This chapter covers the following topics:
* eating disorders

* personality disorders

* sleep disorders

* drug-induced psychiatric syndromes

* pain and psychiatry

* complementary medicines.

Chapter learning objectives

After reading this chapter, you should be able to:

* describe the aspects of the clinical, presentation and management of eating disorders, personality disorders and sleep disorders

* list a range of psychiatric syndromes that are associated with drug treatment.

Key terms

Eating disorders
Iatrogenic illness
Insomnia
Pain
Personality disorders
Sleep disorders

Introduction

Although a great deal of prescribing of psychotropic medication occurs in the context of major categories of mental disorders such as mood and anxiety disorders and schizophrenia, there are many situations where medications are used for other populations. Furthermore, the presence of comorbid medical and psychiatric disease states may also necessitate the use of complex combination medication regimens that involve both psychotropic agents and other drugs. This includes complementary products that a patient/client may elect to use in addition to prescribed medicines. It is not possible to address the entire range of possible scenarios in which health workers might expect to encounter psychotropic drug use, but selected examples or important subgroups are reviewed in this chapter. Additionally, pregnancy, lactation and medication are discussed.

Eating disorders

Eating disorders are a form of mental illness affecting females more often than males. Various forms of eating disorders may be encountered, including anorexia nervosa, bulimia nervosa and binge eating disorder. Each of these disorders is associated with significant psychiatric morbidity and the potential for serious medical complications, both acute and chronic in nature. Key diagnostic features for the three major eating disorders are outlined in Table 12.1.

Table 12.1: Diagnostic features of eating disorders

Anorexia nervosa: persistent mental and behavioural syndromes directed towards the objective of weight loss or thinness, leading to significant weight loss or the absence of expected weight gain during a period of growth. People with anorexia will engage in activities that result in the attainment and maintenance of body weight well below normal limits. Those affected often express an extreme fear of gaining weight. As well as restrictive food and drink consumption patterns, people with anorexia may adopt purging behaviours (e.g. self-induced vomiting, use of laxatives or diuretics) or excessive exercise patterns.

Bulimia nervosa: regular episodes of uncontrolled overeating (binge eating), associated with extreme behaviours directed at reducing or controlling weight (e.g. self-induced vomiting, purging) or fasting. Unlike those with anorexia, bulimic people usually have normal body weight or may be overweight.

Binge eating disorder: recurrent episodes of binge eating in the absence of the regular use of inappropriate control behaviours consistent with bulimia nervosa.

Source: American Psychiatric Association (2000)

It is of interest that the prevalence of eating disorders varies in different societies: in countries and cultures where large body weight is considered to be indicative of beauty or attractiveness (e.g. in South Pacific Islands and parts of Africa), anorexia is almost unknown. Eating disorders are often chronic in nature and are frequently associated with significant denial. The fundamental approach to the management of eating disorders must address long-term engagement with appropriately qualified specialist services, and this may be particularly difficult to attain in the early phase of treatment due to significant denial.

Key elements of the treatment approach should include:

* strategies for a return to normal or near normal weight range appropriate to gender, height and developmental stage

* addressing the underlying family and personal problems that may be contributing to the illness or preventing recovery

* implementation of multidisciplinary team approach to treatment, incorporating psychotherapy, dietician input and, in some cases, pharmacotherapy. Family therapy has been shown to improve the outcome of adolescents still residing with their families. While its status for older people is less certain, it may be helpful in conjunction with individual therapy.

* initiation of strategies to support the families and carers of those affected.

Even when all of these elements are incorporated in the treatment plan, persistent morbidity is common, and mortality is high. Eating disorders may be complicated by significant medical complications such as a Mallory-Weiss tear (injury to the lower oesophagus or upper part of the stomach, which may cause significant bleeding), hormonal disturbances causing disruption or cessation of menstruation, electrolyte disturbances (e.g. hypokalaemia, hyponatraemia, hypomagnesaemia), dehydration and cardiac rhythm abnormalities. Much of the management of eating disorders is undertaken in the outpatient setting, interspersed where necessary with brief admissions to hospitals or other specialised treatment units.

Pharmacotherapy is not considered to be indicated for the intrinsic treatment of anorexia nervosa itself, but antidepressants may be useful in the context of comorbid depression. Antipsychotic medication may be considered in the context of extreme agitation. Nutritional supplements and vitamins may also be needed, and their use should be guided by appropriate specialist input. In contrast, the management of bulimia nervosa does sometimes involve pharmacotherapy in addition to the cognitive approaches that are regarded as first-line treatment. The SSRI antidepressants are the agents most extensively used for this purpose, and are administered at standard starting doses similar to those encountered in other settings, but it appears that higher maintenance doses than those used for depression may be needed after slow up-titration. A cautious approach is needed if using higher dosages of citalopram, in view of the potential for broadening of the Q-T interval.

TINA'S STORY

Tina is a 17-year-old girl who is currently completing her final year of high school studies. She has been brought to see her GP by her mother, who is concerned that 'she eats nothing, and weighs nothing'. Tina is found to be 170 cm tall and weighs 38 kg. She exercises at the gym for an hour every day, and stopped having periods over a year ago. She tearfully exclaims, 'I don't even know why I'm here – there's nothing wrong with me!'

Ask yourself!

Hearing about Tina's case:

1   What other history and investigations might be needed to guide Tina's treatment?
2   Should pharmacotherapy be considered at this stage?

From the consumer's perspective – *How does this feel for me?*

The early stages of the assessment and treatment of eating disorders is often marked by significant denial.

'I couldn't stand being fat like those other girls.'

'I'm only exercising to be healthy – I'm stressed out at school.'

Personality disorders

Personality disorders are psychiatric conditions that are commonly encountered in clinical practice. They are recorded in Axis II of the multiaxial assessment

system of the *Diagnostic and Statistical Manual of Mental Disorders* (DSM-IV-TR).
Often present comorbidly with Axis I disorders, personality disorders are marked
by an enduring pattern of inner experience and behaviour that is noticeably
different from the norm associated with the person's culture and background.
These features are pervasive and inflexible, are stable over an extended period of
time, and can be traced to an onset in late childhood or early adolescence. Usually
grouped into 'clusters' of disorders with shared clinical features, personality
disorders affecting cognition (the personal style of perceiving and interpreting
oneself, others, or events); range, intensity, lability, and appropriateness of
emotional response; interpersonal functioning; and impulse control. Commonly
encountered personality disorders are summarised in Table 12.2.

Table 12.2: Common personality disorders and associated symptom patterns

Cluster A
Paranoid personality disorder: distrust and suspiciousness such where motives are interpreted as malevolent
Schizoid personality disorder: detachment from social relationships with restricted range of emotional expression
Schizotypal personality disorder: discomfort in close relationships, cognitive or perceptual distortions, and eccentricities of behaviour

Cluster B
Antisocial personality disorder: disregard for, and violation of, the rights of others
Borderline personality disorder: instability in interpersonal relationships, self-image and affect, marked impulsivity
Histrionic personality disorder: excessive emotionality and attention seeking
Narcissistic personality disorder: grandiosity, need for admiration, lack of empathy

Cluster C
Avoidant personality disorder: social inhibition, feelings of inadequacy, hypersensitivity to negative evaluation
Dependent personality disorder: submissive and clinging behaviour related to an excessive need to be taken care of

Obsessive-compulsive personality disorder: preoccupation with orderliness, perfectionism, and control

Personality disorder not otherwise specified

Pattern meets the general criteria for a personality disorder and traits of several different personality disorders are present, but the criteria for a specific personality disorder are not met; or

Pattern meets the general criteria for a personality disorder, but not one included in the classification above.

Source: American Psychiatric Association (2000)

It is widely accepted that personality disorders are not amenable to pharmacotherapy interventions, and that non–drug approaches must form the cornerstone of the management in these cases. Medications may be helpful in addressing some common findings such as diminished impulse control, aggression or anxiety. Another way in which pharmacotherapy may assist is in the provision of a targeted intervention for a syndrome that may not necessarily be a part of the personality disorder per se, but may destabilise the symptoms of the disorder (e.g. substance abuse, depression). Brief, tailored pharmacological interventions with drugs such as antipsychotics may assist in cases where there is severe agitation or distress, but benzodiazepines and related agents should be issued with considerable caution because of the risk of substance dependence and/or abuse.

Ask yourself!

1 Counter-transference occurs when the therapist begins to project their own unresolved conflicts onto the patient/client. What factors contribute to counter-transference in clinical teams involved in the treatment of people with personality disorders, and how might this influence the pharmacotherapy that is implemented?

2 Apart from potential for substance dependence and/or abuse, what other problems might arise from the use of medications for people with personality disorders?

Sleep disorders

Sleep disorders are common and, given that sleep is integral to so many facets of normal human physiological function, it is not surprising that sustained sleep disturbance can have profound effects upon physical and emotional well-being. Many medical conditions are associated with sleep disturbance, ranging from fundamental issues such as poorly controlled pain or severe respiratory disease with impaired gas exchange, to underlying disorders such as hyperthyroidism. Many psychiatric disorders such as anxiety disorders or depression have sleep disturbance as a major feature, and the effective management of the underlying illness will often allow an improvement in sleep quality. In addition to the obvious ramifications with respect to quality of life, severe sleep disorders can also have wider implications: for example, daytime somnolence associated with poor sleep secondary to a condition such as sleep apnoea can result in workplace accidents or motor vehicle accidents.

In the DSM-IV-TR (American Psychiatric Association, 2000), sleep disorders are categorised into several groups, including the primary sleep disorders, sleep disorders secondary to a general medical disorder, sleep disorders secondary to the effects of other mental disorders, and substance induced sleep disorders. Poorly controlled symptoms from general medical disorders, for example suboptimally treated pain or dyspnoea, are a very common basis for poor sleep, and naturally the approach to managing this type of sleep disorder is directed at the underlying illness state. Similarly, anxiety, depression and psychotic symptoms may cause sleep disturbance, and the correct management of the underlying disorder will often be accompanied by improved sleep.

Substance-induced sleep disorders

Substance-induced sleep disorders may take many forms. In some cases, it is relatively straightforward to identify sleep disturbances that occur as a result of the use or abuse of substances with stimulant properties. The disruptive effects of drugs such as amphetamine derivatives and cocaine arise as a result of the effects of these agents on serotonin and dopamine receptors in the brain. Stimulant drugs may also distort sleep patterns in other ways. For example, persistent or binge use of these agents may create a situation where the person becomes severely sleep deprived and potentially exhausted. After sustained intoxication, the user will eventually manifest a significant need for sleep (a 'crash'), where they may sleep hours or even days at a time. Interestingly, the characteristic withdrawal symptoms experienced by users after sudden discontinuation of these agents often include excessive drowsiness and lethargy. Some stimulant agents such as nicotine and caffeine are not regarded as illicit drugs of dependence or abuse. Even so, these agents can produce sleep disturbance, particularly if used heavily at or around the time of anticipated sleep. Caffeine is a substrate of the hepatic isoenzyme **cytochrome P450** 1A2, which means that concurrent use of drugs such as fluvoxamine can decrease hepatic clearance and increase serum concentrations, exaggerating the stimulant effect. After smoking cessation, the activity of cytochrome P450 1A2 will decrease, meaning that, unless caffeine intake is decreased, caffeine toxicity with sleep disturbance may be observed. Some sedating agents such as alcohol and benzodiazepines are associated with sleep disturbance during withdrawal – an alcoholic may have no difficulty falling asleep while intoxicated, but may experience sleep disturbance later in the night, after blood alcohol concentrations decline. Finally, many prescribed drugs may cause sleep disturbances with various symptoms – examples include corticosteroids, beta agonists (e.g. salbutamol, salmeterol), pseudoephedrine, theophylline and some antidepressants.

Primary sleep disorders

There are two major types of primary sleep disorders. Dyssomnias are the conditions where the primary complaints involve difficulty in getting enough sleep, problems in the timing of sleep, and complaints about the quality of sleep. Examples of dyssomnias include primary insomnia, narcolepsy, breathing-related sleep disorders and circadian rhythm sleep disorders. Parasomnias are those conditions associated with abnormal behavioural and physiological events during sleep. One example of a parasomnia is sleep terror disorder, which involves recurrent episodes of panic-like symptoms occurring during non-REM sleep. Typically affecting younger people, a child may wake screaming, will be difficult to wake during the episode and will have little memory of it. Other examples include somnambulism (sleep walking), somniliquism (sleep talking), bruxism (grinding of the teeth) and nocturnal eating.

Primary insomnia

Despite the common beliefs held in the general community, primary insomnia is actually quite rare – insomnia is much more commonly a symptom associated with another problem (see above). Inaccurate perceptions of sleep quantity and quality, unrealistic expectations about sleep, and belief that a lack of sleep will be more disruptive than it actually is leads many people to present to their local doctor seeking a 'quick fix' involving the use of hypnosedatives. People who seek help for persistent insomnia need a thorough history and investigation to find evidence for reversible causes, and should be counselled to adopt good 'sleep habits' (refer Table 12.3).

Table 12.3: Sleep habits that may assist with the management of insomnia

Decrease or eliminate caffeine, especially after noon.
Don't use alcohol or tobacco near bedtime.
Avoid heavy meals near bedtime.
Avoid heavy exercise near bedtime.
Establish a regular schedule for retiring and rising.
Have the bedroom at a comfortable temperature; minimise light and noise.
Use the bedroom for sleeping and sex only.
Consider relaxation or meditation approaches.

Where addressing sleep habits does not prove to be sufficient, pharmacotherapy using agents such as benzodiazepines (e.g. temazepam) or other short-acting hypnosedatives such as zopiclone or zolpidem may be tried. General principles to guide the use of these drugs include an approach that uses the lowest effective dose, intermittent dosage wherever possible, short-term use (regular use for only two to four weeks) and the preferential use of agents with shorter elimination half-life, so as to risk less daytime sedation (a 'hangover' effect). For some people, the use of zolpidem may produce serious parasomnias (sleep dysfunction) (refer to those described below) and can create a risk of accidental injury – if this problem is observed, the drug should be promptly and permanently withheld. It is not appropriate to use other sedating drugs such as antipsychotics for the management of insomnia.

Narcolepsy

Narcolepsy is a primary sleep disorder that involves irresistible episodes of daytime sleepiness, attacks of cataplexy (loss of muscle tone that may occur in the context of emotional lability or excitement), and hypnopompic (the threshold of consciousness) or hypnogogic (the state between being awake and falling asleep) hallucinations (respectively, hallucinatory experiences when waking up or going to sleep). Once the diagnosis has been confirmed with polysomnography, it is important to provide counselling with respect to potentially dangerous situations such as driving. Pharmacotherapy options that can be considered include dexamphetamine 5 to 10 mg orally, twice daily (morning and midday), or methylphenidate 10 to 20 mg (immediate-release) orally, twice daily (morning and midday). Another option is to use the non-amphetamine derivative modafinil at a dose of up to 400 mg in divided doses. Antidepressant (SSRIs) may be helpful in treating cataplexy symptoms.

Breathing-related sleep disorders

Breathing-related sleep disorders are most commonly characterised by excessive sleepiness during the day and/or disrupted sleep at night – examples include sleep apnoea where there is restricted air flow and/or brief cessations of breathing. Obstructive sleep apnoea (OSA) is a condition where, because of mechanical disruptions, airflow stops but the respiratory system continues to work, whereas central sleep apnoea (CSA) is a condition where the central respiratory drive is compromised for brief periods during sleep. OSA is the more common form, occurring in 1–2% of population. The person is usually minimally aware of apnoea problem (which may be reported by a sleep partner), and those affected will often snore, sweat during sleep, wake frequently, and have morning headaches. It is a common observation that people with severe OSA have truncal obesity, and may experience episodes of falling asleep during the day. OSA is not treated with pharmacotherapy, but rather with mechanical ventilation assistive devices such as those supplying continuous positive airway pressure (CPAP).

Circadian rhythm sleep disorders

Circadian rhythm sleep disorders are associated with disturbed sleep where the primary problem is due to the brain's inability to synchronise day and night – examples include jet lag and problems encountered by shift workers with changing work schedules. Targeted interventions with short-acting hypnosedatives or agents such as melatonin or agomelatine may provide some assistance.

Other dyssomnias

Restless legs syndrome involves unpleasant sensations in the lower limbs that have variously been described as creeping, crawling, tingling, itching feelings. Restless legs syndrome can delay sleep or wake a person from sleep. Although restless legs syndrome is often idiopathic (arising spontaneously or from an obscure or unknown cause), it may also be secondary to other conditions including normal pregnancy, renal failure, peripheral vascular disease or peripheral neuropathy. Low-dose opioids and other specific pharmacotherapy interventions such as roprinrole or pramipexole may be helpful.

Periodic limb movements in sleep is another dyssomnia that involves repeated, low amplitude, brief, jerky, rhythmic movements in a cycle of approximately every 20–60 seconds. Affecting more men than women and more common among the elderly, this condition may be associated with renal failure, congestive heart failure or PTSD. Low dose l-dopa (e.g. 100/25) may be helpful for movements at the time of sleep onset, whereas controlled-release products are preferred for movements after sleep onset. Massage and cold compresses may also assist. Other pharmacotherapy such as bromocriptine, pergolide or roprinrole may also be trialled under the guidance of a sleep physician.

Drug-induced psychiatric syndromes

Although drug therapy is often an integral part of the management of various mental illnesses, it is also important to acknowledge that medications are an important cause of iatrogenic illness, where morbidity and even mortalities may result directly from the effects of medical treatment (Dukes & Aronson, 2006; Rossi, 2012). The drugs used in the treatment of psychiatric and also general medical conditions can give rise to symptoms that have a primarily psychiatric nature, and thus an important part of clinical review in the mental health setting is to seek evidence for drug-induced psychiatric syndromes. The recognition of these symptoms is important because it can help to prevent the creation of a 'prescribing cascade' (refer to Figure 12.1).

Figure 12.1: Example of a prescribing cascade

SSRI prescribed for Obsessive-Compulsive Disorder

Dosage is often at the upper limit of cited range, commonly associated with severe nausea/vomiting

Metoclopramide prescribed for nausea and vomiting

Dopamine antagonist anti-emetics frequently associated with EPSE, particularly in the elderly

Anticholinergic drug prescribed for EPSE

Drugs such as benztropine are prescribed for EPSE, but have systemic anticholinergic effects

Antipsychotic drug prescribed for delirium associated with anticholinergic drugs

Ongoing antipsychotic drug therapy associated with metabolic disturbance, hyperglycaemia

Drugs for diabetes and hyperlipidaemia prescribed

Drugs such as aspirin, metformin, ACE inhibitor are advocated in evidence-based guidelines

Potential for other serious effects such as GI bleeding, acute renal failure, lactic acidosis

Significant potential for drug–drug and drug–disease interactions in context of polypharmacy

Many examples of drug-induced psychiatric syndromes have been published in international literature, and a range of important examples is provided in Table 12.4. It is also important to note that drug–drug interactions are themselves important sources of morbidity and mortality related to psychotropic medications, and that the interactions may involve medications used for general medical conditions as well as for psychiatric illnesses. For a detailed discussion of psychotropic drug interactions, it is important to refer to a reliable specialist text.

A range of clinically important drug-induced psychiatric syndromes is outlined in Table 12.4.

Table 12.4: Clinically significant psychiatric syndromes associated with medicinal drugs

Drugs linked to depression
Interferons
Retinoids
Clonidine
Mefloquine
Corticosteroids
Verapamil
Oral contraceptives
Some anticonvulsants

Drugs linked to psychosis
Corticosteroids
Some anticonvulsants
Anticholinergic drugs
Antidepressants
Fluoroquinolone antibiotics

Amphetamines and related stimulants

L-dopa and others dopaminergic drugs

Drugs linked to mania

Corticosteroids

Antidepressants

Sympathomimetic amines (e.g. pseudoephedrine)

Drugs linked to anxiety

Corticosteroids

Antidepressants

Xanthines (e.g. theophylline, caffeine)

Amphetamines and related stimulants

Sympathomimetic amines (e.g. pseudoephedrine)

An issue to consider is the possible influence of the environment where the medication is administered on a drug-induced psychiatric syndrome. For instance, high-dose pulse corticosteroid treatment is often administered in the setting of a general medical unit – if an episode of drug-induced mania or psychosis occurs, trained staff may not necessarily be available for patient/client management, and a transfer to a psychiatric unit may be necessary. Another example is the psychosis or severe depression secondary to mefloquine that may occur in a traveller visiting a developing nation where antimalarial prophylaxis is needed; the isolation from medical services may render the problem more dangerous.

ARTHUR'S STORY

Arthur is a 77-year-old man with a history of hypertension and rheumatoid arthritis, but no history of any mental illness at any stage of his life. He was admitted to hospital under the supervision of his rheumatologist for consideration of options in connection with his severe rheumatoid arthritis. After discussion at a consultant ward round, Arthur is given pulse corticosteroid therapy in the form of a bolus intravenous infusion of methylprednisolone 1000 mg. The following morning he is acting very much out of character – loud, garrulous and sexually suggestive towards ward staff. Arthur's wife is in tears – 'he's never been like that, he's just not himself'. The consultation liaison psychiatry team are called in to consult.

Ask yourself!

In relation to Arthur's case:

1   What is the most likely diagnosis?

2   What treatment is likely to be needed and what is the prognosis?

3   Is the syndrome likely to recur upon rechallenge?

From the carer's perspective – *How does this feel for me?*

Many medicinal drugs used in the management of general medical conditions can cause psychiatric syndromes.

Corticosteroids are among the most common causes of mental state changes associated with medicinal drug use.

'He's never like that!'

'What have you done to him? You've poisoned him!'

'Will he get better? I hope he doesn't stay like this.'

Care Plan

The following is an example care plan for the patient/client presented in this chapter. The areas of daily living that are considered include bio-psycho-social factors and the plan is mapped out using the nursing process (Assessment; Planning; Implementation; Evaluation). Remember: the success is in the detail, so be specific about *who, when and what* in the collaborative plan; never include someone in the plan if they were not consulted in the planning process; and always work within a recovery-orientated framework (refer to Chapter 1).

Date: 1 August 2012

Name: Arthur | Case manager: TBA | Consultation: Liaison nurse

Areas of daily living	Assessment of current situation	Goal	Plan (undertaken with patient/client)	Implementation	Who is responsible? (Include only those who have been consulted in the planning process)	Evaluation/ review date
Mental health	No history Corticosteroid-induced psychosis/mania	Stabilise symptoms.	Taper corticosteroid dosage. Introduce a mood stabiliser and/or antipsychotic.	Refer for psychiatric review. Taper corticosteroids to manage corticosteroid-induced psychosis. Introduce mood stabiliser. Constant observation	Treating doctor and team	1/8/12
Social	77-year-old married man	Involve wife in discharge planning after hospitalisation.	Family meeting	Family meeting	Treating doctor to organise	2/8/12

(Continued)

Date: 1 August 2012

Name: Arthur   Case manager: TBA   Consultation: Liaison nurse

Areas of daily living	Assessment of current situation	Goal	Plan (undertaken with patient/client)	Implementation	Who is responsible? (Include only those who have been consulted in the planning process)	Evaluation/ review date
Biological	Hypertension Rheumatoid arthritis Corticosteroid therapy in the form of a bolus intravenous infusion of methylprednisolone 1000 mg. Developed corticosteroid-induced psychosis/mania.	Manage corticosteroid-induced psychosis/mania.	Taper corticosteroid dosage. Introduce a mood stabiliser and/or antipsychotic.	Refer for psychiatric review. Taper corticosteroids to manage corticosteroid-induced psychosis. Introduce mood stabiliser. Constant observation	Treating doctor and team	1/8/12
Environmental	Admitted for rheumatoid arthritis treatment. Lives with his wife.	None identified	N/A	N/A	N/A	N/A
Substance using behaviours	None reported.	N/A	N/A	N/A	N/A	N/A
Risk behaviours	Possible risk of falls.	Reduce risk of falls	Falls assessment	Falls assessment Constant observation until symptoms abate	Nurse	Review every shift change

Pain and psychiatry

Caring for people with comorbid mental illness and significant pain can present a range of challenges for practitioners. Both acute pain and chronic pain syndromes are highly relevant in this regard: the interrelationship between mental illness and pain characteristics can be complex and highly variable, and can have clinical, sociological and legal implications for the individual and practitioner as well as broader populations or health services. A comprehensive discussion of this topic is beyond the scope of a generalist text, but Table 12.5 illustrates a range of potential issues.

Table 12.5: Examples of issues relevant to pain management and psychiatry

Response to analgesia

Some psychotropic drugs can alter the response to analgesia. Pretreatment with opioids in a substitution program can reduce the patient's responsiveness to the analgesia used for acute pain (e.g. postoperative pain) because of tolerance. Naltrexone (used for alcoholism) completely blocks the effects of all opioids.

Other drug interactions

Many psychotropics can interact with drugs used for pain control. In some cases there is a pharmacokinetic interaction: SSRIs can inhibit the metabolism of opioids, meaning that effects are potentiated with the possibility of toxicity (e.g. fluvoxamine can cause potentially lethal methadone accumulation). In other cases effects can be diminished (paroxetine partially blocks the effects of codeine). Other possibilities include pharmacodynamic interactions (e.g. concurrent use of tramadol with many antidepressants may cause the serotonin syndrome), or compounded risk of adverse effects (increased bleeding risk with SSRI + NSAID).

Interplay between mental illness and potential drug-related problems

People with severe, untreated depression may not respond to pain relief as expected – even when given appropriate doses of analgesics, pain may not be properly controlled until the depression has been treated. Those with PTSD are at increased risk of iatrogenic substance use disorders if treated with benzodiazepines or opioids. People with exacerbations of schizophrenia or mania should not be allowed to self-administer analgesia without close supervision. A false or over-valued belief system (characteristic of psychiatric disorders) may lead some patients/clients to forego proven conventional treatments and use complementary products instead, thus contributing to non-adherence.

The issues outlined in Table 12.5 are only examples – particularly when dealing with chronic pain management, the involvement of a mental health team is considered to be essential for sound management.

Complementary medicines

Research suggests that many people who are affected by mental illness use complementary medicines or alternative therapies, but may not necessarily inform the psychiatric team about this (or may report details inconsistently or incompletely). In one small study, a range of 85 different complementary treatments had been used by over half of the subjects during the six months prior to interview (Alderman & Kiepfer, 2003). Of those using these products, a third of those questioned reported that they had not informed their doctor.

Examples of complementary approaches that are used with the intention of affecting mental state or mental symptoms include St John's wort, SAMe (S-adenosylmethionine), passionflower extract, gentian extract, ginkgo products, acupuncture and aromatherapy. It is sometimes overlooked that these types of products can have clinically significant impact upon mental state, comorbidities and the effects of prescribed drugs. For example, use of St John's wort can cause induction of hepatic enzymes to an extent that can actually cause the failure of oral contraceptives.

It is important to ensure that the matter of complementary medicine use is included when taking a comprehensive clinical history. As a rule, it is generally best to request that these products be suspended or at least recorded during hospital inpatient stays.

Drugs in pregnancy and lactation

There are situations in which a woman may be affected by a mental disorder during the course of pregnancy or while breastfeeding, and it is necessary to consider the use of psychotropic drugs as a part of the treatment. The effects of the drug upon the mother and the developing foetus need to be taken into account, and the overall risks and benefits considered in balance. The teratogenic effects of various drugs are different and may vary in accordance with the trimester of pregnancy during which exposure occurs. In some cases the risk is highest during the first and second trimesters (during organogenesis) whereas for other medications exposure late in pregnancy may create the risk of perinatal complications (e.g. bleeding) or drug withdrawal in the neonate. The risks associated with maternal intake of drugs during lactation will largely depend on the extent to which the drug is secreted into breast milk, which is the major determinant of neonatal exposure. Extensive discussion of this complex area is beyond the scope of a generalist text, and where necessary it is appropriate to seek advice from a specialist information centre such as those located in major women's and children's hospitals.

Summary

It is clear that many important forms of psychiatric syndrome occur in addition to those seen in the context of major depression, bipolar disorder, schizophrenia and the anxiety disorders. In some cases, conditions such as personality disorders, eating disorders and sleep disorders occur comorbidly with other psychiatric syndromes. Pharmacotherapy does not always play an important role in the management of these conditions, but clinicians do need to have awareness of the drug therapy options that may prove helpful. In addition, it is important for clinicians to be aware of medications that may cause psychiatric syndromes.

On the Horizon in Pharmacotherapy for Sleep Disorders

One promising avenue for the management of primary insomnia involves the use of a long-established antidepressant, doxepin, which binds histamine H1 receptors with high specificity. At low doses, doxepin selectively antagonises H1 receptors, promoting the initiation and maintenance of sleep. Trials for chronic primary insomnia treated with oral, low-dose doxepin 3 or 6 mg once daily improved wake time after sleep onset, total sleep time and sleep efficiency to a significantly greater extent than placebo (Krystal et al., 2011; Langford et al., 2012) . Unlike the case with benzodiazepine, the effect of doxepin was maintained to 12 weeks without evidence of physical dependence or worsening insomnia after withdrawal.

Ramelteon is a potent and selective human melatonin MT1 and MT2 receptor agonist. Unlike benzodiazepines and other hypnosedatives, ramelteon has no measurable affinity for the GABA receptor complex, and in addition has little affinity for the serotonin 5-HT2B receptor. Its actions at the MT1 receptor are localised in the hypothalamic suprachiasmatic nucleus where it mediates circadian of melatonin. The MT2 receptor is in the hypothalamic suprachiasmatic nucleus and the neural retina and is thought to mediate the effects of melatonin on circadian rhythms. The drug has now been approved in the USA as a treatment for primary insomnia: the recommended dose is 8 mg taken within 30 minutes before going to bed. Ramelteon should not be taken with or immediately after a high-fat meal.

Discussion questions

1   Which pharmacotherapy might be useful for the management of some eating disorders?

2   What are the most common causes of insomnia?

Test yourself (answers in the back of the book)

1   With respect to eating disorders, which of the following statements is most accurate?

   A   There is an equal prevalence among both genders.

   B   Drug treatment is never used as a management option.

   C   Menstrual abnormalities with anorexia nervosa may cause osteopaenia.

   D   Most eating disorders are benign and self-limiting.

2   Pharmacotherapy for personality disorders:

   A   is not regarded as a first-line approach

   B   usually involves a mood stabiliser agent

   C   should include benzodiazepines

   D   none of the above

3   Which of the following agents has been used for the treatment of narcolepsy?

   A   Modafanil

   B   Olanzapine

   C   Donepezil

   D   Diazepam

4   Which of the following agents is most prominently associated with depression?

   A   Amlodipine

   B   Enalapril

   C   Verapamil

   D   Frusemide

5 Which of the following agents has a significant drug interaction with methadone?

A Fluvoxamine

B Bupropion

C Ziprasidone

D Lithium

Useful websites

Australian Psychological Society: *Understanding and Managing Eating Disorders* available at <www.psychology.org.au/publications/tip_sheets/eating>

American Academy of Sleep Medicine: *The International Classification of Sleep Disorders, Revised Diagnostic And Coding Manual* available at <www.esst.org/adds/ICSD.pdf>

What are Personality Disorders? Available at <http://au.reachout.com/find/articles/personality-disorders>

References

Alderman C. P. & Kiepfer, B. (2003). 'Complementary medicine use by psychiatry patients of an Australian hospital' *Annals of Pharmacotherapy* 37(12): 1779–1784.

American Psychiatric Association. (2000). *Diagnostic and Statistical Manual of Mental Disorders*, 4th edn, Text Revision *(DSM-IV-TR)*. Washington DC: American Psychiatric Publishing, Inc.

Dukes M. & Aronson, J. (2006). *Meyler's Side Effects of Drugs: The International Encyclopedia of Adverse Drug Reactions and Interactions*. Amsterdam: Elsevier.

Krystal A. D., Lankford A., Durrence H. H., Ludington E., Jochelson P., Rogowski R. & Roth T. (2011). 'Efficacy and safety of doxepin 3 and 6 mg in a 35-day sleep laboratory trial in adults with chronic primary insomnia' *Sleep* 34: 1433–1442.

Lankford A., Rogowski R., Essink B., Ludington E., Heith Durrence H., Roth T. (2012). 'Efficacy and safety of doxepin 6 mg in a four-week outpatient trial of elderly adults with chronic primary insomnia' *Sleep Med* 13: 133–138

Rossi S. (2012). *Australian Medicines Handbook*. Adelaide, South Australia: AMH Pty Ltd.

Part 3

Advanced Practice and Context

Chapter 13

Adherence and Concordance

Chapter overview

This chapter covers the following topics:

* adherence
* concordance
* compliance
* non-adherence.

Chapter learning objectives

After reading this chapter, you should be able to:

* have a better understanding of the burden of chronic conditions such as mental illness
* know the difference between adherence, compliance and concordance
* identify factors that can influence adherence.

Key terms

Adherence
Concordance
Compliance
Non-adherence

Introduction

In this chapter you will first begin to understand the global burden of disability of chronic conditions, and in particular mental illness and comorbidity. You will then explore the notion of adherence and compliance. Importantly, you will also discover what role adherence can offer on the road of recovery for patients/clients who are prescribed medicines for a mental disorder. You will touch on the concepts of recovery and concordance skills, and how concordance can be brought to life through Anne's and Bob's examples. You will also discover some of the factors that can influence adherence.

The global burden of disability of chronic conditions

Chronic non-communicable diseases such as heart disease, cancer and diabetes are the biggest killers worldwide. Chronic disease accounts for 48% of the global disability (World Health Organization, 2005, p. 39) and accounts for 60% of all deaths worldwide. Chronic conditions affect people of all ages and affect both men and women equally. According to global statistics, chronic disease burden is most prevalent among the poor. This is thought to be due in the main to exposure to a number of vulnerabilities (exposure to poor nutrition, poor access to education, fewer job prospects, etc.). Chronic conditions include heart disease, stroke, diabetes, cancer, chronic respiratory disease and mental illness. Mental disorders were more frequent among people with one of the chronic physical conditions such as diabetes, cardiovascular disease (CVD) and cancer than for those without them (as demonstrated in Australia with recent data showing 28% compared with 18% – Australian Institute of Health and Wellbeing, 2010, p. 167). Alarming statistics are emerging about the projected figures for chronic conditions: by 2030 depression is expected to be the leading burden of disease around the world, jumping from third position as seen in 2004 (World Health Organization, 2008).

According to the World Health Organization 450 million people worldwide are affected by mental or behavioural problems at any time, and one in four patients/clients visiting a health service has at least one mental or behavioural disorder. Alarmingly, most of these disorders are neither diagnosed nor treated

(World Health Organization, 2007, 2011). In Australia, one in five people will experience a mental illness during their lifetime. Some people will experience mental illness once and fully recover, while other individuals will continue to battle with mental illness relapses throughout their lives (Australian Bureau of Statistics, 2006). *Non-psychotic mental illnesses* are conditions in which a person experiences a range of psychiatric symptoms that remain based in reality. Such symptoms include feelings of depression, sadness, and tension or fear that are so disturbing as to affect the person's ability to cope with day-to-day living. Conditions that can cause these feelings include anxiety disorders, eating disorders and depression. Psychotic mental illness consists of *schizophrenia and subtypes of schizophrenia* (this disorder affects approximately 1% of Australians at some point in their lives), *bipolar affective disorder* (this condition affects up to 2% of Australians at some time during their lives), and *some forms of depression*.

During the 1990s there were dramatic advances in the treatment of schizophrenia. Just as the serotonin reuptake inhibitor class of antidepressants has largely replaced the older and more problematic tricyclic antidepressants, a shift in the treatment of schizophrenia is now taking place. The first of the new (postclozapine) atypical antipsychotic medications, risperidone, was introduced in 1994, followed by olanzapine, quetiapine, sertindole and ziprasidone. These medications, known as the new generation of antipsychotics, are better tolerated than the old generation of antipsychotics and provide a greater choice of treatment options for patients/clients. However, medication is only one ingredient on the road to recovery from mental illness since mental illness is diverse in aetiology and treatment. The road to recovery is captured by this personal reflection from a person living with schizophrenia (Wagner, 2004):

> Schizophrenia is, for most people, an uncharted and terrifying shadow-land that they seek to avoid along with the sufferer whose torments, pain and oddnesses so scare them. In the past, such people were put behind the locked doors of asylums. Today they are simply consigned to the anonymity and powerlessness of poverty, and are forgotten. We can't find our way alone, not without the help and understanding so often denied us. In spite of the closets imprisoning us, we still live among you, hundreds of thousands of us. Only with support and encouragement will we ever be able to break open the doors.

Over 60 years ago the *British Medical Journal* reported an association between mental illness and poor physical health (Philips, 1934). Individuals with persistent mental illness are subjected to the long-term effects of antipsychotic medication, have high rates of substance misuse, eat less balanced diets, smoke more, and take less exercise than the general population (Phelan, Stradins & Morrison, 2001). It is well accepted that mental illness is the largest single cause of disability burden and that morbidity and mortality rates from physical illness are much higher for this group than in other populations. Comorbid mental illness and physical illness incrementally worsens health compared with mental illness alone or any of the chronic non-communicable diseases such as cardiovascular diseases, cancers, chronic respiratory diseases and diabetes alone (Edward, Rasmussen & Munro, 2010; Moussavi et al., 2007; Page et al., 2010). In the context of adherence to medications and other treatments, people who experience mental illness in conjunction with a physical illness (a comorbid condition) are presented with many challenges to *sticking to* their treatment regimen!

Moreover, the multiple medical comorbidities such as ischaemic heart disease, diabetes and chronic respiratory illness that are so common among those treated for serious mental illness are themselves conditions that often necessitate the use of complex medication regimens. Evidence-based practice results in the need to initiate a range of treatments to accommodate issues that might arise as a result of the effects of drugs used for the management of mental illness. For example, the consumer who develops hyperglycaemia in association with antipsychotic medication may eventually progress to a diagnosis of type II diabetes mellitus. A diagnosis of diabetes may then require the addition of aspirin and a statin for prevention of cardiovascular disease, an angiotensin converting enzyme inhibitor for nephroprotection, and a hypoglycaemic agent such as metformin or gliclazide. This phenomenon is sometimes referred to as a prescribing cascade: the initial drug (the antipsychotic agent) might have been administered as a single daily dose, but the ensuing complications eventually result in the addition of four or five other medicines and up to seven or eight occasions of medication administration each day. Remembering to take these additional medications and remaining motivated to do so can present a real challenge, and in the case of diabetes there may be an additional complication whereby the condition progresses to an insulin-dependent state requiring multiple daily administrations of parenteral medications. If these challenges are considered in the context of the patient with a severe psychiatric illness causing significant distress and impairment, it is evident that there is a high likelihood that all medications in the regimen (including psychotropic drugs) may not be taken as prescribed. If this in turn creates a destabilisation of comorbid medical conditions, there can be a direct impact upon the stability of the psychiatric symptoms.

The interrelationships demonstrated in the example above clearly illustrate the importance of a holistic consideration of the consumer's medical and psychiatric illnesses, personality characteristics and simultaneous stressors, and the overall effect of these upon functionality and treatment outcomes. The mostly widely used benchmark compendium of the features of these disorders is the *Diagnostic and Statistical Manual of Mental Disorders*, published by the American Psychiatric Association, and currently in its fourth edition (usually referred to as DSM-IV). It is noteworthy that in the introduction of the DSM-IV, a discussion of the term 'mental disorder' acknowledges that this type of terminology 'implies a distinction between "mental" disorders and "physical" disorders that is correctly described as a "reductionist anachronism of mind/body dualism"'.

Mental and physical illnesses are intimately linked, and this is reflected in the multiaxial assessment system that is fundamental to the DSM-IV. In this system, information about psychiatric conditions, general medical conditions, psychosocial issues and environmental problems, and a global assessment of functioning, are linked to create a comprehensive picture that can be used for the purpose of capturing, organising and communicating complex clinical information relevant to the care of those affected by mental illness. Moreover the codes and terms of the DSM-IV are compatible with those of the *International Statistical Classification of Diseases and Related Health Problems* (ICD-10) created by the World Health Organization. The value of this approach is that a common basis for the comparison of the prevalence and incidence of mental illness is available, and that a categorical framework for research and clinical treatment of these disorders has been established.

Although the DSM multiaxial assessment system has primarily been designed by psychiatrists for the use of psychiatrists, this system elegantly facilitates multidisciplinary care. The information that is presented allows a range of other involved clinicians to access a global picture of the issues relevant to a holistic approach to care management, and thus is apposite to the information needs of nurses, psychologists, social workers and pharmacists. The multiaxial system allows the collation of assessment information on five axes or domains of information, allowing various members of the treatment team to participate in the planning of treatment, as is outlined below:

Axis I, information about clinical disorders that includes the various important psychiatric illnesses is documented. Examples of various clinical diagnoses that would be documented in Axis I include dementia; substance-related disorders; schizophrenia; mood disorders, such as major depression; anxiety disorders, such as post-traumatic stress disorder; and eating disorders.

Axis II is used for the documentation of personality disorders and mental retardation, but may also be used for noting prominent maladaptive personality features and defence mechanisms that do not meet the threshold for a personality disorder. The reason for the use of a separate axis to document these conditions is, at least in part, to ensure that appropriate consideration will be assigned to these, even when more florid Axis I disorders may serve to divert the focus of clinical attention. Notable personality disorders that can be documented in Axis II include paranoid personality disorder, schizoid personality disorder, antisocial personality disorder, borderline personality disorder and narcissistic personality disorder.

Axis III is used to describe general medical conditions that are potentially relevant to the understanding or management of the mental disorder in a number of ways. For example, in some cases a general medical condition may be centrally related to the cause of mental symptoms, such as is the case with some forms of epilepsy. Another example would be situations where psychiatric symptoms may be a part of a psychological reaction to a general medical condition, such as the psychological sequelae of knowledge of infection with the HIV virus. A particularly important issue is the presence of an Axis III that might influence choice of drug treatment, or where the use of particular drug therapy may alter the monitoring required to ensure safe and effective drug therapy.

Axis IV Documentation of issues that may be influential in the diagnosis or treatment of mental disorders is noted in Axes I and II. These issues may also influence general medical conditions in Axis III, which in turn may affect the person's overall health and well-being, or else may have a significant effect upon the stability and severity of a mental illness (thus necessitating alterations to drug therapy and monitoring that will be integral to the pharmaceutical care plan). Psychosocial and environmental issues are documented in Axis IV, and information from this domain will be required by staff caring for the patient/client, particularly as it extends beyond elements that merely focus upon drugs and disease states. The DSM-IV lists a number of different categories of issues that would be documented in Axis IV of the multiaxial assessment, many of which have direct relevance to the implementation of care plans. Categories (with examples of issues that could be relevant to the provision of pharmaceutical care) include:

- problems with primary support group, for example health problems in the family
- problems related to the social environment, for example inadequate social support; living alone; difficulty with acculturation
- educational problems, for example literacy challenges
- economic problems, for example poverty or insufficient welfare support
- problems with access to health care services, for example inadequate health care services; unavailable transportation to health care facilities; inadequate health insurance.

Axis V is used to record a measure of the extent of the issues listed in the first four axes upon the functional capacity, with this impact reflected by the Global Assessment of Functioning (GAF) score. The information can be used in both the planning of treatment and the assessment of the effects, and thus again has very direct relevance to the provision of care.

The organisation of information into the axes of the system shows the connections between these domains of information. The use of this system allows a comprehensive and systematic evaluation of each patient/client by all members of the multidisciplinary team, incorporating an integrated consideration of both mental disorders and general medical conditions, the interaction of these with psychosocial and environmental issues, and the effects that these can have upon characteristics of medication usage.

Adherence versus compliance

'Adherence' is a term that superseded the term 'compliance' in the health care nomenclature in the past decade. Historically, patients/clients were considered either compliant or non-compliant with their treatment and/or medication. The term generally refers to prescribed medication regimens and other medical instructions, but historically was used in the context of medication regimens. Being *compliant* inferred that the patient/client was taking their medications as prescribed, and being *non-compliant* meant they were not. The term 'non-compliant' would historically conjure up images of a person wilfully and irresponsibly not taking their medication, and the term 'compliant' held paternalistic connotations for patients/clients and clinicians alike. While the terminology related to taking medications and following medical instructions is the focus of debate, the World Health Organization (WHO) prefers the term 'adherence'. At the WHO Adherence meeting in June 2001 the following definition of adherence was agreed upon as a starting point for further development of the definition: 'the extent to which the patient follows medical instructions' (WHO, 2003, p. 3).

The words 'medical instructions' also remained unclear for many and needed expansion. This definition was further expanded to include the details of what types of medical instructions were considered to be related to adherence, and these include 'taking medication, following a diet, and/or executing lifestyle changes, corresponds with agreed recommendations from a health care provider' (WHO, 2003, p. 3). Globally, adherence to long-term therapies averages 50%. This figure is alarming given that there are a number of symptoms related to mental illness and other chronic conditions that respond well to medication intervention. For instance, an antipsychotic response can moderate combativeness, tension, hostility, hallucinations and delusions in most cases and antihypertensive medications can moderate the risk of hypertension, negating the potential for stroke.

There has been much research examining factors that affect adherence to medication such as illness- and disorder-related factors, personal factors (such as embarrassment related to taking medication, busy lifestyles, low self-esteem and poor motivation), social factors (family, support), cultural or religious beliefs, economic factors (affordability of medications) and treatment factors (ADR knowledge gaps, duration of treatment for chronic conditions, poor symptom management). Poor adherence to therapies translates to poor outcomes for patients/clients. Many of these factors can be the focus of interventions; the nurse or other health professional can engage the patient/client in discussions related to adherence to (or sticking to) their prescribed medication regimen. While medication as a treatment in those who experience mental disorder is important, it is inadequate as a single treatment option to treat the symptoms of mental illness. However, increased adherence can place the patient/client in a stronger position for recovery.

The concept of recovery has been part of the terminology of health services for the last few decades (Edward, Welch & Elsom, in Edward, Munro, Robins & Welch, 2011). The recovery model adopted in such countries as the United Kingdom, Ireland, Australia, New Zealand, the United States and Canada places the patient/client at the centre of care. There is a lack of consensus of the definition of recovery, which can be viewed from many perspectives: a patient's/client's individual and self-determined recovery, the absence of symptoms, a return to the premorbid state of functioning, an ability to fulfil roles and obligations, or a stable level of well-being. Health care providers are well positioned to work with consumers in an alliance towards recovery, using available resources and providing these in a manner that meets the patient's/client's needs. In light of the lack of consensus of the definition of recovery, interventions undertaken by you as a health care worker will need to be patient-centred and individualised.

Concordance

'Concordance' is a relatively new term and is primarily used in health care language and practice in the United Kingdom. Concordance was initially understood to be an agreement relating to therapy and therapeutic discussions. This notion of concordance has since been broadened to include support and communication about treatment. The term 'concordance' has been used incorrectly as a synonym for adherence. In essence, concordance is a *set of skills* to enable mental health workers to be more effective when talking to patients/clients about their medication.

Skills used by the health profession in the process of facilitating concordance are:

* Engaging the patient/client.

* Exchanging information.

* Having advanced knowledge of treatment and treatment options.

* Using advanced negotiation skills.

* Having the ability to mobilise supports for the patient/client.

* Working with the patient's/client's beliefs about treatment and exploring ambivalence.

* Working with the patient/client to look into the future.

Implicit in the practice of concordance is the patient's/client's beliefs about their condition and treatment. The key elements of a concordance approach are working collaboratively and with flexibility, working with the views and beliefs that patients/clients have about medication, and exploring and working towards a resolution of their ambivalence about taking medication. There is an element of *shared decision-making* involved in the process of concordance. Shared decision-making is suitable for long-term decisions, especially in the context of a chronic illness. As you would expect in the process of concordance, the health professional and the patient/client meet for more than one session, and under these circumstances shared decision-making can be an effective method of reaching a treatment agreement (Joosten et al., 2008).

Another concept that has recently been described in medication usage taxonomy is that of medication 'persistence'. This term is essentially used to link the extent of concordance with longitudinal duration. Put simply, 'persistence' is a term that can be used to describe the duration of time that a consumer continues to use the medications in the way (dose, frequency, purpose. etc.) that the medicines were intended for when initially prescribed. The greater the duration and extent of persistence, the better the outcomes that can be achieved in the treatment of serious psychiatric illness. Researchers are now beginning to assemble an understanding of the factors that influence persistence.

These include maintaining an extended period of stable symptom control – what this translates to is that the consumer who is able to maintain good symptom control over an extended period of time will be most likely to continue to take the medication as prescribed. Other positive factors include the experience of personal, daily benefit by the consumer (if they feel that they can perceive benefits from taking the medication as prescribed each day, they are more likely to continue to do so); acceptability of side effects if any (taking into account what is important to the consumer, not just the prescriber or mental health team); and avoiding the use of illicit psychotropic substances such as amphetamines or cannabis. Other particularly important positive influences upon persistence are: the maintenance of supportive interpersonal relationships (meaning that consumers with a supportive spouse, family or carers tend to do better); a stable living environment; and meaningful employment or purposeful volunteering. As such, it is clear that an investment in facilitating these positive outcomes for consumers can improve medication persistence, and ultimately achieve better outcomes for the management of chronic illness – both psychiatric conditions and comorbid medical issues.

ANNE'S STORY

Anne is a 32-year-old single woman who is working part-time in hospitality. Anne has diabetes type 2 and also has a diagnosis of bipolar affective disorder. Anne sees her case manager and psychiatrist regularly and has done so for the past two years. Even though Anne appears to be engaged with regular appointments with her treating team, the case manager has found it difficult to engage Anne in talking about her medication and her intermittent non-adherence. However, Anne said when speaking to her case manager that she did not believe that she needed to take medication once she felt better. She believed that her blood sugar changes were the reason she had mood swings and when her blood sugar was stable then she did not require the medication prescribed for her diagnosed bipolar affective disorder. Anne said that when she experienced 'racing thoughts' she would stop taking the medication for the bipolar affective disorder as she believed this was a sign of having stable blood sugars since she also felt 'very happy' at these times. Anne wants to finish a diploma in information technology but has found that her frequent relapses and subsequent hospitalisations over the past four years have made this difficult. Anne has a close friend called Sara with whom she shares a house. Anne also has a brother, Tim, with whom she has dinner once a fortnight.

Ask yourself!

As Anne's health care worker:

1   What strategies can you utilise to better engage Anne?

2   How can you work with Anne's beliefs about her medication?

3   What supports can you mobilise to help Anne look forward towards her goals?

4   Are there circumstances where characteristics of Anne's use of medications may have a broader impact for others around her?

The student nurse's experience of medication management

With the introduction of **advanced practice** roles in nursing with nurse prescribing rights, the nurse's role in medication management now reaches further than that of administration and monitoring of side effects. What this essentially means for the student nurse is an increased focus and expectation of pharmacology knowledge, advanced drug calculation skills development, and other contextual considerations related to medication therapy for patients/clients. These contextual considerations relate to the pharmacodynamics of medicines, the pharmacokinetics of drugs, standards, legislative considerations particular to the geographical location of practice, and remaining within a scope of practice that is directly related to qualifications (Hemingway, Stephenson & Allmark, 2011). Medications management education is diverse across different tertiary education organisations for nurses, and it is a challenge for these institutions and indeed the students in regard to national standards for registration within Australia.

Ask yourself!

1   What medication management knowledge do I have?

2   What medication knowledge gaps do I have?

3   How can I develop my skills to effectively engage patients/clients in my care?

4   How well do *I* do when I need to take medications (e.g. antibiotics) myself?

BOB'S STORY

Bob is a 24-year-old single man who lives at home with his parents in a semirural area. He has a five-year history of psychosis and a comorbid substance misuse disorder. For the past two years Bob's team has found him difficult to engage and he is non-adherent intermittently. Bob is prescribed 15 mg of olanzapine at night. Bob admits to drinking two to eight cans of beer a day and he says he enjoys five joints of cannabis each day since he believes the joints relax him. Some of Bob's beliefs about his non-adherent behaviours are:

'I don't have a mental illness, so I don't need the medication.'

'The cannabis and alcohol help me relax and relieve my stress.'

As Bob's health care worker you could spend time with Bob looking back over his treatment experiences. You can ask him to begin his story at any point he wished (*this is part of engagement and working collaboratively*). Throughout Bob's story you can reflect back the essence of what he was saying; it is important to use reflection to support self-generated positive accounts about medication (*this is reflective listening, an advanced communication skill*). At the end of the session with Bob it is important to offer Bob the opportunity to clarify points he has made as well as show him you have been listening to him throughout the session. This can occur throughout the session also (*this is known as summarising and is also an important ingredient for engagement*). Each subsequent session with Bob should be linked with the previous session, and you can achieve this by summarising the key points from the previous session. At the end of each session, there needs to be an 'in principle' agreement about the topic for discussion in the coming session (*linking sessions together and agreeing on the topic for discussion in the next session provides structure and focus; with Bob's involvement in deciding the topics to address at each session, you can provide him with a sense of control and ownership over his medication management*).

Care Plan

The following is an example care plan for the patient/client presented in this chapter. The areas of daily living that are considered include bio-psycho-social factors and the plan is mapped out using the nursing process (Assessment; Planning; Implementation; Evaluation). Remember: the success is in the detail, so be specific about *who, when and what* in the collaborative plan; never include someone in the plan if they were not consulted in the planning process; and always work within a recovery-orientated framework (refer to Chapter 1).

Date: Today's date

Name: Bob Young   Case manager: MH Nurse

Areas of daily living	Assessment of current situation	Goal	Plan (undertaken with patient/client)	Implementation	Who is responsible? (Include only those who have been consulted in the planning process)	Evaluation/ review date
Mental health	5-year history of psychosis and a comorbid substance misuse disorder.	Minimise the adverse effects of psychotic symptoms.	Monitor early warning signs of psychosis which are: • feeling more agitated • pacing more • poor sleep • reduced concentration Action: if early warning signs are present • use distraction techniques • call MH Nurse to discuss and organise a possible review of medication.	Develop an early warning signs list with Bob and document this for Bob's record and MH Nurse's record. Bob to keep a list of early warning signs with him and a copy to be attached to the fridge door.	Bob MH Nurse Bob	15/3/12 Ongoing

Social	Lives at home with parents.	Would like to move into own residence.	Develop a budget plan with Bob. With Bob, scope the local rental options in the area of Bob's choice.	Bob and MH Nurse to undertake budget planning. Check local paper for rental options.	Bob and MH Nurse — 4 weeks; Bob — 24 weeks
			Consider shared accommodation options.	Check shared care options.	MH Nurse — 24 weeks
Biological	History of non-adherence to medication/treatment. Bob's beliefs about his non-adherent behaviours are: • 'I don't have a mental illness, so I don't need the medication.' • 'The cannabis and alcohol helps me relax and relieves my stress.'	Improve adherent behaviour.	Discuss with Bob his motivation for, beliefs and ambivalence about adhering or not adhering to medication/treatment. Continue with regular appointments with MH Nurse.	MH Nurse and Bob	Every 2 weeks

Date: Today's date *(Continued)*

Name: Bob Young

Case manager: MH Nurse

Areas of daily living	Assessment of current situation	Goal	Plan (undertaken with patient/client)	Implementation	Who is responsible? (Include only those who have been consulted in the planning process)	Evaluation/ review date
	Prescribed 15 mg olanzapine nocte.	Maintain therapeutic effect of olanzapine.	Maintain therapeutic effect of olanzapine.	Ensure regular appointments for Bob with psychiatrist related to positive effects of olanzapine.	MH Nurse	Every 12 weeks
Environmental	Lives in a semirural area, possible isolation.	Minimise potential for isolation.	Explore with Bob membership to community groups related to Bob's interests.	Develop a list of at least 2 interests of Bob.	Bob and MH Nurse	12/4/12
Substance using behaviours	Consumes 2–8 cans of beer a day.	To reduce the risks associated with risk drinking	Explore Bob's motivations and beliefs related to drinking	Work together to discuss reduced drinking or alcohol drinking cessation.	MH Nurse and Bob	Each appointment
	Intake of 5 joints of cannabis each day.	Reduce the risks associated with cannabis use.	Explore Bob's motivations and beliefs related to cannabis use.	Work together to discuss reduced cannabis use or cannabis use cessation.	MH Nurse and Bob	Each appointment

Some considerations regarding medicines and adherence or non-adherence

For many people who are prescribed medicine there are often many practical matters that can affect their adherence, for example:

* forgetting to take the medication

* lack of access to a chemist to fill prescriptions

* inability to afford the cost of medications

* experience of stigma as a result of side effects of the medication (e.g. movement disorders, weight gain, sexual dysfunction).

Other influencing factors that may contribute to non-adherent behaviours and will need your consideration when you are assessing adherence in your comprehensive assessment of patients/clients in your care may be:

* illness-related factors (denial of disorder, level of disability)

* environmental factors (family view of mental illness, media influence)

* factors related to the treating team (non-collaborative, poor follow-up, irregular medication review)

* factors relate to the treatment regimen (adverse effects, no immediate benefits, route of medication administration, e.g. depot injection)

* personality-related factors (beliefs about mental illness, self-esteem, motivation, fear)

* simultaneous substance use disorders.

Ask yourself!

1 How could you incorporate an assessment for adherent or non-adherent behaviour in your initial assessments when there is no place for it on the form the hospital uses?

2 Why would you undertake an assessment for adherent or non-adherent behaviours if other health professionals on your team do not do it?

3 Make a list of the benefits of knowing about adherent and non-adherent behaviours of the patients/clients in your care.

Summary

In this chapter you read about the global burden of disability of chronic conditions, and in particular mental illness and comorbidity. The combination of chronic conditions can certainly make adherent behaviour a challenge for patients/clients. Additionally, being non-adherent is quite expected. It is well known that only 50% of all people prescribed medication for any condition will be adherent to the medication regimen. A way of testing this theory is to get a group of people (friends, family and colleagues at the staff table) and ask how many of them had been prescribed antibiotics before. Then ask those who put their hand up whether they took the full course of antibiotics as prescribed in every case. You will see that 50% of those with their hands up after the first question will not have their hand up now!

You explored in this chapter the notion of adherence and compliance, especially the role adherence can offer on the road of recovery for patients/clients who are prescribed medicines for a mental disorder. With Anne's story you were able to challenge yourself with the complex issues related to her medications and at times non-adherent behaviour. With the story about Bob, in the section 'How does this feel for me?' there are some examples of using concordance skills to improve adherent behaviour potential, even when there is resistance present. Finally, this chapter presented some factors that can influence adherence for you to consider.

Discussion questions

1 *How* would you incorporate assessment of adherence and non-adherence and use of concordance skills in your routine practice?

2 *Who* can use concordance skills in their practice (e.g. nurse, doctor, pharmacist, psychologist, social worker, occupational therapist)?

3 *What* lessons can you take from the example given of the session with Bob?

4 *What* challenges exist in the use of Consumer Medicines Information (CMI) for patients/clients treated for mental illnesses, and how might these be addressed in an interdisciplinary context?

Test yourself (answers at the back of the book)

1 Comorbid mental illness and physical illness:

A incrementally worsens health compared with mental illness alone

B incrementally worsens health compared with any of the chronic non-communicable diseases such as cardiovascular diseases, cancers, chronic respiratory diseases and diabetes alone

C incrementally worsens health compared with mental illness alone or any of the chronic non-communicable diseases such as cardiovascular diseases, cancers, chronic respiratory diseases and diabetes alone

D incrementally improves health compared with mental illness alone or any of the chronic non-communicable diseases such as cardiovascular diseases, cancers, chronic respiratory diseases and diabetes alone

2 Globally, adherence to long-term therapies:

A averages 80%

B averages 70%

C averages 60%

D averages 50%

3 Concordance is:

A adherence to medication

B a set of skills to enable mental health workers to be more effective in talking to patients/clients about their medication

C compliance to medication outlined by the mental health worker

D all of the above

4 An increased focus on and expectation of pharmacology knowledge, advanced drug calculation skills development and other contextual considerations related to medication therapy for patients/clients:

A is the role of the student

B is the role of the nurse

C is the role of the health care worker

D all of the above

5   Influencing factors that may contribute to non-adherent behaviours, and need
    your consideration in your comprehensive assessment of patients/clients in
    your care, are:

    A   illness-related factors and person-related factors in simultaneous
        substance use disorders

    B   environmental factors and factors related to the treating team

    C   factors related to the treatment regimen

    D   all of the above

Useful websites

Gray, R. *Adherence Therapy Manual* available from <www.academia.
    edu/702928/Adherence_therapy_manual>

World Health Organization: *Investing in Mental Health* available from <www.
    who.int/mental_health/media/investing_mnh.pdf>

References

Australian Bureau of Statistics. (2006). *Mental Health in Australia: A Snapshot,
    2004 –05*. Retrieved 8 January 2008, from <www.abs.gov.au/ausstats/
    abs@.nsf/mf/4824.0.55.001>.

Australian Institute of Health and Welfare. (2010). *Australian Health – The Twelfth
    Biennial Health Report of the Australian Institute of Health and Welfare* (Cat. No.
    AUS 122). Canberra: Australian Institute of Health and Welfare.

Edward K., Rasmussen B. & Munro, I. (2010). 'Nursing care of clients treated
    with atypical antipsychotics who have a risk of developing metabolic
    instability and/or type 2 diabetes' *Archives of Psychiatric Nursing* 24(1): 46–53.

Edward K. L., Munro I., Robins, A. & Welch A. (2011). *Mental Health Nursing:
    Dimensions of Praxis*. Melbourne: Oxford University Press.

Hemingway S., Stephenson J. & Allmark H. (2011). 'Student experiences of
    medicines management training and education' *British Journal of Nursing*
    20(5): 291.

Joosten E., DeFuentes-Merillas L., De Weert G., Sensky T., Van der Staak C. & De
    Jong C. (2008). 'Systematic review of the effects of shared decision-making
    on patient satisfaction, treatment adherence and health status' *Psychotherapy
    and Psychosomatics* 77(4): 219–226.

Moussavi S., Chatterji S., Verdes E., Tandon A., Patel, V. & Ustun B. (2007). 'Depression, chronic diseases, and decrements in health: results from the World Health Surveys' *Lancet* 370(9590): 851–858.

Page K. N., Davidson P., Edward K. et al. (2010). 'Recovering from an acute cardiac event–the relationship between depression and life satisfaction' *Journal of Clinical Nursing* 19(5–6): 736–743.

Phelan M., Stradins L. & Morrison, S. (2001). 'Physical health of people with severe mental illness' *BMJ* 322(7284): 443.

Philips R. J. (1934). 'Physical disorder in 164 consecutive admissions to a mental hospital: the incidence and significance' *BMJ* 2: 363–366.

Wagner P. (2004). *A Voice from Another Closet*. Retrieved 12 February 2005, from <www.schizophrenia.com/newsletter/buckets/ newsletter/197/197pwagner .html>.

World Health Organization. (2003). *Adherence to Long-term Therapies: Evidence for Action*. Geneva: World Health Organization.

World Health Organization. (2005). *Preventing Chronic Diseases. A Vital Investment*. WHO Global Report (No. 0300-5771). Geneva: World Health Organization.

World Health Organization. (2007). *Projected DALYs for 2005, 2015 and 2030 by WHO Region*. Retrieved August 2008, from <www.who.int/healthinfo/ statistics/bodprojections2030/en/index.html>.

World Health Organization. (2008). *The Global Burden of Disease: 2004 Update*. Geneva: World Health Organization.

World Health Organization. (2011). *Mental Health Atlas*. Geneva: World Health Organization.

Chapter 14

Nurse Practitioner and Other Advanced Practice Roles

Chapter overview

This chapter covers the following topics:

* the advanced practice role
* the nurse practitioner
* prescribing medicines in an advanced role.

Chapter learning objectives

After reading this chapter, you should be able to:

* describe an advanced practice role
* discuss the professional pathway towards becoming a nurse practitioner
* describe the nurse practitioner role in the context of the Medicare Benefits Scheme and the Pharmaceutical Benefits Scheme.

Key terms

Australian Nursing and Midwifery Council
Advanced practice
Competency standards for advanced practice
Nurse practitioner
Prescribing formulary
Prescribing medications

Introduction

In this chapter you will explore the concepts of nurse practitioner and other advanced roles in relation to psychopharmacology. Nurses today are able to embark on advanced practice roles and some of these roles enable them to prescribe medications, order pathology tests and make referrals to other health professionals for the patients/clients in their care.

Advanced practice

Advanced practice literally means expanded practice, but still within the scope of the expanded role. Advanced practice incorporates formal education, a high level of autonomy, independent practices and collaborative networks.

Advanced practice is defined by the International Council of Nurses (ICN, 2002) as needing:

> … a registered nurse who has acquired the expert knowledge base, complex decision-making skills and clinical competencies for expanded practice, the characteristics of which are shaped by the context and/or country in which s/he is credentialed to practice. A Master's degree is recommended for the entry level.

Nurse practitioners

The nurse practitioner (NP) role is an advanced practice role in nursing. NPs are registered nurses who have completed a Master's degree and are authorised by the appropriate regulatory body to function independently in an advanced and extended clinical role within a multidisciplinary team context.

Nurse practitioners work in a number of practices including the following examples

* aged care

* chronic disease

* community and primary health care

* emergency care

* mental health

* midwifery

* paediatrics

* oncology

* palliative care

* rural and remote locations.

Nurse practitioner competency standards

The NP competency standards were articulated by the **Australian Nursing and Midwifery Council** in 2006. These standards cover such aspects of the role as extended practice, autonomy, accountability, clinical leadership that advances the profession, clinical care and collaborative networks.

Standard 1

Dynamic practice that incorporates application of high level knowledge and skills in extended practice across stable, unpredictable and complex situations (Australian Nursing and Midwifery Council, 2006): the NP is required to have and to continuously develop expert skills to facilitate comprehensive assessments and health status monitoring, including evidenced-based interventions and appropriate medication prescribing and monitoring in collaboration with the treating team for patients/clients in their care.

Standard 2

Professional efficacy whereby practice is structured in a nursing model and enhanced by autonomy and accountability (ANMC, 2006): the NP is recognised within the context of a nursing model that relates to their area of speciality and is considered a clinical leader in that field. In this context, NPs are able to work independently with a high level of autonomy within the multidisciplinary team.

Standard 3

Clinical leadership that influences and progresses clinical care, policy and collaboration through all levels of health service (ANMC, 2006): the NP is a significant contributor to the evidence base of the profession. NPs have a significant role in adding to the existing knowledge base, informing policy, clinical practice and the ongoing professional development of themselves and others in their team.

Prescribing medications as an advanced nursing practice for NPs

Prescribing medications is no longer the sole domain of medical practitioners and dentists. Prescribing rights have been extended to other health care professionals such as NPs as a way to advance the quality of health care services to patients/ clients and increasing patient/client choice and access within health care. The nurse prescribing and initiating taxonomy builds upon work done by N^3ET in 2005, which examined nurse practitioner prescribing in Australia (Emmerton, Marriott, Bessell, Nissen & Dean, 2005; N^3NET, 2006). The **prescribing formulary** relates to a form of prescribing that is based upon an agreed list of medicines that may be prescribed by an individual or group of prescribers. Details such as dosage, indications and special precautions vary within Australia among the states and territories.

Different prescribing programs have been developed to enable nurses (including enrolled nurses) and midwives to initiate treatment with a limited range of medicines in each state and territory. However, at present, only nurse practitioners (and midwife practitioners in NSW) are authorised to independently prescribe medications. Dependent prescribing occurs when there has been a delegation of authority from an independent prescriber but often involves restrictions related to the scope of the prescribing. No Australian examples of dependent prescribing have been identified at the present time. Dependent prescribing models for the prescription of medicines by nurses have been introduced overseas, including a supplementary prescribing program in the UK.

Nurse-initiated medicines may be administered on the basis of orders written by registered nurses, midwives and enrolled nurses. These generally include Schedule 2 and Schedule 3 medicines and focus on wellness, minor symptom management and parameters of use are usually regulated or governed by institutional policy. These drugs are usually simple to prescribe and have a relatively benign safety profile when ordered for therapeutic use. They are most commonly used for relatively minor complaints such as headache, constipation and dyspepsia, and many are available from supermarkets (some Schedule 2) or community pharmacy outlets (Schedules 2 and 3). However, it is within the scope of practice for NPs to independently prescribe some restricted medicines from Schedule 4, as outlined in each state or territory prescribing formulary. NPs are expected to employ reflective practices to maintain a high level of professional development and accountability in their specific autonomous role.

Ask yourself!

1   How could I undertake formal advanced practice such as becoming a NP?

2   How do NPs ensure accountability in their practice, especially when they are responsible for independently prescribing medicines?

3   What challenges are presented by independent NP prescribing roles in institutional settings such as hospitals?

Medicare Benefits Scheme and Pharmaceutical Benefits Scheme for the nurse practitioner

The Australian government's Department of Human Services is responsible for the development of service delivery policy and provides access to social, health and other payments and services such as the Medicare program. Medicare looks after the health of Australians through the organised delivery of programs such as the Medicare Benefits Scheme, Pharmaceutical Benefits Scheme, the Australian Childhood Immunisation Register and the Australian Organ Donor Register.

In Australia, NPs are eligible under the Medicare Benefits Scheme (MBS) to hold a practice provider number and provide reimbursed services to patients/clients in their care. The MBS schedule states:

> To provide services under Medicare, the legislation requires that a nurse practitioner be a participating nurse practitioner. A participating nurse practitioner is an eligible nurse practitioner who has a Medicare provider number and who provides Medicare services in a collaborative arrangement or collaborative arrangements with one

or more medical practitioners, of a kind or kinds specified in the regulations (Department of Health and Ageing, 2011, p. 814).

Services provided by participating nurse practitioners are covered by MBS items 82200, 82205, 82210 and 82215. These items cover four time-tiered specific types of service that allow the participating nurse practitioner to perform a:

✳ professional attendance for an obvious problem, straightforward in nature, with limited examination and management required (item 82200)

✳ professional attendance for a patient presenting with clinical signs and symptoms with an easily identifiable underlying cause following a short consultation lasting less than 20 minutes (item 82205)

✳ professional attendance for a patient presenting with clinical signs and symptoms with no obvious underlying cause requiring a more detailed consultation lasting at least than 20 minutes (item 82210)

✳ professional attendance for a patient presenting with multiple clinical signs and symptoms with the possibility of multiple causes and outcomes requiring an extensive consultation of at least 40 minutes (item 82215). (Department of Health and Ageing, 2011, p. 817)

Under the MBS a nurse practitioner in their advanced practice role will also be able to refer private patients/clients to a specialist and consultant physician for clinical services, as required. A referral given by a participating nurse practitioner is valid until 12 months after the first service given for the purpose of referral.

The Pharmaceutical Benefits Scheme (PBS) and the related Repatriation Pharmaceutical Benefits (RPBS) scheme are complex, highly developed systems that are used in Australia as mechanisms for the distribution and supply of pharmaceutical drugs to patients/clients. The RPBS was established shortly after the end of World War I, and allows the provision of free pharmaceuticals to returned servicemen and servicewomen. Efforts to establish the PBS commenced in 1944, and met with some opposition from the medical profession at that time. Under Section 15 of the *Pharmaceutical Benefits Act 1947*, the Commonwealth made arrangements to supply free products for immunisation against diphtheria and whooping cough. After the election of a new Commonwealth government in 1949, a limited scheme to provide a list of 139 'life-saving and disease preventing drugs' free of charge to the whole community was conceived and was implemented the next year. The PBS has been maintained, updated and preserved by consecutive federal governments since that time, and subsequently has become very sophisticated in operational terms.

The PBS is now used to regulate the supply of medications in the community setting and also for hospital outpatients and those being discharged from hospitals. Although patients/clients now contribute a copayment towards the cost of the medicines provided, the fundamental principle is to ensure that consumers have access to safe, clinically effective and cost-effective medication treatment at an affordable price. The Pharmaceutical Benefits Advisory Committee (PBAC), comprised of various experts from pertinent fields of medicine, pharmacy and pharmacology, makes recommendations to the federal Health Minister in relation to the range of medications to be listed on the schedule of pharmaceutical benefits; these drugs are made available at a subsidised cost to the Australian public and other citizens of countries with which Australia has a reciprocal health care agreement. The PBAC may also stipulate the conditions or circumstances where a drug may be supplied as a pharmaceutical benefit, for example limiting use to particular disease states or where other therapy has proven to be ineffective. Through the work of the Drug Utilisation Sub-Committee (DUSC) the use of these medications is closely monitored and characterised in the annual publication, *Australian Statistics on Medicines*. The PBS also encompasses other specialised programs such as the 'Closing the Gap' initiative, which was designed to facilitate appropriate access to medicines for Indigenous Australians, and the highly specialised drugs programs that underpin the supply of complex medications by tertiary hospitals.

Under the PBS, prescribers are provided with personalised or non-personalised, colour-coded prescription pads for the purposes of prescribing medicines. The personalised and non-personalised prescription pads for authorised nurse practitioners and midwives have the same look and feel as prescription pads for other prescribers but the colour is different. On the personalised prescription pads the indicator 'NP' for nurse practitioner or 'MW' for midwife is printed after the prescriber number to help the pharmacy identify the prescriber type. On the non-personalised prescription pads, authorised nurse practitioners and midwives indicate their prescriber type by ticking the appropriate box on the prescription form. A new online service called Health Professional Online

Service (HPOS) offers access to Medicare Australia's online services for health professionals through a single entry point. NPs may undertake PBS prescribing limited by scope of practice, and must comply with the relevant state or territory prescribing rights. To prescribe PBS medicines a nurse practitioner must have established collaborative arrangements, and in some cases there are additional requirements. These might specify parameters for a 'continuing therapy only' model, where treatment has been initiated by a medical practitioner or for a shared care model (where the NP and medical practitioner have entered in a formalised arrangement with an agreed plan to manage the care, in a person-centred model of care).

IAN'S STORY

Ian is a 25-year-old man who lives with friends. His family live near his home and are close to Ian. Ian works as an IT person for a company in the city. Ian has a past history of anxiety and panic disorder. He has been seeing his GP regularly for this anxiety. Ian has had a weekend of partying and has taken some ecstasy with alcohol. He is not a regular user of ecstasy but this time experienced panic and a feeling of not being fully 'present in him'. Ian presents to the emergency department of the hospital where you are working as a nurse practitioner.

Ask yourself!

As Ian's health care worker:

1 Describe your first few interventions with Ian.

2 List any medications that may help Ian with his feelings of panic.

3 Discuss the types of educational information that Ian would benefit from knowing, and those that his family and friends would benefit from knowing.

From the consumer's perspective – *How does this feel for me?*

Consumers and/or their significant others may ask you questions about your advanced role based around your scope of practice and these could relate to seeking their own clarification or seeking reassurance. These questions will need to be answered by you in a sensitive and honest manner in order to reassure and maintain the therapeutic alliance you have developed with the consumer and/or their significant others.

Some of these questions may include:

'I didn't think nurses could prescribe medications. Are you sure you are able to do this?'

'Have you spoken to my doctor before you referred me for some more tests? Usually my doctor is the person that does this, not the nurse.'

'I am not sure you are meant to be changing my medication prescription. Are you allowed to do this?'

A person-centred approach to NP prescribing in the context of mental illness

To provide a truly person-centred approach in the provision of NP prescribing services, many considerations need to be taken into account. The primacy of the needs of the patient/client must be taken into account, and prescribing must be undertaken in a way that ensures that no aspect of the care provided is compromised by the implementation of NP prescribing. This involves the NP ensuring that they have acquired an appropriate knowledge base and skill mix, in particular as these relate to the pharmacology of psychotropic drugs and the need to consider the potential impacts of prescribed drugs used for mental illness relating to the stability of comorbid medical illness. Another principle of paramount importance relates to effective interprofessional communication. NPs involved in prescribing for patients/clients with mental illnesses need to ensure that medical practitioners involved in the care of the patient/client are aware of the full range of medications prescribed and the rationale for the details of treatment selection. The NP can also benefit from interprofessional collaboration with pharmacists, who can contribute expertise and knowledge in relation to both the prescribing processes and the psychopharmacology of the drugs.

Ask yourself!

1   Under what specific circumstances would it be advantageous for a patient/client to have medications prescribed by a NP for the management of a mental illness?

2   When might autonomous NP prescribing present challenges for continuity of care, and the safe and effective use of psychotropic drugs?

Summary

Nurse practitioner and advanced practice roles are important in facilitating leadership in health care, increased accessibility of clinical services and greater choice for consumers. These roles have an important place in the future of health care service provision and professional advancements in the health care arena. An increased level of autonomy and accountability means that clinical outcomes for patients/clients meet, and often exceed, standards for competency, providing patients/clients with an expert resource as they progress through the health–illness continuum in an often under-resourced health care system.

Discussion questions

1   Describe the challenges for the nurse practitioner and advanced practice health care worker.

2   Define autonomy and accountability and how these influence practice when prescribing medicines such as psychoactive medicines.

3   Describe the contributions to practice, patient/client and the profession in the nurse practitioner and advanced practice role when working with a patient/client who is prescribed psychoactive medications.

Test yourself (answers at the back of the book)

1   Nurse practitioners work in a number of practices including:

   A   aged care and chronic disease

   B   community and primary health care

   C   mental health

   D   more areas than those listed above

2   NP standards cover such aspects of the role as:

   A   extended practice, autonomy and accountability and clinical leadership that advances the profession, clinical care and collaborative networks

   B   extended practice that advances the profession, clinical care and collaborative networks

C   extended practice, autonomy and accountability that advances the profession

D   extended practice and clinical leadership that advances the profession, clinical care and collaborative networks

3   The prescribing formulary relates to a form of prescribing based upon an agreed list of medicines that may be prescribed by an individual or group of prescribers. Details are included such as:

A   dosage and special precautions that vary within Australia from state to state and territory

B   dosage, indications and special precautions that vary within Australia from state to state and territory

C   dosage and indications

D   special precautions since they vary within Australia from state to state and territory

4   Nurse initiated medicines may be administered on the basis of orders written by registered nurses, midwives and enrolled nurses. These generally include:

A   Schedule 1 and Schedule 3

B   Schedule 2 and Schedule 4

C   Schedule 2 and Schedule 3

D   Schedule 1 and Schedule 5

5   Services provided by participating nurse practitioners are covered by MBS items:

A   82200, 82207, 82210, 82215

B   82223, 82205, 82210, 82215

C   82211, 82205, 82210, 82215

D   82200, 82205, 82210, 82215

Useful websites

Australian Health Professional Online Services available at <www.medicareaustralia.gov.au/hpos/index.jsp>

Australian Government Department of Health and Ageing: *The Pharmaceutical Benefits Scheme* available at <www.pbs.gov.au/pbs/home>

References

Australian Nursing and Midwifery Council (2006). *National Competency Standards for the Nurse Practitioner.* Australian Nursing and Midwifery Council.

Department of Health and Ageing. (2011). *Medicare Benefits Schedule Book.* Canberra, Australia: Australian Government Department of Health and Ageing.

Emmerton L., Marriott J., Bessell T., Nissen L. & Dean L. (2005). 'Pharmacists and prescribing rights: review of international developments' *J Pharm Pharm Sci* 8(2)S: 217–225.

ICN Nurse Practitioner/Advanced Practice Nursing Network. (2002). Retrieved 28 October 2011, from http://66.219.50.180/inp%20apn%20network/practice%20issues/role%20definitions.asp.

N³NET. (2006). National Nursing & Nursing Education Taskforce: National Nurse Prescribing Glossary. Melbourne, Australia: National Nursing & Nursing Education Taskforce.

Test Yourself Answers

Chapter 1

1 B

2 C

3 D

4 C

5 A

Chapter 2

1 D

2 D

3 A

4 D

5 B

Chapter 3

1 D

2 B

3 B

4 D

5 A

Chapter 4

1 B

2 C

3 C

4 C

5 A

Chapter 5

1 B

2 D

3 A

4 B

5 D

Chapter 6

1 C

2 C

3 D

4 B

5 B

Chapter 7

1 D

2 A

3 D

4 C

5 B

Chapter 8

1 B

2 C

3 B

4 B

5 A

Chapter 9

1 D

2 D

3 C

4 C

5 D

Chapter 10

1 B

2 C

3 B

4 D

5 C

Chapter 11

1 C

2 A

3 A

4 C

5 A

Chapter 12

1 A

2 C

3 B

4 B

5 D

Chapter 13

1 C

2 D

3 B

4 D

5 D

Chapter 14

1 D

2 A

3 B

4 C

5 D

Glossary of Terms

Absorption – The means by which a drug enters the body after administration.

Adherence – The extent to which clients take medications as prescribed by their health care providers.

Administer – To give a medication to a patient/client. It may include some activity to prepare the medicine to be administrable.

Advanced practice – The degree of autonomy enjoyed by a mental health nurse practitioner, in the form of extended and expanded practice.

Adverse drug reaction – An unintended and unwanted effect of a drug.

Adverse event – An unintended and harmful event that can cause patient harm; this may include adverse drugs reactions or other forms of iatrogenic harm.

Ageing – Advancing in life.

Anticholinergic – Describes a substance that opposes or annuls the physiological action of acetylcholine.

Antidepressant – A drug that is used for the treatment of major depression, as well as a variety of other, unrelated mental disorders.

Antipsychotic drug – A medication used for some types of mental disorders.

Anxiety – A mental state or symptom characterised by uneasiness, unrest and apprehension. Not always indicative of a mental disorder.

Anxiety disorders – A range of clinically significant mental disorders where various manifestations of anxiety are the primary symptoms, causing distress and impairment not better accounted for by the effects of a general medical condition or the effects of a substance.

Attention deficit/hyperactivity disorder (ADHD) – A syndrome of disordered learning and disruptive behaviour that is not caused by any serious underlying physical or mental disorder and is characterised primarily by symptoms of inattentiveness or symptoms of hyperactivity and impulsive behaviour.

Australian National Medicinal Drug Policy – In Australia, a policy framework designed to allow timely access to required medicines at a cost affordable to individuals and the community, ensuring medicines meet appropriate quality, safety and efficacy standards, the maintenance of a responsible and viable medicines industry in Australia, and the achievement of Quality Use of Medicines.

Australian Nursing and Midwifery Council – The independent accrediting authority for nursing and midwifery under the National Registration and Accreditation Scheme. It sets standards for accreditation and accredits nursing and midwifery courses and providers.

Autism spectrum disorders – Lifelong developmental disabilities characterised by marked difficulties in social interaction, communication, and restricted and repetitive interests and behaviours. The word 'spectrum' is used because the range and severity of the difficulties people with an autism spectrum disorder experience can vary widely.

Autonomy – An ethical principle that relates to allowing people to 'self-rule' and make decisions for themselves.

Beneficence – An ethical principle that relates to 'doing good' and to the ethical theory of utilitarianism (which maintains that effort should be directed to achieving the greatest amount of good because the most people would benefit).

Bipolar I disorder – An affective disorder primarily characterised by episodes of elevated mood (mania), usually interspersed with periods of major depression.

Bipolar II disorder – An affective disorder primarily characterised by episodes of major depression, often interspersed with periods of mood elevation (hypomania or mania).

Child and adolescent psychiatry – A discipline that encompasses the clinical investigation of biological, psychosocial, genetic and environmental factors in child and adolescent psychiatric disorders.

Client – A person receiving mental health care in the community setting.

Compliance – The process of complying with a schedule of treatment.

Cytochrome P450 – A family of hepatic enzymes involved in drug metabolism.

Dependence – A syndrome where a person needs to take a drug to function or to avoid adverse consequences. Abruptly stopping the drug may cause withdrawal symptoms. A related term is 'drug addiction': the compulsive use of a substance despite its harmful effects.

Dispense – To prepare, and distribute for administration, medicines to those who are to use them.

Drug distribution – When used in connection to pharmacokinetics, the reversible movements of drug within the body, usually from one compartment to another.

Drug elimination – The various ways in which a drug irreversibly leaves the body.

Drug interaction – A clinical phenomenon whereby the effects of one drug are altered by the concurrent administration of another.

Dual diagnosis – Comorbidity of mental disorders and substance use disorders.

Eating disorder – Any of several psychological disorders (as anorexia nervosa or bulimia) characterised by serious disturbances of eating behaviour.

Electroconvulsive therapy (ECT) – A treatment used for major depression and some other forms of mental illness. It involves the induction of seizures by the application of an electrical current to the brain via the scalp.

Ethical decision-making – A decision-making process based on principles intended to allow choices based on sound ethical frameworks and principles.

Ethical principles – Factors and frameworks to use when considering the ethical actions to be taken in any given situation.

Euthymia – An affective state whereby mood is neither significantly depressed or elevated ('normal mood state').

Extrapyramidal side effects (EPSE) – Side effects that are common with antipsychotic medications, as well as with a few other types of medications. Extrapyramidal symptoms are usually divided into different categories. Dyskinesias are movement disorders, whereas dystonias are muscle tension disorders.

Generalised anxiety disorder (GAD) – A disorder characterised by at least six months of persistent and excessive anxiety and worry.

Half-life – The time required for the plasma concentration to decrease by 50% from its original value.

Iatrogenic illness – Illness induced inadvertently by a physician or surgeon or by medical treatment or diagnostic procedures.

Insomnia – Abnormal inability to obtain adequate sleep.

Involuntary treatment – Treatment provided in the context where a person's mental condition is impaired to an extent that their capacity to understand their disorder is compromised and the disorder may have a negative impact on the person's judgement and safety, taking into account situations where the person may present a risk to themselves and/or others.

Justice – An ethical principle based upon concepts of equity and fairness, relating to non-discriminatory actions.

Major depressive disorder – An affective disorder characterised by recurrent major depressive episodes in the absence of episodes of mood elevation, not better explained by the effects of another mental disorder, use of substances or general medical conditions.

Major depressive episode – A clinically significant episode characterised by affective disturbance in which the prominent symptoms relate to depressed mood.

Mechanism of action – The underlying physiological processes through which a drug produces its actions.

Medication administration – The means by which a medicinal drug is administered to a patient.

Medication calculations – Mathematical processes used to ascertain the correct amount of drug to be administered to a person, considering the drug's individual characteristics.

Medication-related problem – A research and clinical term used to define situations where people may be exposed to one of eight categories of actual or potential medication-related harm.

Medicinal drug – A drug that is used with the intention of producing therapeutic effects to treat or prevent a medical outcome (as opposed to illicit or recreational drugs).

Mental Health Act – Jurisdictional legislative framework underpinning principles of assessment, treatment and care of people with mental illness and those who may be influenced by them.

Metabolic impacts – The consequences of some antipsychotic medications: weight gain, hyperglycaemia, hypertension and hyperlipidaemia.

Metabolism – A process occurring in various organs (most importantly the liver) whereby a drug is converted to a metabolite (a compound that usually has less pharmacological activity than the parent compound, and is easier to excrete in the urine).

Mood disorder – A mental disorder where the primary features relate to persistently abnormal affective states.

Mood stabilisers – Drug treatments used to promote the maintenance of euthymia and to reduce the frequency and intensity of episodes of affective disturbance associated with mood disorders.

Non-maleficence – A broad ethical tenet based on the principle that treatments and interventions should not cause avoidable or anticipatable harm to a person.

Nurse practitioner – A registered nurse with the education and experience required to perform in an advanced clinical role. A nurse practitioner's scope of practice extends beyond that of a registered nurse.

Obsessive-compulsive disorder (OCD) – A mental disorder where the person may have obsessions (which cause marked anxiety or distress) and/or compulsions (which may relieve anxiety).

Pain – A state of physical, emotional, or mental lack of well-being or physical, emotional, or mental uneasiness that ranges from mild discomfort or dull distress to acute, often unbearable agony. May be generalised or localised.

Panic disorder – A disorder involving recurrent panic attacks with persistent concern about their implications. May be accompanied by agoraphobia (anxiety about and/or avoidance of situations or places that might be difficult to leave without embarrassment or excessive inconvenience).

Patient – A person receiving treatment and care in the hospital or other close direct-supervision setting.

Pharmacodynamics – The scientific discipline used as a basis to understand the effects (either therapeutic or harmful) of drugs in the body and the effects arising from concurrent administration of more than one drug.

Pharmacokinetics – The pharmacological science addressing the disposition of drugs and their metabolites in biological systems.

Pharmacological management – Care intervention aimed at reducing the number of, or rationalising the use of, as many medications as possible.

Pharmacology – The scientific and clinical discipline that addresses the effects of drug substances.

Pharmacotherapy – Management with a medical drug that is directed at treating, curing or preventing the manifestation of a disease state.

Polypharmacy – The practice of administering many different medicines, especially concurrently, for the treatment of the same disease.

Positive symptoms – Symptoms that are an excess or distortion of a person's normal functioning, such as formal thought disorder, hallucinations or delusions.

Post-traumatic stress disorder (PTSD) – A disorder that occurs after exposure to a traumatic event. It may be characterised by mentally re-experiencing the event accompanied by symptoms of hyperarousal and/or avoidance of circumstances or cues that the affected individual associates with the event.

Prescribing formulary – A circumscribed list of the medicines that are normally available at a particular health care location such as a hospital or pharmacy, and that are approved for use in that setting or by a specific prescriber.

Prescribing medications – The act of providing instructions for the dispensing of medications, usually in writing by an authorised prescriber after clinical assessment of a specified patient/client.

Psychosis – A condition in which a person experiences a misinterpretation of reality as a result of impaired cognition and emotional, social and communicative behaviours.

Psychotropic drug – A drug that acts in the central nervous system, and which may influence perception, mood, consciousness, cognition or behaviour.

Quality Use of Medicines – A systematic approach to the use of drugs in a way designed to promote judicious selection of treatment, safe and effective use of medicinal drugs, and ensuring that patients/carers have knowledge and skills to use medicines safely.

Receptors – Cellular structures that interact with drugs to produce pharmacological responses.

Recovery framework – A framework central to all mental health services, addressing the facilitation of recovery and wellness, a philosophy of hope and partnership with patients/clients and their carers, and understanding consumers in the context of their whole selves and not just their illness or disorder. It embraces respect for individual rights, allowing patients/clients to set their own goals, and focuses upon strengths rather than symptoms.

Relapse – The recurrence of symptoms after a period of recovery from mental illness.

Renal clearance – A process whereby a drug is eliminated from the body by various processes that take place in the kidneys.

Serotonin syndrome – Sometimes also referred to as serotonin toxicity, a syndrome caused by a drug-induced excess of serotonergic activity, with clinical manifestations such as neuromuscular excitation, autonomic stimulation and mental status changes.

Sleep disorder – A persistent sleep problem that causes the patient/client significant emotional distress, and interferes with their social or occupational functioning.

Substance abuse – A maladaptive pattern of substance use leading to clinically significant impairment or distress.

Substance dependence – The compulsive physiological need for and use of a habit-forming substance (such as heroin, nicotine or alcohol) characterised by tolerance.

Substance-induced anxiety disorder – Characterised by prominent anxiety attributable to the direct effects of substance intoxication or withdrawal

Tardive dyskinesia – Irregular, stereotypical movements of mouth, face and tongue, and choreoathetoid movements of the fingers, arms, legs and trunk.

Tic disorder – A habitual, usually unconscious quirk of behaviour or speech.

Index

abbreviations (medications) 94–7
  medications errors cause 94
  recommended terms 95–7 *tab 5.3*
absorption (drugs) 48–50, 51 *fig 3.1*
abuse
  alcohol 216–17 *tab 9.2*
  child abuse 240
    childhood sexual abuse as
      PTSD basis 168
  sexual 168
  substance 142, 213, 232
accountability 26–42, 328–9
acetylcholinesterase (AChe) inhibitor
  drugs 261
act utilitarianism 35
actions (drug) *see* pharmacodynamics
addition 79
adherence 201–3
  case study 317
  compliance versus 312–13
  disability and chronic conditions,
  global burden of 306–12
    Axis I, II and III 310
    Axis IV 311
    Axis V 311–12
  medicines considerations 321
  WHO definition 312
administration
  drugs 55
    antipsychotics 190–4
    checking before administering—Six
     Rights 83–5
    drug schedules 86–7
    inpatients 89–94
    national inpatient medication
     charts 89–94
    oral 48–9
    parenteral 49–50
    patient's own medication 98
    pharmaceutical care
     continuity 98–9

    rectal 48–9
    safe/unsafe abbreviations 94–7
  electroconvulsive therapy 120 *fig*
   6.2, 121–2
adolescents
  major depression in 251–3
  mental illness in 239–54
  psychiatric syndromes 242 *tab 10.1*
  weight considerations 81
adverse drug reactions (ADRs) 8, 17,
  65–8
  action for 104 *fig 5.3*
  idiosyncratic adverse effects 66
  Naranjo questionnaires 67–8
  screening during assessment 70–1
  Stevens–Johnson syndrome 67 *fig*
   4.2, 141
Adverse Drug Reactions Advisory
  Committee 103
affective blunting 185
age 64
ageing, physical effects of 258–60
agomelatine 128
agonists 63
agoraphobia 164
akathisia 195
alcohol 16, 213, 214 *tab 9.1*
  abuse 216–17
  alcoholism treatment 232
  alcohol-use disorders 157
  concentrations 215
  intervention best practice
   216–17 *tab 9.2*
  standard drink definition 215–17
  thiamine deficiency 218
alogia 185
alpha-adrenergic blockade 188–9
Alzheimer's disease 261
  vaccination development 273–4
amphetamines 186, 214 *tab 9.1*
  crystal methamphetamine 225

anaesthesia
  ECT use and   121–2
  ketamine   146
analgesia   297 *tab 12.5*
ankylosing spondylitis   260
anorexia nervosa   281 *tab 12.1*
antagonists   63
anticholinergic effects   66, 189
anticonvulsive drugs   127, 177, 201
antidepressants   128–34
  action duration   134
  anxiolytic onset of   162
  causing serotonin syndrome   126
  choice of   128–34
  consumer view primacy   124–5
  controversies in use   252 *fig 10.1*
  discontinuation syndrome   134
  initiation
    augmentation agent addition
      128–9
    use at standard dose   128
  merits of   124
  methadone levels and   224
  properties   129–32
  selection of, treatment choice
    considerations   125 *fig 6.3*
  selective serotonin reuptake
    inhibitor   125
  standard daily doses   133 *tab 6.6*
  tricyclic antidepressants   7, 9, 10 *tab
    1.1*, 125–6, 128, 133, 165
antiepileptic drugs   220
antipsychotic drugs   9, 103, 138–9, 170,
  187–94, 307
  adverse effects   194–200
    clozapine side effects   190, 198–9
    extrapyramidal side effects   66,
      190, 194–6, 261
    metabolic side effects   196–8
    Q-Tc segment prolongation
      199–201
    sedation   200
    sexual dysfunction   200
  atypical   189–90
  dosage and administration   190–4
  drug interactions with   200–1
  first-generation   188–9

clinical effects   189 *tab 8.4*
  prescribing considerations
    191–4 *tab 8.5*
  second-generation   188–90
  treatment phases   191 *fig 8.2*
  typical   188
anxiety
  association with other disorders   153
  psychopathology, non-indicative
    of   151–2
  self-medication   152
  state anxiety   152
  trait anxiety   152
anxiety disorders   7, 124
  antidepressants, anxiolytic
    onset of   162
  associated comorbid substance
    disorders   157
  commonly encountered anxiety
    disorders and treatment
      generalised anxiety disorder   161–3
      obsessive–compulsive disorder
        174–6
      panic disorder   164–7
      post-traumatic stress disorder
        167–74
  diagnosis and management
    principles   159–60 *tab 7.2*
  non-pharmacological treatment
    of   154–6
  part of life, not always an illness
    151–3
  pharmacological management   156–7
  pharmacotherapy, general principles
    156–60
  prevalence rate   151
  substance-induced anxiety
    disorder   152
  treatment combinations, merits
    155–6
arthritis   259–60
Asperger's syndrome   250
assessment
  ADRs screening   70–1
  alcohol and   216
  of pharmacodynamics   70–1
  of pharmacokinetics   55

atomoxetine   245
attention deficit/hyperactivity disorder
  (ADHD)   242–9
    in children/adolescents   242 *tab* 10.1
    diagnostic criteria   243 *tab* 10.2
    treatment, after evaluation   244
    treatment of   244–6
      controversy in   246–7
Australian Medication Management
  Plan   98–9
Australian Medicines Handbook
  [publication]   14
Australian National Medicinal Drug
  Policy   11–15
    elements   14–15
Australian Nursing and Midwifery
  Council   328
Australian Prescriber [publication]   14
Australian Statistics on Medicines (ASM)
  [publication]   8, 332
Australian Therapeutic Goods
  Administration (TGA)   169
autism spectrum disorders   250
autonomy   30, 328–9
autonomy (ethical principle)   35
avolition   185

'bagging'   122
barbiturates   9
Beers list   265–71
    abridged version   266–9 *tab* 11.2
behaviour
    abnormal   240
    disorganised   184–5
beneficence (ethical principle)   35
benzodiazepines   9, 157–8, 161–2
    alcohol withdrawal and   217
    clinical aspects   162 *tab* 7.3
    hazards   159 *fig* 7.1
bereavement   113–15
best practice, guidelines and
  standards   14
binge eating disorder   281 *tab* 12.1
biological treatment   6
bipolar affective disorder   307
    bipolar I disorder   117–18
      diagnostic criteria   118 *fig* 6.1

bipolar II disorder   118
    diagnostic criteria   118
case study   143
children and   252–4
elevated mood, conditions associated
    with   116–18
management
    of depression in   140–1
    of mania/hypomania   138–40
modafinil   147
pharmacotherapy for   138–47
psychosis feature   182–3
riluzole   147
tamoxifen   147
treatment
    general principles   138–47
    maintenance mood stabiliser
    141–3
blood   50–1
    blood dyscracias   198–9
bones and joints   259–60
brain
    cerebrolysin   273
    children's neurodevelopment   240
    damage to   240
    'decade of the brain'   7
    dendrites   61
    dopamine hypothesis and
      schizophrenia   185–6
    electroconvulsive therapy   119–23
    melatonin synthesis   255
    nervous system and   259
    neurons—brain cells   61
    neurotransmitters   61 *fig* 4.1, 61–4,
    120, 186
      effects of nicotine on   219
    of older people   259
    organic brain syndromes   182–3
breathing-related sleep disorders   289–90
bright light therapy   123
bronchodilators   263
buccal administration   85
bulimia nervosa   281 *tab* 12.1, 283
buspirone, clinical aspects   163 *tab* 7.3

caffeine   214 *tab* 9.1, 286–7
cannabis   214 *tab* 9.1, 221–2

capacity
  legal 32–3
  mental 181
capsules 48–9
carbamazepine 139–42
cardiac system 265 *tab 11.1*
cardiovascular disease (CVD) 262–3, 306
care *see* health care
care plans 247–9
  adherence and concordance 317–20
  anxiety disorders 171–3
  law, ethics and accountability 38–43
  mental illness 247–9
  mental illness in special
    populations 294–6
  mood disorders 135–7, 143–5
  for older people 274–6
  pharmacodynamics 72–4
  schizophrenia 203–7
  substance use disorders 228–31
cataplexy 288–9
central nervous system (CNS) 50, 265
  tab 11.1
  extrapyramidal side effects
    mediation 194–5
  neurodevelopment 240
  of older people 259
  receptor blockade 189–90
  see also brain; nephron;
    neurotransmitters
central sleep apnoea (CSA) 289
cerebrolysin 273
charts
  medication charts 99
    national inpatient medication
      charts 89–94
chemical restraint 33
children
  child abuse 168, 240
  general psychiatry for
    bipolar affective disorder 253–4
    major depression in 251–3
    psychosis 253–4
  mental illness in 239–54
  neurodevelopment 240
  psychiatric syndromes 242 *tab 10.1*
  self-description 239–40
  vulnerability of 16

weight considerations 81
chlorpromazine 7, 188
cholinesterase inhibitors 261
chronic conditions 306–12
chronic obstructive pulmonary disease
  (COPD) 262–3
cigarette smoking 201
  cessation programs 220
  complications 220
  COPD and 263
  see also nicotine; tobacco
circadian rhythm sleep disorders
  289–90, 300
clearance 51, 54, 134
clients 6
  condition/treatment, beliefs
    regarding 314
  educating 55
  with poor dentition 122
  right individual 83
clinical disorders 310
clinical leadership 329
clinical trials 65, 241, 263–4
clozapine, side effects 190, 198–9
cocaine 214 *tab 9.1*, 222–3
cognitive behavioural therapy
  (CBT) 118–19, 154, 165, 252
cognitive disorders 260–2
  pharmacotherapy for 273–4
Commonwealth Department of Health
  and Ageing 272
communication
  between health care sectors 157
  interpersonal 19–20
  potential harm reduction and 89–94
community-based health workers, patient
  care information, relaying 14
comorbid substance disorders 157
comorbidities 262–4, 308
competency standards
  Standard 1 328
  Standard 2 328
  Standard 3 329
complementary medicines 298
compliance 140
  adherence versus 312–13
concordance 313–15
  case study 315

confidentiality   28
    legislative variation   31
consent   28
consequential ethics   37
Consumer Medicines Information
    (CMI)   14, 71, 105
context
    adherence and concordance   306–21
    anxiety disorders   151–77
    mental disorders, legal and strategic
        context for   27–8
    mental illness
        in children and adolescents
            239–54
        in special populations   281–99
    mood disorders   112–48
    nurse practitioner and other advanced
        practice roles   327–34
    older people   258–76
    psychoses   181–208
    psychotropic drug use   4–22
    substance use disorders   213–32
continuity (of pharmaceutical care)   98–9
convulsions
    anticonvulsive drugs   127, 177, 201
    electroconvulsive therapy and
        119–20
corticosteroids   263
corticotropin releasing factor   170
Council of Australian Health Ministers,
    Pharmaceutical Reforms agenda
    13–14
crystal methamphetamine   225

dangerous drugs, recording of   88–9
decision-making
    ethical   36–7
    legal capacity and   32–3
    shared   314
delirium   262
'DELIRIUM' mnemonic   262
delusions   181–2, 182 tab 8.1, 184–5
dementia   260–2
dendrites   61
denial   282
deontology   36–7
dependence   8
deprescribing   269–70

depression   307
    children/adolescents, major depression
        in   251–3
    depressed mood, conditions associated
        with   113–15
    dose–effect association with
        cannabis   221–2
    drugs linked to   292 tab 12.4
    major depressive disorder   113–14
        drug therapy for   10 tab 1.1
        general principles of treatment for
            123–5
        psychosis feature   182–3
    transcranial magnetic stimulation   123
    vagal nerve stimulation   123
depression pharmacology   146–7
diabetes mellitus   197, 201
Diagnostic and Statistical Manual of Mental
    Disorders (DSM-IV)   181–2, 213,
    283–4, 286, 309–10
    Global Assessment of Functioning
        (GAF) score   311
    multiaxial assessment system
        Axis I, II and III   310
        Axis IV   311
        Axis V   311–12
        categories   311
'DIGFAST' mnemonic   118 fig 6.1
disability, global burden   306–12
disability support   21–2
discontinuation syndrome   134, 166
    case study   134–5
discrimination   32, 36
disease states   64
    multiple diseases–multiple
        medicines   260
disinfection   99
disorders
    anxiety   124, 151–77
    attention deficit/hyperactivity   242–9
    autism spectrum   250
    bipolar disorder   117–18,
        138–47, 182–3, 252–4, 307
    cognitive   260–2, 273–4
    comorbid substance   157
    dysthymic disorder   115
    eating   124, 281–3
    'high prevalence'   112, 151

learning   242
major depressive   112–14, 182–3
mood   6, 112–48
personality   283–5, 310
pervasive development   242
psychiatric, attention deficit/
   hyperactivity disorder   242–9
sleep   285–90
substance/substance use   142, 170,
   213–31
tic   242, 250–1
distribution (drugs)   50–1, 51 *fig 3.1*
volume of distribution   50–1
division   79
documentation   85
of personality disorders/mental
   retardation   310
of POMs   97
Domiciliary Medication Management
   Review (DMMR)   272
donepezil   261
dopamine   222–3
hypothesis   185–6
dosage   250
antidepressants, standard daily
   doses   133 *tab 6.6*
of antipsychotics   190–4
based on body weight   64
dosage errors   81
dose–effect association between
   cannabis and depression/
   anxiety   221–2
drug calculations, correct
   formulae   81–2
increasing   49
older people, lower dose for   258
overdose   17, 128–34
   case study   21–2
   deliberate   128
right dose   83–4
subtherapeutic dosage   17
doxepin   299
drug calculations, correct formulae
   81–2
drug interactions   8, 17, 21–2, 53, 69–70,
   125–7
pharmacodynamic interactions
   69, 125–6
serotonin syndrome   126

drug therapy   10 *tab 1.1*
Drug Utilisation Sub-Committee
   (DUSC)   332
drug-induced psychiatric
   syndromes   290–4
clinically significant syndromes
   associated with medicinal drugs
   292–3 *tab 12.4*
'prescribing cascade' example
   291 *fig 12.1*
drugs
absorption   48–50
actions/activity   188
   ageing process, influence of   258
   pharmacodynamics   59–75
administration   55
   case study   56
   drug calculations   81–2
   routes   48–9
   therapeutic effectiveness   55
adverse drug reactions   8, 17, 65–8
   ADR profiles   66
   case study   21–2
amphetamines   186
anticonvulsive   127, 177, 201
antidepressants   7, 9, 10 *tab 1.1*,
   124–5, 128–34, 162, 165, 252
   see also tricyclic antidepressants
antiepileptic   220
antipsychotic drugs   9, 103,
   138–9, 170, 187–94
benzodiazepines *see* benzodiazepines
bound/unbound   51
for children   241
chlorpromazine   7, 188
comorbid substance disorders   157
concentration of   50
dangerous drugs, recording   88–9
dependency, diagnostic criteria
   219–20
design foundation   63
distribution   50–1
dosage   49, 64
dose range   84
drug diversion   245–6
drug-related harm *see* iatrogenic illness
effects   115 *tab 6.2*
   anticholinergic effects   66
   long-term effects of   269–71

drugs (*cont.*)
    monitoring   101–4
    physiological and biochemical *see*
     pharmacodynamics
    placebo effect   64, 156
    significant first pass effect   49
    see also adverse drug reactions
  efficacy monitoring   101–4
  elimination of *see* elimination
  half-life   54
  illicit   16
    cannabis   214 *tab 9.1*, 221–2
    ecstasy   126, 223, 333
    MDMA   126
  interactions   17, 200–1, 297
   tab 12.5
  of low therapeutic index   64
  mechanism of action   61
  medicinal   16, 292–3 *tab 12.4*
  metabolism of *see* metabolism
  movements, within body *see*
   pharmacokinetics
  multiple drug treatment   66
  'new drugs'   188
  non-steroidal anti-inflammatory
   drugs   70
  older people and   271–4
  pharmacological action   60–75
  postmarketing surveillance
   process   65
  in pregnancy and lactation   298–9
  prescription drugs/medication
   87–8, 213
  profiles   66
  psychosis, as possible cause of   183
   tab 8.2
  psychotropic   4–22
   volume of distribution   51
  reactions   16
  relative availability of   157–8
  reserpine   188
  response
   factors influencing   64
   psychological   64
  schedules   86–7
  side effects   65
   extrapyramidal side effects   66

  susceptibility to   264–5
  tachyphylaxis   158
  tolerance   158
  used in electroconvulsive therapy
   122–3
  'washout' period   63, 134
dual diagnosis   213, 227
dyssomnias   290
dysthymic disorder   115
dystonic reactions (dystonia)   195

eating disorders   124, 281–3
  case study   283
  diagnostic features   281 *tab 12.1*
ecstasy   126, 223
  case study   333
education
  drug calculations education   81–2
  medications management   316
  psychoeducation   119, 155
  regarding pharmacodynamics   71
  regarding pharmacokinetics   55
electroconvulsive therapy (ECT)   6,
  119–23
  administration   121–2
  anaesthesia and   121–2
  associated risk
   complications   121
   pre-existing conditions   120–1
  associated stigma   119
  drugs used in   122–3
  electrode application   120 *fig 6.2*
  mode of action   119–20
  neurotransmitters, effect on   120
  teratogenesis, risk of   121
elimination   51–4
  elimination half-life   54
  excretion   47
  hepatic drug elimination   52–3
  mechanisms
   metabolic elimination   52
   renal excretion   52
  metabolism   47
  plasma clearance   51, 54
  renal drug excretion   53–4
endogenous compounds   62–3
  agonists/antagonists   63

enzymes   63
  activity   52
  hepatic enzyme induction   69–70
  hepatic enzyme inhibition   70
  inhibition of   63
equity   36
errors
  dosage errors   81
  medication administration error   83–5
    causes   94
    due to labelling/packaging   97
ethics   26–42
  clinical trials, children and   241
  ethical decision-making   36–7
  ethical principles   34–6
    autonomy   30, 35
    beneficence   35
    justice   36
    non-maleficence   35–6
  ethical theories   36–7
    deontology   36–7
    libertarianism   35
    natural law   37
    paternalism   35–6
    teleology   37
    transcultural principles   37
    utilitarianism   35
euthymia   139
evaluation
  of pharmacodynamics   71
  of pharmacokinetics   55
excretion   47
exploitation   32
extrapyramidal side effects   66, 190,
  194–6, 261
  manifestations   195–6
eyesight   259

fairness   36
falls   271–4
  falls risk assessment   271
fasciculations   122
first pass effect, significant   49
first-generation (typical)
  antipsychotics   188–9
    nature of clinical effects   189
      tab 8.4
fluoxetine   252

*Fourth National Mental Health
  Plan: An Agenda for Collaborative
  Government Action in Mental Health
  2009–2014*   27–8
freedom   33
funding
  availability of, adoption of research
    models condition   13–14
  Commonwealth Department of
    Health and Ageing   272

galantamine   261
gastrointestinal (GI) system   265 *tab 11.1*
gastrointestinal side effects   261
gastrointestinal tract   48–9
  gut mucosa   49
generalised anxiety disorder (GAD)
  symptoms   161
  treatment for   161–3
    drug therapy, clinical aspects
      162–3 *tab 7.3*
genetic disposition   184 *fig 8.1*, 240
Global Assessment of Functioning
  (GAF) score   311
glucose tolerance (impaired)   197
government
  Australian, Fourth National Mental
    Health Plan   27–8
  Federal government policy
    initiatives   14
  New Zealand
    Te Kōkiri Plan   28
    Te Tāhuhu Plan   28
guanfacine   254
guardianship   28
gut-wall metabolism   49

half-life   54
half-life agents   158–9
hallucinations   181–2, 182 *tab 8.1*,
  184–5, 223, 289
  hallucinogens   214 *tab 9.1*
hand hygiene   99
harm
  to 'do no harm'   35–6
  drug-related   272
  iatrogenic harm contributor—
    oxycodone   225–6

harm (*cont.*)
  potential for   269
  potential harm reduction   89–94
  self-harm   141
health care
  considerations
    people with substance use
      disorders   227–31
    prescribing considerations   191–4
      tab 8.5
    treatment choice
      considerations   125 *fig 6.3*
    weight considerations   81
  continuum   13
  planning *see* care plans
  reform funding   13–14
  service delivery initiatives   14
heart disease   262–3
hepatic drug elimination   52–3
  hepatic enzyme induction   52–3,
    69–70
  hepatic enzyme inhibition   53, 70
heroin   224
Hippocrates   4 *fig 1.1*, 4–5
  non-maleficence   35–6
Home Medicines Review
  (HMR)   272
human immunodeficiency virus
  (HIV)   224
human rights   28
  restriction of   30–1
hyperglycaemia   197
hyperprolactinaemia   197–8
hypertension   262–3
hypnogogic   289
hypnopompic   289
hypomania/hypomanic episode   138–40
  diagnostic features   117 *tab 6.3*

iatrogenic illness   18
  HMR reduction of   272
  oxycodone   225–6
idiosyncratic side effects   66, 189
IH (inhalation) administration   85
immune system   265 *tab 11.1*
inflammation, non-steroidal
  anti-inflammatory drug   70

information
  checks against prescription orders   83
  clinical disorders information   310
  neurotransmitters   61 *fig 4.1*, 61–4,
    62 *tab 4.1*
  patient care   14
  patient/client information   71
  relaying of   14
  self-description   239–40
  sources of   14
inhalants   214 *tab 9.1*
injections   49–50
  injected heroin   224
  intramuscular   50
    sites   101
  monitoring drug efficacy and
    effects   101–4
  safe injection techniques, general safety
    principles   99–103
  subcutaneous   50, 101–2 *fig 5.2*
insomnia   7, 287–8
interactions (drug)   8, 17, 21–2, 53,
  69–70, 125–7, 200–1
International System of Units (SI)   82
interpersonal therapy   118–19
intervention
  early   21–2, 27–8
  intervention best practice for alcohol
    abuse   216–17 *tab 9.2*
  psychological   251–2
  recovery framework and   20–1
  specific medical   160, 186–7 *tab 8.3*
  symptom-based   159
  therapeutic, electroconvulsive
    therapy   122
intoxication   115 *tab 6.2*, 225, 286
intradermal administration   85
intramuscular (IM) administration   85
intramuscular injections (IMI)   50,
  101–2 *fig 5.2*
  sites   101
intravenous administration   49–50, 85
involuntary treatment   28–33
  case study   38–43
  criteria   28–9
  Initial Orders   29–30
  initiating   29–30

interim involuntary treatment
order 29
role of family/carers 30
isolation 33

joints and bones 259–60
justice (ethical principle) 36

kidneys 53–4, 258, 265 *tab 11.1*
nephron 53 *fig 3.3*
Korsakoff psychosis 182–3, 218

labelling (medication) 97
checks against medication orders 83
lactation 298–9
lamotrigine 141, 253
language, plain language 71
law 26–42
documentation—legal
requirements 85, 88–9
legal capacity 32–3
legal obligations to inform 103
legislation regarding NPs 330–1
mental disorders, legal and strategic
context for 27–8
Mental Health Acts 27–33
natural 37
psychostimulant drugs—legal
requirements 245
leadership, clinical 329
learning disorders 242 *tab 10.1*
legislation *see* law
Lhermitte's sign 166
libertarianism 35
Librium 7
lithium 9, 54, 70–2, 139–42, 253
toxicity of 142–3
features 143 *tab 6.7*
liver 52–3, 258
lupus *see* systemic lupus erythematosis

maintenance mood stabiliser 141–3
major depressive disorder
conditions associated with depressed
mood 115 *tab 6.2*
diagnostic criteria (abridged) 114
tab 6.1
lifetime prevalence rate 112
psychosis feature 182–3

symptoms 115
terminology 113
Mallory-Weiss tear 282
management
anxiety disorders, pharmacological
management of 156–7
co-occuring mental and alcohol-use
disorders 217
of depression in bipolar
disorder 140–1
of insomnia 288 *tab 12.3*
of mania/hypomania 138–40
medicines, medicines management
pathway cycle 19 *tab 1.3*
medicines management
pathway cycle 18 *fig 1.2*
professional roles 19 *tab 1.3*
student nurse's experience 316
of nicotine-dependent people 220
pain 297 *tab 12.5*
of schizophrenia 186–7 *tab 8.3*
self-care management strategies 21–2
service provision–paediatric mental
illness 241
mania/manic episode 138–40
case study 143
diagnostic features 116–17 *tab 6.3*
'DIGFAST' mnemonic 118 *fig 6.1*
drugs linked to 293 *tab 12.4*
mood stabilisers versus antipsychotic
drugs 138–9
safety issues 138
symptoms 138
marijuana *see* cannabis
mathematical skills 79–81
conversion 79–82
decimals 80
metric system 82
percentages 81
units
conversion 80–3
International System of Units 82
mechanism of action 61
Medicare Benefits Scheme 330–3
medication
adherence/non-adherence 321
antipsychotic medications 9, 103,
138–9, 170, 187–94

medication (*cont.*)

Australian Medicines Handbook   14

bulletin   14

classification of, New Zealand   87–9

complementary medicines   298

disinfection   100

failure to receive   17

indication   16–17

information   83

Consumer Medicines
Information   14

labelling and packaging   83, 97, 259

non-click lock containers   260

right medication   83

long-term effects of   269–71

management, student nurse's
experience   316

medication charts   99

medication lists   265–71

medication management process   18
fig 1.2

medication orders   83

right medication   83

medication-related problems   13,
16–18

categorisation system   16–17 *tab 1.2*

medications management
education   316

misadventure, people at risk of   13

multiple diseases–multiple
medicines   260

national inpatient medication
charts   89–94

nurse-initiated   329–30

patient, client and carer
education   104–6

patient's own   98

'persistence'   314–15

Pharmacy-Only Medicine   88

prescription medicine   87–8, 225–6

Quality Use of Medicines   11–15

recording dangerous drugs   88–9

restricted medicine (Pharmacist Only
Medicine)   88, 330

right medication   83

for schizophrenia treatment   186–7
tab 8.3

selection of   13, 17

self-medication   152

sensitivity to   259

side effects, susceptibility to   264–5

strength of   83–4

trials   124–5

withholding   84

medication administration

calculations   78–106

basic mathematical skills   79–81

checking before
administering   83–6

different schedules of drugs   86–7

drug calculations   81–2

continuity of pharmaceutical
care   98–9

documentation—legal
requirements   85

labelling and packaging   97

right route   85

safe injection techniques, general safety
principles   99–103

safety and

general safety principles   99–103

safe/unsafe abbreviations   94–7

medication-related problems   13, 16–18

categorisation system   16–17 *tab 1.2*

medications, abbreviations   94-7, 170

Medicines Act 1981 (NZ)   87–8

memantine   262

memory impairment   122, 259

mental disorders

documentation of   311

legal and strategic context for   27–8

management of   310

physical disorders, distinction   309

treatment of   5–6

mental health

effect of cannabis on   221

legislation   27–33

Mental Health Acts   27–33

mental health care availability   31

mental health law

Australian   26

legal context for treatment   26–42

New Zealand   27

Mental Health Acts   27–33

mental health promotion   20–2
Mental Health Review Board   29–30
mental health services, strategic
   plans   27–8
mental illness   240
   attention deficit/hyperactivity
      disorder   242–9
   autism spectrum disorders   250
   in children and adolescents   239–54
      nature of   241
   non-psychotic   307
   people with   213–26
   potential drug-related problems
      and   297 *tab 12.5*
   psychiatry
      general   251–4
      special issues   239–42
   psychotic   307
   service provision–paediatric mental
      illness   241
   in special populations   281–99
   tic disorders   250–1
mental retardation, documentation
   of   310
metabolic elimination (drug
   metabolism)   52
metabolic impacts   141–2
metabolic side effects   196–8
metabolism   47, 51–4
   children, effect on   240–1
   drug metabolism
      in children   240–1
      pathways   52 *fig 3.2*
      tobacco smoking influence   220–1
   gut-wall   49
   metabolic derangement   253
   metabolic side effects   196–8
   presystemic   49
metabolites   51–2, 54
methylphenidate   245
metric system   82
misadventure, people at risk of   13
modafanil   254–5
monoamine oxidase inhibitors
   (MAOIs)   7, 9, 63, 126, 128, 165–6
   properties   130
   standard daily doses   133 *tab 6.6*

mood disorders   6, 112–48
   bereavement   113–15
   bipolar disorder, general principles of
      treatment for   138–47
   elevated mood   116–18
      bipolar I disorder   117–18
      bipolar II disorder   118
   mood disturbance spectrum
      conditions associated with
         depressed mood   113–15
      conditions associated with elevated
         mood   116–18
   non-pharmacological
      treatment   118–23
   pharmacotherapy for   123–36
mood stabilisers   66, 138–9, 253
morbidity   157, 183–4, 221, 282
   medication-related   272
mortality   183–4, 221, 282
movement disorders   253
multidisciplinary care   18–20
   case study   21–2
multiplication   79
myalgia   122
myocardial infarction   262–3

Naranjo questionnaires   67–8
narcolepsy   288–9
National Inpatient Medication Chart
   (NIMC)   89–94, 94 *tab 5.2*
National Medicinal Drug Policy   13
   objectives   12
National Mental Health Policy and
   Plan   11
National Mental Health Strategy   11–12
National Prescribing Service   14
National Statement of Rights and
   Responsibilities   11
natural law ethics   37
negative symptoms   185
   exacerbation by
      pharmacotherapy   185
neglect   240
negligence   28
nephron   53 *fig 3.3*
neuroleptic malignant syndrome   196
neurotransmitters   61 *fig 4.1*, 61–4,
   186, 219

neurotransmitters (*cont.*)
    D-cycloserine and   177
    effect of ECT on   120
    enzymatic degradation and   63
    neurotransmitters, receptors and
        functions   62 *tab 4.1*
    N-methyl-D-aspartate (NMDA)   262
neutropaenia   198–9
nicotine   213, 214 *tab 9.1*, 219–21,
    286–7
    see also cigarette smoking
non-discrimination   36
non-drug therapies   154
non-maleficence (ethical principle)   35–6
non-pharmacological treatment
    for anxiety disorders   154–5
    of mood disorders
        electroconvulsive therapy   119–23
        psychological theory   118–19
non-psychotic mental illness   307
non-steroidal anti-inflammatory drug
    (NSAID)   70
nurse practitioners (NPs)   81, 327–8
    case study   333
    competency standards
        Standard 1   328
        Standard 2   328
        Standard 3   329
    education, drug calculations
        education   81–2
    MBS and PBS   330–3
    prescribing, person-centred
        approach   334
nursing practice *see* practice

obsessive–compulsive disorder   174–6
    case study   175–6
    features   174–5 *tab 7.6*
    treatment of   175
obstructive sleep apnoea (OSA)   289
older people
    ageing, physical effects of   258–60
    Beers list   265–71
    bones and joints   259–60
    brain and nervous system   259
    case study   270, 293–4
    cognitive disorders   260–2

comorbidities   262–4
drugs and   271–4
ECT use   121
eyesight   259
falls and   271–4
multiple diseases–multiple
    medicines   260
organ system function,
    declining   258
side effects, increasing susceptibility
    to   264–5
vulnerability of   16
weight considerations   81
opioids   214 *tab 9.1*
    heroin, regulated opioid
        replacement   224
oral administration   48–9
    factors altering absorption   54–5
organ systems   258
organic brain syndromes   182–3
osteoporosis   67, 198, 271
overdose   128–34
    deliberate   128

packaging (medication)   97
pain
    management   297 *tab 12.5*
    psychiatry and   297–8
panic disorder   164–7
    case study   166–7
    clinical features   164 *tab 7.4*
    diagnostic feature   165
    treatment for   165–6
parasomnias   287
parenteral administration   49–50, 85
Parkinsonism   189, 195
paternalism   35–6
patients
    care plans   72–4
    compliance   140
    condition/treatment, beliefs
        regarding   314
    dignity of   31
    education   55, 71
    inpatients, national inpatient
        medication charts   89–94
    patient care information   14, 71

person-specific factors, ADRs and   66
   with poor dentition   122
   right individual   83
patient's own medication (POMs)   98
periodic limb movements   290
personal protective equipment
   (PPE)   83, 99–100
personality disorders   283–5
   common disorders and associated
      symptom patterns   284–5
      tab 12.2
   documentation of   310
pervasive development disorders, in
   children/adolescents   242 *tab 10.1*
pH   49
PHARMAC   15
Pharmaceutical Benefits Advisory
   Committee (PBAC)   332
Pharmaceutical Benefits Scheme
   (PBS)   8, 330–3
pharmaceutical care, continuity
   of   98–9
Pharmaceutical Reforms   13–14
Pharmacist Only Medicine   88
pharmacodynamic drug interactions   69
pharmacodynamics   59–75
   biochemical effects   47
   case study   71–2
   interactions   126–7
   nursing practice and
      assessment   70–1
      education   71
      evaluation   71
   physiological effects   47
   science of drug actions   60–70
      adverse drug reactions   65–8
      drug interactions   69–70
      receptors   61–3
pharmacokinetics   47–8
   drug absorption   48–50
   drug distribution   50–1
   drug elimination   51–4
      excretion   51–4
      metabolism   51–4
   interactions   126–7
   nursing practice and   54–5
   science of drug movements   47–8

pharmacology
   for bipolar affective disorder   147
   depression pharmacology   146–7
   for schizophrenia   208
pharmacotherapy   6, 121
   for alcohol dependence   217
   antidepressants and overdose   128–34
   case study   21–2
   drug interactions   125–7
   general principles of treatment
      anxiety disorders   156–60
      bipolar affective disorder   146–7
      cognitive disorders   273–4
      major depression   123–5
      on the horizon anxiety
         disorders   177
      schizophrenia   208
      substance abuse   232
      substance use disorders   232
   for OCD   175
   palliation of schizophrenia   183–4
   problems associated with use   16
   psychotropic   18–20
      professional roles   19 *tab 1.3*
Pharmacy-Only Medicine   88
phencyclidine   214 *tab 9.1*
physical restraint   33
placebo effect   64, 156
plasma   50–1
   clearance   51, 54
   concentration   54
   drug plasma levels   64
   plasma proteins   51
PO (by mouth) administration   85
policy
   Australian National Medicinal Drug
      Policy   11–15
   Federal government policy initiatives,
      QUM funding   14
   New Zealand drug policy   15
   No Wrong Door Policy   227
   tobacco use and   220
polypharmacy   200, 264, 271
polysubstance   214 *tab 9.1*
populations
   ageing   260
   antidepressants, use in   124

populations (*cont.*)
  ECT and special populations   121
  Indigenous   217
  special, mental illness in   281–99
  vulnerable   16
positive symptoms   184–5
postmarketing surveillance process   65
post-traumatic stress disorder
  (PTSD)   167–74
  case study   170–1
  characteristic symptoms   168–9
    tab 7.5
  childhood sexual abuse as basis   168
  reducing likelihood of   177
  treatment of   169–71
practice
  adherence and concordance   306–21
  advanced   327
    prescribing medications—NPs
      advanced practice   329–30
  dynamic   328
  'evidence vacuum'   241
  law, ethics and accountability   26–42
  medication administration and
    calculations   78–106
  nurse practitioner and other advanced
    practice roles   327–34
  pharmacodynamics   59–75
    assessment   70–1
    education   71
    evaluation   71
  pharmacokinetics   47–56
    assessment   55
    drug administration   55
    education   55
    evaluation   55
  psychotropic drug use, history and
    context   4–22
  recovery-oriented   21–2
pregnancy   298–9
prescribing formulary   329
prescribing/prescription
  advanced nursing practice—
    NPs   329–30
  Australian Medicines Handbook   14
  Australian Prescriber   14
  deprescribing   269–70

legal obligations to inform   103
  National Prescribing Service   14
  NP prescribing   329–30, 334
  for older people   273 *tab 11.3*
  postmarketing surveillance
    phase   9–10
  'prescribing cascade'   308–9
    example   291 *fig 12.1*
  prescribing considerations—
    antipsychotics   191–4 *tab 8.5*
  prescription errors   81
  prescription medicine   87–8, 225–6
  prescription orders, checks
    against   83
  psychotropic prescribing   9–11
  right dose   83–4
prescription medicine   87–8, 213
presystemic metabolism   49
primary insomnia   287–8
primary sleep disorders   287–90
*Principles for the Protection of Persons with
  Mental Illness and for the Improvement of
  Mental Health Care*   31–2
problems
  drug-related   181
  medication-related   16–18
    categorisation system   16–17 *tab 1.2*
    prevalence   13
  see also iatrogenic illness
profile (pharmacokinetic)   47
propofol   122
proteins, enzymes   63
psychiatric illnesses   221
  in children/adolescents   242 *tab 10.1*
psychiatric syndromes, drug-
  induced   290–4
psychiatry   11
  general   251–4
  pain and   297–8
  pain management   297 *tab 12.5*
  societal stigma   240
  special issues   239–42
psychoeducation   119, 155
psychological factors   64
psychological interventions   251–2
psychological theory   118–19
psychological treatment   5–6

psychopharmacology, paediatric, on the
  horizon   253–4
psychoses
  adherence   201–3
  antipsychotic medications   187–94
    adverse effects   194–200
    drug interactions with   200–1
  case study   228
  crystal methamphetamine and   225
  drugs as possible cause of   183 *tab 8.2*
  drugs linked to   292–3 *tab 12.4*
  features—delusions and
    hallucinations   181–2, 182 *tab
    8.1*, 184–5
  Korsakoff psychosis   182–3
  links with cannabis   221–2
  psychosis—set of symptoms   181–3
  schizophrenia   183–7
  subclassification   182–3
psychosis   7
psychostimulant drugs   250
  case study   247
  safety concerns with use in
    children   244 *tab 10.3*
psychotherapy   155
psychotic mental illness   307
psychotropic drugs   6
  administration   48–9
  case study   21–2
  children, effect on   240–1
  medication-related problems   16–18
  mental health service provision
    recovery framework   20–2
  multidisciplinary care   18–20
  policy
    Australian National Medicinal
      Drug Policy   11–15
    New Zealand drug policy   15
  prescribing, major changes   9–11
  Quality Use of Medicines   11–15
  treatment
    biological   6
    historical aspects   6–9
    psychological   5–6
  use: history and context   4–22
psychotropic pharmacotherapy   18–20
  professional roles   19 *tab 1.3*

Q-Tc segment prolongation   201
Quality Use of Medicines (QUM)
  11–15
  achievement of   14–15
  key issues   13
  policy initiatives funding   14
  principles   12

ramelteon   299–300
receptors   50, 61 *fig 4.1*, 61–3
  neurotransmitters, receptors and
    functions   62 *tab 4.1*
  receptor blockade   189–90
recording, dangerous drugs   88–9
recovery   313
  mental health service provision
    recovery framework   20–2
      guiding principles   21
recovery-oriented practice   21–2
rectal administration   48–9, 85
rehabilitation   21–2
relapse, prevention   21–2
renal drug excretion   53–4
renal system   265 *tab 11.1*
  drug excretion   52
Repatriation Pharmaceutical Benefits
  (RPBS) scheme   8, 331
research
  models arising from   13–14
  regarding prevalence of medication-
    related problems   13
reserpine   188
Residential Medication Management
  Review (RMMR)   272
respiratory system   265 *tab 11.1*
restless leg syndrome   290
restraint   33–4
  case study   38–43
retardation
  growth   245
  mental
    in children/adolescents   242
      tab 10.1
    documentation   310
rheumatoid arthritis   260
  case study   293–4
rights

rights (*cont.*)
  exercise of 32
  human 28, 30–1
  The Six Rights 83–5
risk
  ADRs/side effects 65
  of antipsychotic drug treatment
    201–2
  associated with cigarette
    smoking 220
  associated with ECT 120–1
  falls risk assessment 271
  medication administration error,
    Six Rights and 83–5
  of pharmacotherapy 121
  respiratory depression 224
  of stroke 263
  of teratogenesis 121
risperidone 250, 307
rivastigmine 261
rule utilitarianism 35

safety
  Beers list 265–71
  mania/manic episode sufferers 138
  personal protective equipment 83, 99
  psychostimulant drug use with
    children 244 *tab 10.3*
  safe injection techniques 99–104
  safe/unsafe abbreviations 94–7
schedules/scheduling
  drug schedules 86–7, 87 *tab 5.1*
  toxicity and 86
schizophrenia 183–7
  assessment—individual
    perceptions 185
  biological theory 185–6
  cannabis and 221
  case study 202–3
  diagnostic criteria 184–5
  genetic disposition for 184 *fig 8.1*
  management of 186–7 *tab 8.3*
  morbidity/mortality
    associations 183–4
  prevalence rate 183–4
  Q-Tc segment prolongation
    199–200

symptoms
  assessment 185
  negative 185, 188
  positive 184–5
  treatment 307
    medications 186–7 *tab 8.3*
    of symptoms 186–7
scleroderma 260
screening 70–1, 216
seclusion 33–4
second-generation (atypical)
  antipsychotics 189–90
sedation 200, 262, 288
  sedatives 214 *tab 9.1*
seizures 158
  electroconvulsive therapy and 120
selective serotonin reuptake inhibitors
  (SSRIs) 7, 125, 165, 201, 250, 283
  clinical aspects 163 *tab 7.3*
  drug interactions examples
    127 *tab 6.5*
  fluoxetine 252
  properties 129
  as PTSD first-line treatment 169
  standard daily doses 133 *tab 6.6*
self-description 239–40
self-determination 35
self-harm 141
self-medication 152
self-rule 35
sensitivities 70–1, 259
serotonin syndrome 126, 223
  diagnostic criteria 126 *tab 6.4*
sexual abuse 168
sexual dysfunction 200
side effects 65
  extrapyramidal side effects 66
significant first pass effect 49
Six Rights, The 83–5
  case study 85–6
skin preparation 99–100
SL (sublingual) administration 85
sleep disorders 285–90
  breathing-related 289–90
  primary 287–90
    breathing-related sleep
      disorders 289–90

circadian rhythm disorders 289–90

dyssomnias 290

insomnia management, sleep habits and 288 *tab 12.3*

narcolepsy 288–9

primary insomnia 287–8

substance-induced 286–7

societal stigma 240

sodium valproate 139–42

St John's wort 126, 298

state anxiety 152

Stevens–Johnson syndrome 67 *fig 4.2*, 141

stress, corticotropin releasing factor 170

stroke 262–3

subcutaneous administration 85

subcutaneous injections 50

substance abuse 142, 213, 232

substance dependence 213

psychosis and 227

substance disorders

classification of

substance abuse 142, 213

substance dependence 213

substance use disorders

care considerations 170, 227–31

case study 226

people with mental illness and 213–26

substance-induced anxiety disorder 152

psychosis feature 182–3

substances

classes, diagnosis associated with 214 *tab 9.1*

definition 213

substance-induced sleep disorders 286–7

subtraction 79

suicide 21–2, 123

case study 134–5

suicidal behaviour 239

suicidal ideation 128, 221

surveillance, postmarketing surveillance process 65

susceptibility 264–5

medication implications 265 *tab 11.1*

suxamethonium 122

systemic circulation 48–50

systemic lupus erythematosis (lupus) 260

tablets, enteric-coated 48–9

tachyphylaxis 158

tardive dyskinesia 103, 195–6, 251

Te Kōkiri: New Zealand Mental Health and Addiction Action Plan 2006–2015 28

Te Tāhuhu–Improving Mental Health 2005– 2015: The Second New Zealand Mental Health and Addiction Plan 28

teleology 37

therapeutic effect 55, 60

medication, right time 84

therapy

bright light 123

cognitive behavioural therapy 118–19, 154, 165

drug therapy for major depression 10 *tab 1.1*

indication without 16

interpersonal therapy 118–19

national therapeutic guidelines 14

non-drug 154

psychoeducation 155

'psychological therapies' 154

psychological treatment 155

psychotherapy 155

thiamine deficiency 218

tic disorders 250–1

in children/adolescents 242 *tab 10.1*

Tourette's syndrome 250–1

tobacco 16

toxins 220

tolerance (to drugs) 158

Tourette's syndrome 250–1

toxicity 47, 53–5, 61, 124

cigarette smoking 201, 220

drug accumulation 258

haematological 199

lithium and 142–3

features 143 *tab 6.7*

toxicity (*cont.*)
  medication, right time   84
  methadone levels and   224
  overdose and   128
  serotonin toxicity   126, 223
TP (topical) administration   85
trait anxiety   152
transcranial magnetic stimulation
  (TMS)   146
transcultural ethical theory   37
treatment
  of ADHD   244–7
  adherence to planned treatment
    approach   71
  antipsychotic drug treatment   201–3
  bipolar affective disorder, maintenance
    mood stabiliser   141–3
  degrading   32
  drug therapy for GAD   162–3
    tab 7.3
  electroconvulsive therapy   119–23
  general principles of treatment, major
    depression   123–5
  initiating   329
  involuntary   28–33
  non-drug   119
  non-pharmacological treatment
    anxiety disorders   154–6
    electroconvulsive therapy   119–23
    of mood disorders   118–23
    psychological theory   118–19
treatment
  of obsessive–compulsive
    disorder   175
  for panic disorder   165–6
  of post-traumatic stress disorder
    169–71
  psychological treatment   155
  psychotropic drug treatment
    biological   6
    modern   6–9
    psychological   5–6
  of schizophrenia symptoms
    186–7, 307

transcranial magnetic
  stimulation   123
treatment phases—
  antipsychotics   191 *fig 8.2*
tricyclic antidepressants   165
  properties   129
  standard daily doses   133
    tab 6.6
tricyclic antidepressants (TCAs)   7, 9, 10
  tab 1.1, 125–6, 128
tryptophan   255

urine   53–4
US Food and Drug Administration
  (FDA)   169
utility/utilitarianism   35

vagal nerve stimulation   123, 146
Valium   7
ventilation, mechanical   122
vision *see* eyesight
volume of distribution   50–1

washout time   63, 134
Webster packs   259
weight
  dosage
    estimation   64
    prescription errors   81
  weight gain   196–7
Wernicke's encephalopathy   218
withdrawal   158, 166
  alcohol   216–17
  crystal methamphetamine   225
  heroin   224
  tobacco   220
World Health Organization (WHO)
  adherence definition   312
  definition of safe injection   99
  disinfection   100
  *International Statistical Classification of
    Diseases and Related Health Problems*
    (ICD-10)   309
  mental/behavioural disorders   306–7

zopiclone   170